No Period. Now What?

No Period. Now What?

A Guide to Regaining Your Cycles and Improving Your Fertility

Nicola J. Sykes, PhD,
with Stephanie Buckler, Esq.,
and Lisa Sanfilippo Waddell, LCSW

Antica Press
Waltham, MA

Book updated March 2019, October 2023. We have revised some text to be more aligned with Health At Every Size© paradigms, updated the partner chapter to be more inclusive, and added links (in the ebook) to a number of relevant blog posts on the the No Period. Now What? website. October2023 updated information on supplements, progesterone use during pregnancy, and ovulation tracking. If you purchase the paperback from other than noperiodnowwhat.com, email anticapress@gmail.com with a copy of your receipt to get a link for the ebook. Links (Amazon US) to other books and supplements that we have come across and find helpful for those working to recover can be found at http://noperiod.info/resources.

Antica Press LLC

Creative Commons License

No Period. Now What? by Nicola J. Sykes, Stephanie G. Buckler and Lisa Sanfilippo Waddell is licensed under a Creative Commons Attribution-ShareAlike 4.0 International License.

http://creativecommons.org/licenses/by-sa/4.0/

Second edition published 2024. Original publication 2016.

Cover design by Mallory Blondin

ISBN-13: 978-0-9972366-2-0
ISBN-10: 0-9972366-2-0

1. Health and Fitness--Women's Health. 2. Health and Fitness--Infertility.

A huge thank you to the hundreds who have contributed to this book; quotes, data, thoughts, experiences, references … you know who you are, and you have played an enormous role in getting this project to fruition.

We would particularly like to thank Mallory Blondin for the cover design and other images, Nico's Mom Helen Herold for copy editing on many of the early chapters, Clare Geraghty and Sharon Olofsson for poring through multiple versions of every chapter doing incredibly thorough copy editing, and Deanna Balas, Megan Langer, and Katrina Green for hours of content editing. As well as many more friends who helped along the way with suggestions and opinions. The book is worlds better for your thoughtful comments and critiques. We would also like to thank Shanta Samantha Gyanchard, Greta Jarvis, and Florence Cleanis for assistance with altering some language from the first edition that was less body positive / Health At Every Size aligned, Kate Albarella RDN for assistance with the PCOS chapter, and Lisa Powell for thoughts on the partner support chapter. Clearly, it takes a village, and we have been blessed with being part of an incredibly supportive and helpful group.

An even bigger thank you to our spouses: Mark, Aaron, and Jim, without whom we never could have found time to get this project completed.

Thanks too to our children: Antony, Timmy, Cam, Lee, Devorah, and fur babies Wubby, Buster, and Cowgirl for being understanding about their Mommies needing to spend "a few minutes" on the computer.

Publisher's note: This publication is designed to provide accurate and authoritative information in regard to the subject matter covered. It is sold with the understanding that the services of a competent medical professional will be sought with regards to your personal situation.

Consult with Dr. Nicola Sykes, PhD: http://noperiod.info/appointments for guidance on diagnosis, individualized recovery plans, and supplements/medications.

Visit www.NoPeriodNowWhat.com
for more information and blog posts on a variety of topics.
Find our Support Group at http://noperiod.info/Support,
support for getting pregnant at http://noperiod.info/TTC,
and follow on Instagram @NoPeriodNowWhat

Contents

List of Illustrations..ix
List of Tables x
Prologue..xiii

Part 1:
Hypothalamic Amenorrhea
Nuts and Bolts

1. No Period? 3
2. Factors in HA: What You Eat 15
3. Factors in HA: Exercise and Stress...23
4. Diagnosis..31
5. Hypothalama-WHAT?? 43
6. The HA/PCOS Conundrum 55
7. Brittle Bones and Other Health Consequences of HA 73

Part 2:
The Recovery Plan—Changing Your Habits and Your Life

8. You Want Me to Eat WHAT?? The HA Recovery Plan 95
9. Putting Recovery Into Practice 113
10. What to Expect..125
11. Expanding… Mentally and Physically 139
12. The HA Recovery Plan: Exercise Changes 155
13. There Is More to Life Than Exercise..................................169
14. Running Toward Recovery..179
15. Partners in Recovery 189
16. Recovering Natural Cycles 209
17. Tracking Ovulation and Family Planning 219
18. Still No Period?!..235
19. Luteal Phase...255

Part 3:
When it Takes More Than an "Oops" to Get Pregnant

20. When You Need a Jump-start 269
21. Popping Pills to Ovulate: Oral Medications 281
22. Shooting up: Injectables 301
23. Medicated Ovulation and Beyond 319
24. In Vitro Fertilization 329

Part 4:
What Comes Next?

25. I'm Pregnant—Now What?? 349
26. Pregnancy Loss 365
27. Postpartum, Cycling, and Conceiving Again 383
28. Long-term Health 397

Part 5:
Stories of Hope

29. The Road to Recovery 415

Appendix 491
List of Abbreviations 495
References 499
Index 537

List of Illustrations

BMI range in survey respondents 7
Weight loss in survey respondents 8
Underfueling 18
Common calorie-averse eating behaviors 19
Total intake, taking exercise into account 25
Exercise among survey respondents 26
Average exercise intensity among survey respondents 27
Survey respondents' hormone levels during HA 35
Control centers in the brain 45
Reproductive hormone levels through the menstrual cycle 46
Hormones and hunger control 49
Interrelationship between nutrition and reproduction 53
Types of bone 76
Subclinical eating disorder symptoms 97
Eating behaviors during HA and after recovery 98
Physical symptoms during HA and after recovery 127
Luteal phase and exercise 162
Intercourse timing and the chance of pregnancy 221
Fertility Friend chart 230
LH during and after HA 236
Number of cycles to achieve conception 272
Ovulation after a non-ovulatory medicated cycle 286
Cycles after miscarriage to achieve another pregnancy 380
Cycle resumption and breast milk production 389
Number of ovulations to achieve subsequent conception 395

List of Tables

Hormones and expected results 34
Additional hormones and expected results..40
Hormonal levels in PCOS 58
Physical symptoms in PCOS...59
Hormonal levels in HA and PCOS..60
Physical symptoms in HA and PCOS..61
Effects of PCOS treatment options on hormones and ovulation..............68
Survey respondents' bone density results...76
Change in bone markers at different energy levels 78
Clover's DXA results 2006-2014 82
Recommended daily caloric intake 102
Resumption of menstrual cycles and weight changes...............................105
Menstrual status in women starting a running program..........................161
Pregnancy rates by cycle day of ovulation 215
Ovulation with naltrexone therapy..248
Suggested supplement or oral medication protocols 249
Normal number of antral follicles 277
HAers with low AMH..278
Ovulation and pregnancy with oral medications......................................285
BMI, ovulation, and pregnancy when using oral meds 286
Suggested oral medication protocols 290
Effect of Clomid timing on lining thickness and pregnancy rate 294
Cycle day of ovulation 297
Effect of ovulation CD on pregnancy rate in injectable cycles................309
Intercourse and IUI timing for pregnancy..320
Factors potentially affecting pregnancy viability 373
Natural cycles after miscarriage 378
Route taken to next pregnancy after miscarriage.....................................379
Length of breast milk production compared to cycle resumption 390
Method of conception for first and subsequent pregnancies...................395
BMI and response to oral fertility drugs 493

Prologue

> "I MORPHED FROM the last one chosen in gym class to an exercise fanatic, getting two to three hours of exercise a day by the time I was in graduate school. I went from eating whatever I felt like to limiting my calories each day in an attempt to lose my love handles and get myself in shape for a healthy, easy pregnancy and delivery. Yeah … not so much. It's hard to get pregnant when you've lost your period."
>
> *-Nicola, a.k.a. Nico*

Is your period missing? Are you ready to find out why and what to do about it? Well, you've come to the right place. We, the authors (Nico, Steph, and Lisa), have all experienced the same problem, known as hypothalamic amenorrhea (HA), and overcome it—just as you will. We met through an online support forum (that we will refer to as "the Board") where it became our mission to provide knowledge of how to recover, as well as support those going through the process. We helped hundreds recover and get pregnant (when desired). Over time it became clear that there were gaping holes in the available information about HA that our experiences prepared us to fill.

Therefore, we set out to create a book that would:

1) provide a thorough understanding of why your periods have stopped
2) detail steps on how to recover your menstrual cycle
3) discuss methods for getting pregnant after recovery
4) lead you through what to expect while pregnant, after having a baby, and with your long-term health

5) provide hope and inspiration from others' experiences to help guide you

In each chapter, we will share our individual stories and thoughts, as well as firsthand testimonies from Board contributors, highlighted as seen below. First, a brief introduction to our own encounters with HA.

> *Nico*: I discovered my period was AWOL when I was in my early thirties and wanted to start a family. Apparently getting pregnant was not going to be as easy as I had thought. My Ph.D. training from M.I.T. led me to research showing that I needed to gain back some of the weight I had recently lost and cut my exercise. But there were so many unanswered questions. How much weight? What level of exercise was acceptable? How long would it take? Would I be able to beat this? Why did I have to undo all my hard work when others could cycle and get pregnant at the drop of a hat?
>
> I started my blog "No Period Baby" around this time, and began posting on the Board (over 5,000 posts), in hopes of sharing my research with others looking for answers and guidance. My desire to help has now culminated in this book.

> **Stephanie (Steph)**: Joining the Board helped me realize that my eating and exercise habits were preventing me from getting my period. While I had recently recovered from an eating disorder of 15 years, I still wasn't eating enough to properly fuel my marathon training. With support and advice from the community, I made lifestyle changes. Those changes, along with a little help from oral medications, led to my pregnancy. I was already a motivational speaker helping others overcome eating disorders; now I had a new mission—to spread awareness about the impact of absent periods and the plan for recovery.

> *Lisa*: Like Nico and Steph, I also lost my monthly cycle as a result of overtraining and undereating. After 10 years of wonky periods and at least 13 more years of *no* periods, finally a five-month "all in" effort allowed me to recover completely normal cycles at 41 years old—something I thought might not be possible. Being a competitive runner most of my life and working in the fitness industry for over 20 years, I understand the *need* for exercise and food control all too well. But my story isn't nearly as important as the lessons I have learned during and after my journey to recovery—lessons you too will learn. Our hope is that you will be inspired by the truths in this book, and equipped to take responsibility for *your* recovery.

> **Additional contributors**: This book would not be possible without the incredible community of women from the Board who are either recovered or working toward recovery. Throughout the chapters, you will find an abundance of firsthand experiences and testimonies from these women that will inspire you to find your way.

Our stories may resemble yours, but if not, don't let that put you off. HA usually results from a combination of undereating, (over)exercising, weight loss, stress, and genetics, so your exact recipe is unique. Whatever your particular situation, our research and observations will offer solutions. In addition, quotes and data from over 300 women who have experienced HA provide further insight and hope. These women spent hours filling out detailed information on three comprehensive surveys because they yearn to help those following in their footsteps... you! To start, we'll provide selected descriptive information on these survey respondents so you can get to know them better. Results from the survey are referenced throughout the book.

- Our respondents are from all over the US and world—36 different states are represented, along with Canada, the UK, Australia, Belgium, Switzerland, New Zealand, France, Bermuda, and China. This is why you may notice different slang in some of the testimonies.
- Those who took the survey were between the ages of 19 and 44, with 90% between the ages of 25 and 39.
- The age at which the first period was experienced (before it disappeared) was between 9 and 17 years old, with an average of 13. Three women never had a natural period.
- At some point before losing their periods, 66% had regular cycles between 21 and 30 days long (average of 28); 25% did not have regular cycles; 9% did not recall.
- The median number of months without a menstrual cycle was 15, with a range of 3 months to 20 years. A quarter had been without a cycle for 10 months or less; another quarter had no periods for more than three years.
    - o Note that this is the time from when respondents realized their period was missing to their next period or start of fertility treatments–*not* since beginning the recovery process. Many go for years without a period, not seeing it as an issue until trying to conceive, and only then making changes.

- Natural cycles were regained by 53% of our survey respondents prior to pregnancy.
    - Among these, 60% regained cycles within six months of following the Recovery Plan, and 90% recovered cycles within a year. Since publishing the first edition of this book in 2016, the median time to recovery has decreased (likely due to the availability of the "All In" guidelines, http://noperiod.info/time2)
    - Whether our respondents' periods returned or not was not dependent on the length of their amenorrhea. (http://noperiod.info/time)
- In order to get pregnant more quickly, 47% chose to use fertility treatments in conjunction with our Recovery Plan. After their first child was born, 79% of these women regained natural cycles (and/or got pregnant naturally). After their final child was weaned, 98% cycled naturally.

We are confident that the data from our survey, as well as the accounts of those who participated in the online forum will help educate you, prove that the Recovery Plan works (part 2), and encourage you to try it for yourself. We hope that you too will be able to examine the evidence, apply it, and become another success story.

Part 1: Hypothalamic Amenorrhea Nuts and Bolts

1
No Period?

> *Nico*: I WAS READY to get pregnant. I had just finished my PhD, had a new job with excellent benefits, the timing was perfect. The last of my birth control pills came with a thrill of anticipation: baby making and pregnancy! I was in the best shape of my life, pregnancy and delivery were going to be a breeze; all the ducks were in their assigned spots. Except one... no fertile signs and no period.

What does it mean when your period is missing? Sometimes absent flow is cause for celebration—less mess, no cramps, and more stable emotions. But as you learn more about the health repercussions of no menstrual cycles, and particularly when you want to get pregnant, there's no reason for festivity.

A missing period means that your reproductive system is not working. This can be caused by a condition called hypothalamic amenorrhea[1], (also known as hypogonadotropic hypogonadism) the focus of this book. It's pronounced hi-po-thah-lam-ic a-men-or-ree-ah. This term is quite a mouthful, which is why we often just write or say "HA" (with each letter pronounced separately, not "ha" as in a laugh). We also use the term "HAers" to indicate those diagnosed with HA rather than writing "people diagnosed with HA" over and over.

The name of the condition tells us the symptom (amenorrhea, a missing period) as well as the cause (the hypothalamus, one of the control centers in the brain). The hypothalamus receives input from all over the body in the form of hormones and chemicals, then responds by making hormones that affect other organs such as those involved in reproduction. There is constant feedback and adjustment to keep the body in a stable, healthy state. But sometimes things go wrong. A signal gets overridden, a hormone level gets too high or low, and the hypothalamus can't keep balance any more. One sign of this is an absent period.

Another cause of missing periods is polycystic ovarian syndrome[2] (PCOS). HA and PCOS present with similar symptoms, but because lifestyle modifications to address each are essentially opposite, misdiagnosis is problematic. The similarities (which we will cover in detail in chapter 6) are a missing period, and sometimes what the ovaries look like when examined using ultrasound as well as high AMH levels. The differences consist of the hormonal picture, physical symptoms, and day-to-day behaviors. If you have been told you have PCOS, but do not exhibit any physical symptoms of PCOS and lost your period only after decreasing food intake, increasing exercise amount and/or intensity, dropping some weight, or experiencing times of high stress, the more accurate diagnosis may very well be HA (http://noperiod.info/HAvsPCOS2).

Variables Involved in Hypothalamic Amenorrhea

There are many components that can cause this hypothalamic shutdown including energy balance, food restrictions, weight loss, exercise, stress, and genetics. For each person experiencing HA, the combination and level of each factor is different. It is also important to note that the absolute amounts of food, exercise, and stress that cause HA vary widely depending on the individual. In the vast majority of cases, the primary driver is an energy deficit from undereating and overexercising, **regardless of body size**. But that is far from the only way to acquire HA. Psychological stress alone can cause HA, but more often, stress combined with undereating, food restrictions, and/or exercise is the culprit. Weight loss, even years in the past, can predispose one to HA; couple weight loss with a stressful event or a change in eating habits and periods shut down. Genetics play a part too, perhaps explaining why one person will lose their period while another with similar physique and habits does not.

Energy. Energy balance is essential to survival. The energy we consume in the form of food fuels critical functions: pumping the heart, energizing the brain, and keeping cells working[3]. After that, fuel is provided for "nice-to-haves" such as growth of hair, nails, immune cells, and bones, as well as keeping body temperature up. Finally, the most expendable: fat storage and reproduction.

Keeping these systems working optimally requires energy, using fuel every second even when just spending the day in bed ("resting metabolism"). Daily activity, like walking from your bed to the bathroom, or jiggling your legs, expends additional energy on muscle movement, and planned exercise demands even more than that.

The bottom line is *our bodies need food* in order to function in a healthy way. Calories keep blood circulating, provide fuel for the brain, allow our immune systems to do their job, and support many other functions[4].

If one is not taking in enough calories to fuel at least the essentials and nice-to-have functions in addition to any physical movement being performed (planned exercise as well as normal daily movement), the body will adapt to the energy deficit by suppressing as much as possible to continue surviving. It will use the fuel provided to energize the most important functions, leaving others like the reproductive system, temperature regulation, and cellular growth and regeneration un- or under-fueled[5]. It may even need to rely on fat stores to fuel the more essential processes. So if our bodies are lacking sufficient fuel for all bodily functions, what suffers?

- **The reproductive system.** A reduction in body fat percentage often leads to celebration and positive feelings based on society's current body ideals ("I'm getting thinner! I'm more 'attractive'! I have a six-pack!"). But remember that while body fat is decreasing, the reproductive system is getting less fuel too. A body doesn't want to spend energy on making babies when there isn't enough to go around—reproduction is one of the most energy-intensive processes a female body endures, but it is not a necessity and will therefore shut down if fuel is lacking. Your body is wise and focuses energy where it is needed most.

- **Body temperature.** Another process that can be neglected is body temperature maintenance. A common complaint among those who have lost their periods is feeling cold all the time. This occurs because your body has chosen not to spend its limited supply of energy on keeping you warm—it has better things to do with that fuel.

- **Other areas.** Your body may also choose not to spend energy on the growth of hair, nails, immune cells, and bones. Is your hair dry and brittle (http://noperiod.info/hair)? Do your nails break easily? Do you get sick often? Have you had a bone scan revealing low bone density? In addition, your digestive system slows down as it attempts to extract every last calorie from the food you consume. Do you suffer from constipation? All of these are signs that your systems are not fully fueled. Your body chooses survival over comfort when forced to make a choice.

Are you getting enough fuel?

Food choices. It is also important that your fuel is coming from a variety of different sources: protein, fat, and both complex and simple carbohydrates (carbs). Each type of nourishment sends signals that work in concert to support the function of the hypothalamus. In the 1990s a low-fat diet was all the rage; then it was the Zone and Atkins diets promoting minimal carbohydrates; now in the twenty-first century there is a focus on eliminating processed foods and sugars, and "intermittent fasting." Any limitation of nutrient sources can lead to a restrictive mindset and psychological issues as well as removing signals our hypothalamus relies on to indicate appropriate resources. Couple this with energy restriction, and hypothalamic shutdown can occur.

Are you restricting the food groups you consume?

> **Steph**: When I was diagnosed with HA, I was in love with carbs. After all, I was a runner and "needed" lots of carbs for quick energy. Proteins and fats were present in my diet but I just didn't love to eat them like I did my granola bars. When I found out I had HA, I was not surprised and attributed it to my history of anorexia. What baffled me was when I was told that my *current* eating habits were contributing to not getting a period. I felt like I ate a TON, and all the time—how could I have HA?! Well, apparently, what I was eating was still not enough to support my body. I had a deficit of over 500 calories per day. Equally as important, I was not eating enough proteins and fats. I had no variety. I ate a lot of granola but that's about it. I needed proteins and fats to kick my hormones into gear.

Weight and weight loss. An additional factor that can play a part in missing periods is current weight and body fat percentage, as well as weight loss history. There are two important points we want to make on this topic. First, **it is completely possible to lose your period at any weight**, although it is more common to do so in those with an underweight or low-normal body mass index (BMI*). Second, losing a significant amount of weight (10 lb or more), even years in the past, makes an absent cycle

---

* BMI = weight (kg) / height (m)^2 OR weight (lb) * 703 / height (in)^2

more likely. People generally think of losing a period as something that only happens to the super-skinny or underweight (i.e., anorexic), but that is not reality. Among our survey respondents (see prologue and appendix for more information), people discovered missing periods across a large range of BMIs, with a median of 19.0 (meaning half the respondents had a BMI below this number and half had a BMI above).

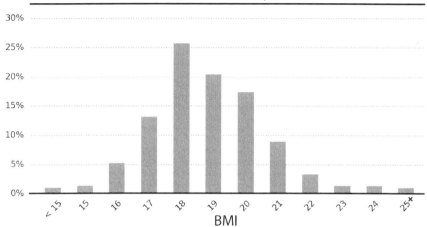

BMI range in survey respondents when absent periods were noticed (data from 286 participants). The percentage of survey respondents at each BMI is illustrated. When people realized their periods were missing, only 33% were at an "underweight" BMI of <18.5, with 7.5% at a BMI of 22 or above. In the years since initial publication of this book, it has become even more clear that any one in any body size can experience HA.

Lots of people get stuck on the BMI argument; "My BMI is 'normal,'" or even, "I'm in a larger body ... so there's no way I have a problem." However, there is no magic number for BMI—no number below which you will automatically lose your period or above which you will definitely have monthly cycles. BMI is just part of the equation. Focusing on BMI also means that medical professionals can miss diagnosing HA accurately, not understanding that absolute weight is only a very small part of what causes HA.

Weight loss—recent or even years in the past—can predispose you to losing your period. We were surprised upon analyzing our survey data (see prologue) that **over three quarters (82%)** of our survey respondents had lost more than 10 lb prior to discovering their periods were missing.

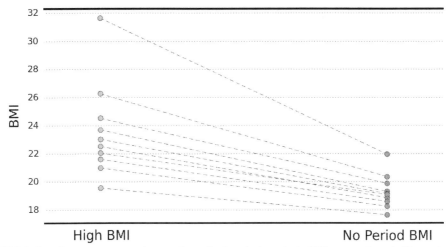

Weight loss in survey respondents prior to losing their periods (272 respondents). Change in BMI for survey respondents who lost more than 10 lb prior to losing their periods is shown. The points on the left show the highest reported BMI; on the right is the BMI at which missing menstrual cycles were noted. Each line represents 10% of the group. The median BMI when periods were lost was 19.0; the median pre-weight-loss BMI was 22.8.

The median weight loss was 21.4% of body weight. That is a substantial change, and many continue to limit caloric intake for fear of re-gaining some or all of the weight lost.

Generally speaking, those who are in smaller than average bodies are engaging in the restrictive behaviors we mentioned, consciously or unconsciously. There have been plenty of disagreements regarding this issue; some will say, "I'm naturally thin," or "I have a small frame." This may be true—but what's also true is that they aren't getting their period. This suggests that their bodies don't agree with their assessment.

Did you ever lose more than 10 lb?

Stress and psychology. Researchers have found that those who have HA tend to have "higher levels of perfectionism" than people without HA[6]. That description rings true for many of us. We set goals for ourselves, and do everything in our power to achieve them. This trait often serves us well—helping us to reach career goals and achieve appearance and exercise aspirations, for example. But the pressure we put on ourselves to meet those high expectations can also lead to a great deal of stress. Then there are the normal day-to-day stressors that life can throw at us involving family, friends, work situations, etc. Stress can be useful in some situations, but when it is chronic and particularly coupled with exercise, it can lead to changes in our brain that suppress the hypothalamus and menstrual cycles.

Clinical studies of two methods of treating amenorrhea support this effect of psychological stress. One group used cognitive behavioral therapy (CBT) to treat the subjects over 20 weeks. In the CBT group, 88% regained their periods by the end of the intervention, as opposed to 25% in the non-treated group[7]. In the second study, a single treatment with hypnotherapy induced return of menstrual cycles in 9 out of 12 participants within 12 weeks[8]. Recovery of cycles through these therapies (in women with relatively normal weight, eating, and exercise habits) suggests that stress can indeed play a role in the loss of periods, and offers avenues for exploration in addition to the eating and exercise Recovery Plan (part 2).

What are your stress levels like? How much do you try to control your eating, exercise, and other factors in your life?

> Nina: I do not think we should overlook the importance of stress management. We are all different with varying set point weights and outside stressors contributing to our HA. Part of what leads us to thin weights and overexercising is the need to control, restrict, and worry about certain aspects of our life (you could say type A). I think that stress plays a big role in the recovery process and if we don't consider that and focus on weight only, we miss the boat on some things.

Exercise. Exercise is another piece of the puzzle that comes into play in two ways: First, by decreasing the number of calories available to the body[9]; second, by increasing the stress hormones, including cortisol[10].

As far as the energy part of the equation goes, many of us don't eat enough to compensate for the exercise we perform, which means we operate at a caloric deficit. When exercise is coupled with energy restriction like this (intentional or not), many of the hormones that regulate our monthly cycles are at abnormal levels within just a few days[11]. You may be thinking, "But I fuel my body. I eat when I am hungry and stop when I am full. I eat more on days I exercise." (Or you might already recognize that you are not eating enough.) Note that hunger signals may not account for exercise as well as we think they do. In multiple research studies where people were told how much to exercise and later given an unlimited buffet to eat from, they ate more than when they had not exercised—but not nearly enough to compensate for all the calories they had burned[12]. So even when not consciously restricting, their bodies were not getting enough fuel when eating as dictated by hunger cues. The eating deficit was considerable, particularly if the diet was low fat[13], probably because low-fat foods are as filling as their full-fat counterparts, without sufficient calories. For example, you can get just as full from plain, raw vegetables as if you were consuming them doused in a calorie rich dressing or a dip. There are also many who practice some form of intermittent fasting; not eating for 12-16 hours of the day because it is supposed to help with hormonal health (not strongly supported by medical research[14]). However, this leads to a large energy deficit each day, even if someone overall is consuming sufficient calories. This has also been correlated with missing periods[15] (http://noperiod.info/energy-balance).

> **Steph**: My relationship with food and exercise changed after I recovered from my eating disorder. Instead of running to burn calories, I was running for enjoyment and I loved it. I thought I was fueling adequately. But I was burning hundreds of calories through exercise, and even when satiated I was still not eating enough to account for my activity. I knew that if I ran an hour, I would have to compensate with added fuel, but I wouldn't do the same for cross-training, which left me at a persistent caloric deficit. Ultimately, I thought I was getting enough, but I wasn't.

The second way exercise can affect menstrual cycles is through increases in stress hormones like cortisol[16]. In a study where women began a running program with increased caloric intake to theoretically offset the energy burned by running, 80% showed signs of menstrual abnormalities within two months[17]. In addition, a multitude of studies have found that stress hormones are increased in those with HA[18], driving home the point that both psychological and exercise stress can have effects on cycles.

How much are you exercising? Are your workouts well-fueled?

Genetics. We all seem to know people who are thin, run marathons, and get pregnant "when their partners simply look at them." It feels unfair that we are afflicted with seemingly sensitive reproductive systems, while others can appear to follow exactly the same lifestyle and have no problems at all. But we are each unique, with a different physical makeup and a different set of challenges to face. Many are also on birth control pills that mask absent cycles. There's no point in comparing. It is likely that our genes play a part in determining the sensitivity of our reproductive systems to energy deficits and stress. A study of people who had lost their periods found mutations (small changes in DNA) in genes controlling the reproductive system, but no mutations were found in normally cycling controls (some of whom were exercising as much as those with amenorrhea)[19]. Since only seven genes were tested, it seems reasonable that there could be mutations in those or other genes that might predispose us to endocrine sensitivity and losing our periods. It's not much, but it does help to answer the "Why me?" question to some degree.

Completing the HA Equation

In some, just one of the factors we have described is sufficient to cause menstrual cycles to stop. In others, a combination of factors is involved, and often, behaviors that would not be a problem on their own create a magnifying effect. The clearest example comes from a study where monkeys were subjected either to exercise with dietary restriction (one hour per day with a 20% reduction in calories), stress (moving to a new cage with different neighbors), or both. Out of eight monkeys subjected to just a move, only one had an abnormal cycle. Of nine monkeys in the exercise plus dietary restriction group, one experienced menstrual abnormalities. However, in the group subjected to the combination of energy restriction, exercise, and move stress, 7 of 10 experienced at least one abnormal cycle[20]. Stress along with reduction in available energy had a much larger effect than either stress or energy reduction alone. Synergy.

What might the combination be for you?

No Period...Not Healthy!

Aside from fertility issues, there are other reasons the absence of a period is problematic. When you're not getting your period it means that your estrogen levels and your other reproductive hormones are low and not increasing through the month as expected, with profound effects. Short term, amenorrhea can be associated with thinning or loss of hair, brittle nails, and skin problems. You know the "glow" of pregnancy people talk about? It comes from an increase in estrogen. But when your estrogen is low, your skin may be dull and dry. Low estrogen can also cause nonexistent libido, and dryness "down there." Longer term, it can lead to brittle bones and fractures, cardiac disease, and an increased risk of dementia and early cognitive decline (a lot more on these health effects in chapter 7).

On top of all this, you can't get pregnant when you're not ovulating or getting your period—except potentially with medical help. Even then, success cannot be guaranteed if you are still overexercising or undereating for your body. Moreover, fertility treatments are never as easy as "the old-fashioned way," not to mention the stress and cost, which can compound if you have to go through multiple cycles because your body isn't ready. If you haven't at least started to work on recovering your missing period naturally before pregnancy by getting your body to a healthy place, it can also lead to potentially worse physical issues down the line. These include stress fractures for you, and preterm delivery and low birth weight for your baby[21]. It can also lead to a much more mentally challenging pregnancy, as you struggle to deal with the weight gain and changing shape that comes with adequately nourishing yourself and your growing child.

Birth Control Pills

Did you know that birth control pills (BCP) or injections can completely mask the lack of an actual menstrual cycle? Many think that because they get a bleed on birth control, everything is fine. They may have read or heard about how not getting a period is a sign of overexercise, undereating, or stress, but since they bleed every month, they believe it's not an issue for them. But in truth, birth control pills provide synthetic hormones that stimulate an artificial period that is not an accurate indicator of your health.

Let us rephrase that, because it's important: **if you're getting your period only because you're on birth control, it doesn't count.**

A BCP-induced monthly bleed tells you nothing about your health. If there are other points in this chapter and the next two that sound familiar and have you nodding your head as you read along, well, keep reading. Chances are if you want to get your period after stopping birth control you'll benefit from following the Recovery Plan.

On the other hand, if you stopped taking BCP already and are not getting your period, you should know "post-pill amenorrhea" is not an evidence-supported diagnosis[22]. You and your doctor should investigate potential causes for your amenorrhea rather than waiting.

> *Mallory:* I questioned the "your body just needs time to regulate after being on the pill for so long" that my doctor gave me as an excuse for months. As soon as I upped my calories and cut out the intense exercise, bam, I got my period that same month! I quickly gained to be in the

> "fertile zone" and that got me my cycles back, although they are somewhat irregular right now. I've also noticed lots of other healthy changes other than just being able to ovulate. Missing periods are definitely not just from being on the pill especially if your BMI is low. Even if you aren't trying to get pregnant right now, conquering HA before more damage is done to your body, your bones, and your mental processes, will make you better off!

Parting Thoughts

You may already suspect a link between your menstrual cycle and how much and what you're eating, your weight or body fat, and/or your exercise patterns. You are probably right. Be aware that even in cases where there is clearly food restriction and overexercise, health care professionals are often under the impression that unless you are anorexic, your habits are fine; however, a large body of research suggests otherwise.

For others—those who are in normal or larger bodies, who consume a standard diet without restriction, or exercise moderately a few days a week—it can be harder to come to terms with these issues causing your absent period. In our experience, however, there usually is some connection based not upon any one factor, but a mix.

The silver lining is that there is a road to recovery and health (and babies, if you so desire). It is not an easy path to follow—it takes commitment and a willingness to sit with the uncomfortable—but when you are ready, we have laid it all out for you in this book.

> *Lisa*: Light bulb moment! Ate clean, exercised (even if moderately in society's eyes), lost a little (or a lot of) weight, then added some stress, and BAM—you have yourself a missing monthly period. Like me, some of you will still question if not getting a period is a result of your eating and/or training habits, which at this point is referred to as denial or, point blank, an unwillingness to do what it takes to recover. I can absolutely relate to both. I refused to be uncomfortable, which is a key first step in recovering from being bound by exercise and food restriction, or any other addiction for that matter. Learning to embrace discomfort is a valuable lesson that can be carried over into every aspect of our lives, because really, in order to thrive we need to get to a place where we can be OK with life not being OK. I can guarantee you there will be a day when the uncomfy will come knocking on your door and you will either pull out some very useful coping skills collected during this time or you will look the other way and continue to run, overtrain, eat "perfectly," not

eat, overeat, etc. If you don't change the direction you are going, you will most definitely end up where you are heading... think about that.

2
Factors in HA: What You Eat

THROUGHOUT OUR LIVES we are bombarded by messages stressing the importance of physical appearance. It starts young; preschoolers comment on people being "fat" because they absorb the message pushed by society that skinny is "good" and "beautiful," and fat is, well, not. The pressure to be thin is amplified as we reach middle school; Nico remembers with horror how she and classmates ostracized and teased one girl who was larger. We comment on the appearance of politicians, reporters, and athletes, as if looks have something to do with job performance. When we see a young girl, we compliment her dress, her hair, and how pretty she is—not her intelligence, knowledge, empathy, creativity, or any of the other countless attributes that make up a whole complex individual.

As we enter our teen years, the importance of being small is further impressed on us through messages about what to eat and what not to eat. Words spin in our heads: *"Low calorie," "Low fat," "Diet to achieve your perfect body," "Lose those last 10 pounds", "Eat clean," "Carbs are bad"* etc., leaving us constantly concerned about what we're eating and what we look like. We are bombarded with the message that in order to be happy, respected, and successful, we must be thin.

> **Ami**: My husband met me at my heaviest weight and we couldn't keep our hands off each other. Then I got skinny—what I thought was sexy—and we only hit the bedroom like twice a month. He always wanted to, but I felt self-conscious, anxious, etc. He has said on many occasions after seeing super ripped girls how awful that looks—why do I want to gross

> my husband out? It really is just the pressure of society and comparing to others' sizes that makes us feel inadequate.
>
> *Lisa*: For me (and others) the disordered eating/over-training conundrum didn't begin with the societal pressures described above, but rather as a coping mechanism for some of life's serious curveballs. Exercise started out as a simple escape from a family member's long-term battle with bipolar disorder and schizophrenia. Leaving the house and walking for hours passing time allowed me to temporarily dissociate from the chaos. Add to that a nasty divorce and custody battle between my parents, and that is when my issues with food became a useful tool. Food was another way to escape and occupy my unsettled mind. With all that said, the over-training and undereating evolved into not only an unhealthy coping skill for life, but also a way to control my physique—seemingly the only thing I felt I could control.

So what do we do in order to attain society's standards, or to cope with other issues beyond our control? We might eat low-calorie foods, eliminate fats, try the latest "in" diet, or count calories until we have them memorized. Or perhaps we deny ourselves a treat here or there, limit portions, skip dessert and have dressing on the side. We may be hungry, tired, edgy, and unhappy, or even feel relatively normal, depending on whether we limit our food and how severe the restrictions are. Whatever the case, we often train ourselves to tune out our body's signals as we work to reach or maintain the size we think of as "healthy." However, ignoring our body's cues is *not* healthy. Over the years, our perception of what is healthy has been distorted, leading to negative physical and psychological effects.

Eating Habits and HA

> *Steph*: After completing intensive treatment for an eating disorder, I was in strong recovery, on the right track physically and mentally, and no one seemed concerned about my weight anymore. I was eating what seemed like a healthy amount for my needs and was generally following a meal plan that my nutritionist modified at the end of my treatment a year earlier. I thought I was satisfied and well-fueled as I trained for my first marathon. However, if I had been honest with myself, I would have realized I remained hungry after eating and my stomach was grumbling well before mealtime. I would have realized that eating lots of low-calorie granola bars just because I liked them was not necessarily giving my body what it

> needed. And I would have known that even though I thought I was on the right track, there was still work left to be done.

A wide range of eating patterns is found in those with HA. Typically, there is restriction in some form. Common scenarios include:

- Some, like Steph, have put in an incredible amount of mental and physical effort to recover from an eating disorder; they have gained weight and have their mental demons cowering in a corner. But perhaps there are some lingering tendencies that have led to less-than-healthy eating patterns and habits over time.
- Others (Nico for example) have taken society's messages to heart, often without realizing. This leads to following the "health plan" of losing weight and subsisting on the bare minimum.
- Or you have Lisa, who was overtraining and undereating as a way of exerting control over her life.
- Another group was at one point in a larger body and lost a significant amount of weight. Maintaining a "too-thin-for-them" weight often leads to the same physical effects (sometimes paired with a restrictive mindset). The weight loss can be years in the past, but the hormonal system remembers and a susceptibility to loss of the menstrual cycle is created.
- Others learn and incorporate information about alternative eating plans—such as a Zone, Paleo, whole food, or raw food diets—sometimes losing weight and sometimes not. They continue over time with constrained food patterns and choices, unaware that the reduced variety (and possibly calories) is not meeting their bodies' needs.
- Next are people who unconsciously undereat because they simply aren't aware of their true caloric needs—especially those who exercise a lot.
- The final (small) group comprises those who truly are meeting their caloric needs; in this case, other factors that we will discuss are the primary culprit for missing periods.

Which category do you fit into?

Typically, those with HA are undereating, whether consciously or not. Our survey respondents averaged 1481 calories per day, with a range from 300 to 2500. The standard recommendation for someone trying to lose weight is 1500 to 1800 calories per day[1]—almost half of our calorie counters were consuming less than that (see part 2 for HA Recovery recommendations).

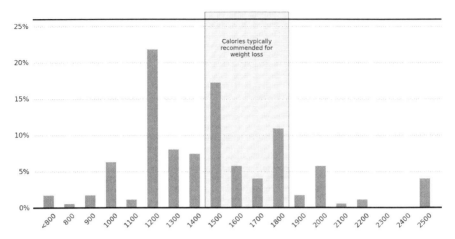

Underfueling. This figure shows the number of calories survey respondents (174 participants) planned to eat each day around the time they realized they were not getting their periods.

Many of us with HA, regardless of where we fall on the spectrum of adequate fueling, exhibit some disordered eating behaviors—often not enough to classify as an eating disorder, but yet at the same time decidedly not "normal." For example:

- Do you have forbidden foods or food groups you don't allow yourself to eat?
- If you eat one of those, do you feel guilty and anxious afterward?
- Is your eating dependent on your exercise—you allow yourself to go out to dinner only if you go to the gym to burn off the extra calories or skip other meals?
- Do you cook separate meals for yourself?
- How about avoiding social gatherings because you don't want to deal with the food or people asking you why you're not eating?
- Have you trained yourself to ignore your hunger—getting pleasure out of not "caving in"?

These behaviors are often found in people trying to control their weight; we show those that are most commonly mentioned by our survey respondents on the next page. How many of these describe you? If you're not sure, sometimes a more objective measure can help. Take the Eating Attitudes Test (EAT-26) online at www.eat-26.com. A score of 20 or above indicates an eating disorder, but you can exhibit disordered traits even if your score is lower. Is your score close to 20, or even higher? (If it is above 20, you might need to seek professional help in addition to the support and advice we will offer.)

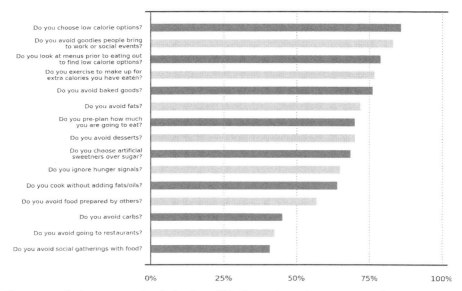

Common calorie-averse eating behaviors. This figure shows the percentage of survey respondents (323 participants) who, when reflecting on their former behaviors, selected "always" or "often" in response to the questions on the left. Compare these results to those who are recovered, in chapter 8. The difference is remarkable!

> *Nico:* When I went on my (in hindsight, completely unhealthy) diet, my daily menu tended not to change much; I'm a creature of habit. I'd have a granola bar and skim milk for breakfast, usually on my way to an early morning workout, followed by a diet soda when I was feeling peckish later in the morning. I became an expert at ignoring the grumbling in my stomach and learned that if I blocked it out long enough, the hunger eventually subsided. I'd avoid eating when someone brought in treats for group meetings or birthdays. I ate the same lunch just about every day (buffalo chicken wrap with one slice of American cheese—to this day when I go back to visit the cafeteria the staff know that's what I get); I liked it, and I knew how many calories it had. Another diet soda also helped fill me up so I no longer needed the French fries I used to get. I'd satisfy my sweet tooth by having a small piece of someone else's cookie. When I was eating at home, everything I ate and cooked was low fat. I'd fry with no oil, and never put dressing or butter on anything.

If you engage in some or many of the behaviors listed, you might already have an inkling they are contributing to your missing period. If you truly have "normal" eating habits and particularly if you are not what our society would consider "slim," you might be struggling to understand why your body is not cooperating. Keep in mind that as we discussed in chapter 1, there are a multitude of factors that combine to cause the shutdown of menstrual cycles.

Perhaps Not so Healthy

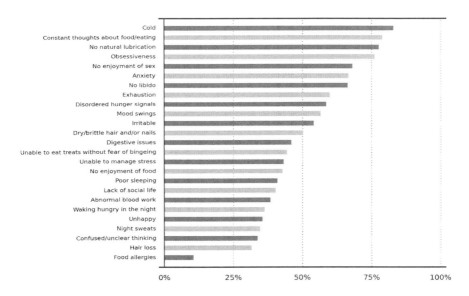

Signs and symptoms you might experience along with no period. This figure shows the percentage of survey respondents(324 participants) who selected that they "always" or "often" feel the symptoms indicated on the left, as compared to those who selected "rarely" or "never." As you can see, more than 50% of respondents always or often exhibited the first 11 symptoms. For a quick, but useful assessment, walk down the list, consider the symptoms and think about how often you experience each. A comparison of the same symptoms after recovery can be found in chapter 10.

Nico thought she was doing all the right things to help with pregnancy and delivery; one frequently reads that losing weight makes it easier to get pregnant. Lisa believed her clean eating and training regimen were good for her. And Steph was certain she was doing a great job fueling her running. But even as we thought we were healthy, we each experienced signs telling us that all was not well.

If you have also experienced some of these signs, you may have habits and thoughts about eating that are leading you to control your intake and not provide your body with enough food to sustain your daily activities.

Summary

In our quest to achieve society's ideals of being thin and healthy, some of us have fallen prey to restrictive, regimented, and controlling attitudes about what and how much we eat. In many cases, the lifestyle we think is so good for us actually has many negative health effects, including shutting down our reproductive cycles.

Do any of these physical symptoms describe you?

- amenorrhea (no period)
- osteopenia or osteoporosis (low bone density as found by DXA scan)
- stress fractures or other broken bones
- feeling cold all the time
- no libido or lubrication
- tired
- being awoken by hunger in the middle of the night or early morning hours
- brittle hair, nails, skin problems
- bowel issues

How about these eating behaviors and thoughts?

- counting calories; restricting to a certain number; feeling anxious if you exceed that amount
- limiting your portion sizes; deciding how much you will eat before you even start your meal
- avoiding certain foods or food groups
- exercising to compensate for "overeating"
- passing on food at social occasions, or avoiding social occasions altogether
- cooking separate meals for yourself
- eating "clean" or having strict food rules

If you're experiencing more than just one or two of the physical symptoms, your body is trying desperately to tell you something. Perhaps you're controlling your eating in some of the ways we describe; perhaps you aren't and *think* you are eating plenty. Regardless, through the rest of this book, we will help you continue to understand what your lifestyle is doing to your body and mind, and teach you how to break away from harmful habits and regain freedom, true health... and your period.

> Lisa: At this point, I'm betting some of you are in a place where you can't relate to the listed habits or physical symptoms (yet), but you are not cycling regularly, if at all (which is why this book piqued your interest). You may currently believe you are uber-healthy with your lean-machine-clean-eating self, but the fact of the matter is you may be undereating. I know I was. You've heard the term "ignorance is bliss," right? I enjoyed it for a long time, so deep in the disorder that I had tunnel vision and was unable to recognize my self-neglect. I actually became quite numb emotionally, too. Now I'm paying the piper. My hope for you is that before you choose to "turn off," or ignore the symptom of not getting a period, you will begin to understand some of the basic physiology of your body and the correlation between a regular menstrual cycle and good health.

3
Factors in HA: Exercise and Stress

"Exercise is good for you!" is a mantra hammered into our brains from an early age. In school, we had the Presidential fitness challenge* and were taught to always lead an active lifestyle. As we got older, messages promoting exercise were all over the media, often leading to the idea that if some exercise is good, more is better. When did you get involved in exercise? Did you participate in sports growing up, or discover the pleasures of exercising after high school or college? Did you get hooked by the "runner's high"? Or if you're the type that doesn't run unless you're being chased, was there another kind of exercise that captivated you? Once you started, you might have branched out into weight lifting and other cross-training, or perhaps classes like aerobics, CrossFit, Zumba, or spin. Often, though, the exercise schedules that start innocently as ways to get moving and healthy evolve into intense training without much recovery time. Or exercise becomes a way to burn off calories to maintain a lower weight. Exercise to this degree can negatively affect your reproductive system, especially if you are not adequately fueling and resting. For most with HA, overexercise is a culprit in their missing period. However, even a moderate exercise schedule can play a part in suppressing your reproductive system.

> *Nico*: I love to exercise. Toward the end of grad school, I set a goal of being able to do 10 pull-ups of my own body weight, and was getting

---

* The Presidential fitness challenge, developed in the 60's is a series of physical tests taken each year during grade school, designed to test overall fitness and teach children about the importance of daily activity.

> pretty close. I loved feeling strong, limber, and healthy. But what was not so healthy was limiting my fuel at the same time I was pushing myself in the weight room along with all the other exercise I was doing. On top of lifting weights three times a week, I played ice hockey three to five times, biked to and from work a couple of days, played squash with my coworkers for two to three hours at a time, and volleyball for another three to six hours a week. On Saturdays and Sundays my husband and I would play golf at a very hilly course and walk the whole way (about seven miles) to get more exercise. Sundays we'd play 90 minutes of hockey first!
>
> I hardly ever took a day off. I loved the exercise and camaraderie of team sports. I loved seeing the long-term improvements in my strength. True, sometimes I'd wake up early for hockey and not want to get out of bed, but once I'd managed that part it was fun. Biking home with already sore legs after playing hockey or lifting weights earlier that day also took some mental prodding, but I enjoyed it once I got started. Or I told myself I did.
>
> Looking back, I cannot believe I managed all this on the small amount of fuel I was allowing myself. In retrospect, it's no wonder my body rebelled by saying, "No way are you making a baby when you're treating me like this!"

Exercising Too Much?

Just as with eating, different exercise patterns can play a role in loss of your period. Common scenarios include:

- Some don't do any formal exercise at all. (For this group, other factors are involved.)
- Another group exercises moderately: perhaps an hour at a time, three to four days per week.
- The next group comprises the daily exercisers: an hour or more each and every day with very few rest days.
- And then there are the exercise overachievers (ahem, Nico!): multiple types of exercise in a day, for many hours.

The problem with exercise lies both in how much you are exercising and whether you are eating to support that exercise, as well as how it affects you mentally. Do you have a need—a compulsion—to exercise? Take a look at your life and your habits. Are you organizing your life around exercise instead of the other way around? Are you grumpy if you don't get your daily exercise in? Do you tell yourself that exercise is for stress relief, but find that fitting exercise in is actually causing stress? Two questionnaires (among many) to help you assess the possibility of an exercise addiction include the Exercise Addiction Inventory (EAI)[1], and the Obsessive Exercise Questionnaire (OEQ)[2].

Even if you are not a compulsive exerciser, and are taking plenty of rest days, exercise can still play a part in missing cycles. First by burning calories—if daily intake is not enough to cover both the energy burned by exercise and the energy needed by the body for daily living, periods can stop[3]. Among our survey respondents who counted calories, many were surviving on *way less* than even the recommendations for ongoing weight loss (1500-1800 calories per day)[4].

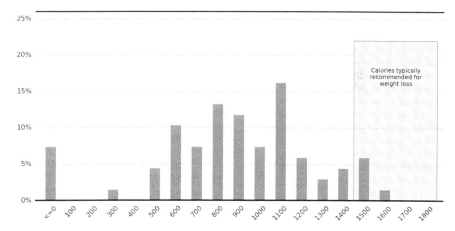

Total intake, taking exercise into account. This figure shows net calories; the number of calories survey respondents (68 participants) were consuming each day after exercise-burned calories were subtracted. The light gray box shows the standard recommendation of 1500 to 1800 calories per day for weight loss. You can see that our respondents who provided calorie information were not eating a sufficient amount for their exercise; in fact, almost everyone was netting fewer calories than the bare minimum recommended for ongoing weight loss*.

The second effect of exercise, as we've mentioned, is to increase levels of cortisol, a hormone associated with stress that can ultimately result in absent cycles[5]. Frequent intense workouts absolutely elevate cortisol levels[6], but moderate exercise coupled with mental stress, and even no exercise but high stress can have the same effect[7]. Along with the amount of fuel being

---

* Only about 20% of our respondents provided information about exercise calorie estimations for each day. Tracking to this level suggests these are likely members of our group who were more restrictive, so the graph may underestimate average daily caloric intake. Regardless, the point is that exercise impacts the calories available for a body's daily functioning.

consumed, this helps explain why those who are not overexercising can still lose periods. Especially, as we have mentioned, because every body reacts differently to the changes in hormones.

The data below from our survey will help you see where your exercise habits fall compared to others with absent periods. Of our survey respondents, nine (3%) classified themselves as non-exercisers. Among the remaining 300, a majority exercised more than five days a week (5.8 was the average), and for 1 to 1.5 hours each session. These averages are high, but there are also many who exercised much less (or not at all) and still lost their periods. As a comparison, after HA recovery the average person was exercising 4.5 days a week, for 45 minutes each session.

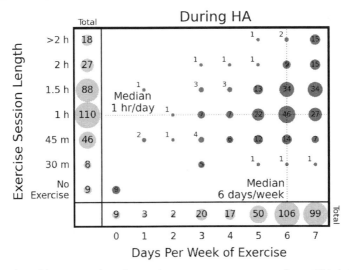

Days per week and hours per day of exercise among survey respondents. This bubble chart shows the exercise habits of our survey respondents when absent periods were discovered. The area of each circle corresponds to the number of respondents. The light gray circles indicate the number of people at each exercise session length and days per week of exercise. For example, 106 respondents (out of a total of 306) were exercising six days per week when missing periods were discovered; only 9 did not exercise.

We also asked about the intensity of exercise at a time *before* periods went missing as compared to when amenorrhea was active, using a scale in which:

- 0 was sitting, breathing, and talking normally, heart rate 40–69
- 5 was moderate exercise: a very fast walk/jog, can carry on a conversation, heart rate 140–149
- 10 was highest intensity exercise: a personal record pace, can't talk, gasping for breath, heart rate 190+

The comparison of average intensity when periods were present to when they were absent is rather striking. The survey respondents were generally pushing themselves much harder when they lost their periods than they had at times when they were still cycling ($p < 1\times10^{-12}$*).

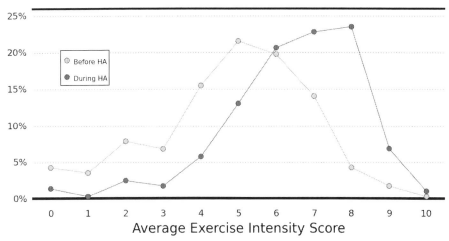

Average exercise intensity among survey respondents. This figure indicates the percentage of survey respondents (278 participants) selecting each average intensity score for the time before they lost their periods (light gray) as compared to when their periods went missing (dark gray). Before period loss the most common average exercise intensity was 5, with most between 4 and 7; with loss of period, the most common average intensity was 7–8, with most between 5 and 8.

> **Stacey S:** When working, I used to get up at 5:45 a.m. and run to the gym to be there when it opened (6:30... I know, how provincial!) and then do 30 minutes of weights. Perfectly timed and executed without fail. Then we went traveling and I had to be a bit "flexible"... my husband lost count of the times he woke up at 7 a.m. to find me at the bottom of the bed (some rooms were very small) doing squats with his backpack on, buck naked (I had limited clothing and his bag was heavier). I incorporated cardio by running up and down the hotel stairs (I put clothes on for that) and sometimes by doing the circuit routine that I had devised the night before...

Female/Male Athlete Triad OR Relative Energy Deficiency in Sport

Have you heard of the "female/male athlete triad"? If so, you've probably noticed that what we have described sounds quite similar. The athlete triad is a combination of:

---

* See the appendix for more information about *p*-values.

1) disordered eating
2) low bone density
3) suppression of the hypothalamic–pituitary–gonadal (HPG) axis

Many athletes (a term used very loosely to describe any person who exercises)[8] experience this cluster of issues. The triad was originally rather stringent, comprising women with diagnosed eating disorders, bone density so low it was defined as osteoporosis, and amenorrhea. More recently, however, it has been recognized that each of these characteristics exists along a continuum and in all genders. You can be at a different point along the range for each of the three components at any given time. In the last few years, others have argued for a more inclusive name for the syndrome that highlights the underfueling aspect, leading to adoption of the term "Relative Energy Deficiency in Sport[9]," as well as the change to Female/Male Athlete Triad.

> *Lisa*: The female athlete triad. It's an interesting term, reflective of what we have discussed so far. When diagnosed with Triad, some of us respond with concern, "Oh shoot… better get this under control," while others tend to equate it with elitism, as if it's another trophy to hang our hats on. For me being labeled triad was a way to stick my head in the sand, proving I didn't have some sort of eating disorder like "those other women." I remember feeling pretty cool when diagnosed with it because I had trained so hard and eaten so strictly. But basically, I had done nothing more than neglect my health.

> *Jenni*: Whenever I see people training to compete in figure or body-building competitions I want to warn them that losing your period isn't a joke. When I was with my trainer and at my lowest, I remember laughing about how I hadn't had a period in almost a year, and deep down, I think I may have even been proud of it, like, "My body fat is too low to have a period, good job, me!!!" BAHHHH, I wanna punch the old me in the throat.

Summary

Many of us exercise not only for the assumed health benefits, but also to help keep our weight in check. But despite what we hear and read, it is possible to take the exercise too far, particularly in combination with the amount we're eating. It doesn't seem possible, but too much exercise (or sometimes even just a moderate amount), often along with not enough food (whether intentional or not) can negate many of the benefits of exercise by robbing you of your period.

Do any of these exercise behaviors or thoughts describe you?

- taking few, if any, rest days
- feeling compelled to exercise and anxious when unable to do so
- using exercise to control your weight, including adding extra exercise to make up for food you feel like you "shouldn't" have eaten
- choosing exercise over hobbies or socializing
- using exercise as a stress outlet or to deal with difficult times

Perhaps none of these fit your situation. As we've mentioned, there are a people who lose their periods with what seems like a very reasonable amount of exercise—three to four days a week or less, and only moderate intensity, or no exercise at all. Keep in mind first that exercise we see as moderate can absolutely have an effect on cycles, and second that when combined with other variables (energy intake, stress, genetics, etc.) the impact on our systems can be magnified.

There *is* hope—folks from each of the categories we have described have followed the Recovery Plan (part 2) and either restored cycles or responded better to treatment (and regained cycles after pregnancy).

> *Lisa:* Are you nodding your head in agreement or finding many of your thoughts being echoed throughout these pages? If so, I am secretly excited because the goal of this book is to provide truths and coping skills that will help you regain your overall health, fertility, and well-being, resulting in recovery. Even if you're *not* nodding in agreement or finding much of this relatable, I encourage you to keep an open mind, especially if you aren't getting your period, exercise regularly, and/or restrict your eating. I was in the latter group—skeptical and unable to see that my behaviors and actions were contributing to not getting a period—in denial. My hope is that you'll stick around long enough to consider the possibility that this might be you, too.

4
Diagnosis

WHEN YOU GO to your doctor and say, "I'm not getting my period," there's a standard workup they will do. There are many potential reasons for amenorrhea, which can include polycystic ovarian syndrome (PCOS), hypothalamic amenorrhea (HA), hyperprolactinemia (high prolactin, which suppresses ovulation), chromosomal or physical abnormalities, or ovarian failure[1]. Because of all these different causes, it is important to see a doctor to rule out some of the less common issues. You might start with your primary care physician, or obstetrician/gynecologist (ob-gyn), or perhaps be referred to an endocrinologist or reproductive endocrinologist (60% of our survey respondents took the "RE" route). At this point it doesn't matter very much what type of doctor you see since the diagnostic tests are fairly standard. Before we get to the tests, though, we will talk a bit more about the varying types and causes of amenorrhea. Let's start with a very basic distinction:

- Primary amenorrhea occurs when you have never gotten a natural period (without intervention like birth controls pills or hormone replacement)—1% of our survey respondents.
- Secondary amenorrhea is when you have had a natural period in the past but are not currently cycling.

The issues causing primary amenorrhea are often completely different from the HA we are discussing in this book, and care should be coordinated by a knowledgeable doctor. In some cases, the amenorrhea is due to chromosomal abnormalities like Turner syndrome (when an X chromosome is missing or abnormal). In others, periods may not occur because of anatomic abnormalities such as an absent uterus, or excess tissue that prevents bleeding[2]. One scenario in which primary amenorrhea is not so different from HA, however, is when girls who are serious athletes starting from a young age do not get their period in an expected timeframe. This is essentially HA, and everything we will discuss in the remainder of the book applies in this case.

There are also a multitude of causes of secondary amenorrhea. For example, Asherman's syndrome (scarring in the uterus that prevents bleeding) can be a culprit. Autoimmune disease, various medications, and thyroid issues, among others, can also cause periods to cease. However, *if what we've discussed in previous chapters applies to you to any degree, chances are that the diagnostic path will lead to hypothalamic amenorrhea.*

We will discuss many of the steps and tests that should be performed to check if you have HA, but the short version is that when you have HA you will likely have some or all of the following[3]:

- low luteinizing hormone (LH)
- low estradiol with normal or low-normal follicle stimulating hormone (FSH)
- thin uterine lining (less than 4 mm)
- polycystic appearing ovaries (chapter 6)
- a history of weight loss, restrictive or "clean" eating, and/or frequent exercise

> *Nico*: The hardest part for me about all the diagnostic stuff was how long it all took. It felt like it was one baby step forward, and then wait, wait, wait… then one more baby step. And more waiting.
>
> After going off the pill in July 2004, I waited to get my period, which didn't happen. So I went to see my primary care doctor in October. She did a bit of blood work to check my thyroid function, and prescribed some Provera (synthetic progesterone) to see if that would cause a withdrawal bleed (often referred to as the "Provera challenge," http://noperiod.info/provera). No such luck. Next, I scheduled an appointment with my ob-gyn. That finally happened in November. When I saw her, she wanted to try the Provera challenge again, drew some blood, and said I needed an ultrasound. The scan had to be done through the radiology department, so it was scheduled for a few days later (luckily still in November). I got the all-clear from that, albeit with a thin lining. Since I'd

> now failed the Provera challenge twice, the next test was a brain MRI to see if it was a pituitary tumor causing my issues. Nope. After that, I took estrogen and progesterone in December to try and trigger a bleed that way. My period came in January. I was happy to see blood FINALLY, but wasn't thrilled that it had taken a lot of hormones to get there.
>
> My ob-gyn called in January to say that I had hypothalamic amenorrhea, and referred me to an RE who could help me get pregnant. I was supremely lucky to get in just a few weeks later! She ordered yet more blood work to help rule out PCOS, and another ultrasound. Finally, after those results came back, she agreed that I did have HA, and we could move forward with fertility treatment. Lifestyle changes wouldn't do anything, she opined, as my cycles had been irregular as a teenager. Little did she know! But that's a story for another chapter…

Your workup should start with your doctor taking your history, doing a physical exam, and drawing some blood (be prepared for them to take quite a few vials). The clinician should ask about[5]:

- your cycles in the past
- galactorrhea (milk in your breasts when you aren't pregnant or nursing)
- birth control history
- recent stressful events
- eating and exercise habits
- recent weight loss
- medication use (some drugs such as opioid pain relievers like OxyContin or tramadol, or antipsychotics such as Thorazine or Compazine can cause menstrual irregularities)[6]

In the physical exam your doctor will check your breasts, feel for your uterus and ovaries (to rule out physical abnormalities), and look for hair in places it doesn't belong (this is called hirsutism and can be associated with PCOS).

Assuming a normal physical exam, your doctor will order a urine test to rule out pregnancy, and send your blood off. He or she should be checking FSH, LH, prolactin, and thyroid stimulating hormone (TSH). It is not recommended to test estradiol (E_2) as part of the latest protocol for evaluating amenorrhea; however, many doctors do still order this test. The next page shows normal results along with those you are likely to receive if you have HA. We have also included some abnormal results that might indicate other underlying issues.

Hormones and expected results

Hormone	What does it do?	Normal result*	Typical result in HA	Other abnormal result
Follicle stimulating hormone (FSH)	Helps eggs mature	Normal (3.0–20.0 IU/L)†	Low normal to normal	High; diminished ovarian reserve/premature ovarian insufficiency
Luteinizing hormone (LH)	A spike causes the mature egg to release (ovulation)	Normal (2.0–15.0 IU/L)	Low to low normal	LH > FSH may be suggestive of PCOS or imminent ovulation (especially if not tested during menstruation)
Prolactin	Stimulates milk production; suppresses FSH, LH, and E_2	Normal (0.0–20.0 ng/mL)	Normal	High may indicate a pituitary cyst or benign tumor‡
Thyroid stimulating hormone (TSH)	Drives secretion of thyroid hormones triiodothyronine (T3) and thyroxine (T4), which help control metabolism	Normal (0.3–3.0 mIU/L)	Normal	High (hypothyroidism) or low (hyperthyroidism). Preferred range is between 0.5 and 2.5 when trying to get pregnant[7].
Sex Hormone Binding Globulin (SHBG)	Protein made in the liver that binds sex hormones and inhibits function; prevents exposure to androgens	Normal (40-120 nmol/L)	Normal to high normal	Low to low normal is associated with PCOS; leads to higher free androgen
Estradiol (E_2)	Secreted by maturing eggs; drives changes in FSH and LH levels	Normal (20–150 pg/mL)	Low to low normal	High may indicate imminent ovulation

* We have listed the standard ranges. You should ask for the reference ranges from the laboratory that performed your testing in order to compare your results.
† Many REs will perform additional testing with an FSH above 12 IU/L as this can be indicative of diminished ovarian reserve.
‡ If your prolactin is high, you should get an MRI to look for a cyst or tumor on your pituitary gland. DO NOT FREAK OUT! These are not uncommon, and almost always benign.

In our experience, the result that most accurately predicts HA is a low LH level, although it is possible to have HA with a normal LH level. To illustrate this, on the next page we show the LH and E_2 levels in our survey respondents who provided information. LH was the most diagnostic; below normal (< 2.0 IU/L) in almost three-quarters of survey respondents. LH often increases with recovery.

- Estradiol was below normal for about half the respondents (< 20 pg/mL). As we mentioned, E_2 is no longer included in diagnostic criteria for HA and often does not change much with recovery. We include these data because it is still commonly tested.
    o As an example of the irrelevance of E_2, Nico's level was 34 pg/mL when tested during HA, 27 on the natural cycle when she got her first positive pregnancy test and more recently, 23 after she'd been cycling regularly for a year.
- FSH was distributed evenly between 0 and 9 IU/L (not shown), so not much help in diagnosis. However, a low FSH suggests a more severe degree of HA (see below).
- SHBG has recently been found to be high in concert with HA and suggested as a potential marker for HA[4]

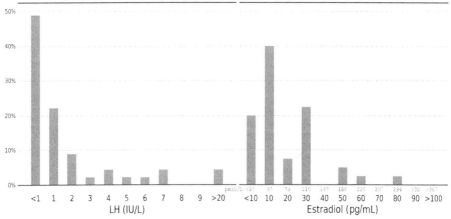

Survey respondents' hormone levels during HA. This figure shows the LH (45 participants) (*left*) and estradiol/E_2 (40 participants) (*right*) levels of our survey respondents who provided information. LH was < 2 IU/L for 72% of respondents, with a median of 1.6 IU/L—a low result like this is commonly seen in cases of HA. Two respondents with suspected PCOS had levels > 20 IU/L. E_2 levels were also generally at the low end of normal, with a median of 19 pg/mL.

In addition to the blood tests and physical exam, another common diagnostic tool is the "Provera challenge," http://noperiod.info/provera. Your doctor will give you a prescription for Provera (or something similar), which is a synthetic version of progesterone. In a normal menstrual cycle, progesterone rises after ovulation to prepare the uterus for a fertilized egg. If no pregnancy occurs, progesterone drops and a period ensues. Provera mimics this cycle. You'll take it for anywhere from 5 to 10 days to see if you bleed after you stop. The standard protocol is to wait two weeks to see if there is any spotting or bleeding, although among our survey respondents, all but one person who got a withdrawal bleed did so within eight days. About 18% (48/256) responded to Provera (i.e., they got a bleed). This indicates a less severe degree of HA. No bleed suggests a more suppressed reproductive system without adequate estrogen to build a uterine lining—in other words, full blown HA. The degree of HA is based on response to Provera and Clomid[8]:

- HA degree 1 (least severe): You bleed after taking Provera and Clomid.
- HA degree 2 (moderately severe): You bleed after taking Provera but do not respond to Clomid.
- HA degree 3 (most severe): You don't get a withdrawal bleed after taking Provera.

If you do not bleed in response to Provera, your doctor may then have you take estrogen for three to four weeks, combined with Provera during the last week. This is different from the Provera challenge described above; the estrogen works to thicken your lining so you have something to shed after you take the Provera. A bleed tells you that are no blockages, uterine scarring, or anatomic abnormalities preventing bleeding. You will already know this if you were recently getting bleeds on birth control, so taking the estrogen/progesterone combination can be unnecessary. If you haven't recently had a bleed and do not menstruate after the estrogen/progesterone combination, your doctor will investigate further to determine if there are other concerns. Sometimes we are told this estrogen/provera combination will "jumpstart" our menstrual cycle, but this is inaccurate.

It is also common to have an ultrasound during the diagnostic process. Look out—this will be a vaginal ultrasound, which can be unnerving if you're not expecting it. Your practitioner will put a condom with some ultrasound jelly onto an ultrasound probe and gently insert it into your vagina. It can be a bit uncomfortable as the probe is twisted around to look at your uterus and ovaries from the correct angles. The sonographer will be looking for any abnormalities, measuring the thickness of your uterine lining, and checking how many follicles you have and how they're distributed in your ovaries. Follicles are little sacs that contain your eggs. During a menstrual cycle you start off with a number of small follicles that are stimulated by FSH; as they grow, one begins to dominate and shuts down the others. Eventually your LH surges, the mature egg is released by the ovaries, and starts on its journey to your uterus. The ovaries of HAers are often classified as "polycystic" because there are frequently many small follicles present on an ultrasound due to lack of ovulation. If your ovaries truly are *polycystic* (meeting the actual definition provided in chapter 6), you may meet the diagnosis of polycystic ovarian syndrome (PCOS). However, if the first few chapters of this book have resonated with you, it is highly likely that you either do not have PCOS, or have HA in addition. Additional blood tests should be performed to rule out or confirm PCOS (chapter 6).

After all these hurdles are cleared, you may get a diagnosis of "hypothalamic amenorrhea (HA), also known as hypogonadotropic hypogonadism (HH)."

> Lisa: I remember when I was diagnosed with HA at 39 (this is after ten years of absent periods, mind you). The first time any of my doctors actually mentioned HA was during an annual visit with a new ob-gyn. After taking a quick history she told me to kick back, watch some Oprah, and eat ice cream. Dr. B assured me that my cycles would return and I would hopefully build back some bone density. Honestly, I didn't believe her. And I certainly didn't trust that living an "unhealthy lifestyle" like the one she was suggesting was the solution. Never mind the fact that I was living an unhealthy lifestyle at the time. How did I not see that? Denial! I refused to entertain the idea that simple weight gain and reduced exercise were the keys to recovery. Can you relate?
>
> I rocked on neglecting my health for another two years while slowly gaining an understanding and accepting the possibility of having HA. I finally saw an RE secretly hoping to find another solution for no period. He was the first doctor to come straight out and say, "Oh, you absolutely have hypothalamic amenorrhea and this is why." He reiterated everything I had learned from the Board, which was further confirmed through blood work and the typical thin uterine lining.

OK, so you have a diagnosis. Now what? If a doctor, a friend, or something you read on the Internet has suggested you may have PCOS as well, you should make sure to read chapter 6 when you get to it (this is super important because HA is often misdiagnosed as PCOS). Chapter 5 will cover hypothalamic amenorrhea in more depth. In the meantime, it is very normal to have mixed emotions once you figure out the root of your issue. Steph and some of our survey respondents describe their feelings after being diagnosed with HA:

> Steph: Walking into that first RE appointment, I had a sick feeling—you know, the pit-of-your-stomach kind. I didn't know what the diagnosis

was going to be, but I had a pretty good idea of what I was going to be told to do about it. Even though I knew it was coming, even though my body had been all but screaming at me for months prior to the diagnosis, when the doctor actually said the words, I shut down. I crossed my arms and got ready to argue with him big time. I didn't want to believe him; I couldn't believe him. And then after everything, I went to my car and I cried and cried. I felt sorry for myself. I felt cheated. I had already recovered from an eating disorder and now this? What?! Even though I knew the diagnosis was coming, that did not make the news any easier, and it took time for me to accept the changes I had to make.

Sara: I was initially relieved to work out what was "wrong" with me, as PCOS (my original diagnosis) didn't make sense. Then I felt angry for getting myself in that predicament in the first place. And then I became very frustrated and impatient trying to make the lifestyle changes. Now I view it as a blessing that has taught me so much about myself, but the initial stages were very difficult.

Amy S: I was not surprised—I knew deep down that this would manifest when I went off the pill. What I did not realize was how much of a struggle it would be to force myself to confront my "body hatred." It was really hard and I was scared about what I had done to my body. I was angry at myself too for what I had done and for having feelings of inadequacy even when faced with this disorder, and terrified that I would never have children. But it was the hardest and best thing I have had to conquer in my life.

Jessica V: Annoyed, like "These people just want to make me gain weight. No one understands me, etc., etc." Irrational thinking that made sense to my warped mind at the time.

Tammy: Relieved, then began to excitedly plan my recovery. Thankful that it was a condition that I could do something about.

Helen: I was never diagnosed. I self-diagnosed and recovered from the advice on the Board! My docs all said "unexplained"! Grrrrr.

Shyanne: Overwhelmed, but also glad it wasn't PCOS anymore. Glad that (because of the Board) I knew I could start right away about doing something about it. I didn't feel helpless.

Danielle: Shocked and upset that 10 years ago I mentioned to my ob-gyn at the time that I didn't get periods. Her response was that most athletes don't get them and I'm fine and most likely ovulating. She said you don't need to bleed to ovulate. And told me not to worry. So I didn't! [Note that this doctor was incorrect—if you ovulate you will get a period unless there are anatomic abnormalities; see chapter 5.]

Emily S: I felt a little "broken" but at the same time glad to have a label that we could begin to address and treat. I think most with HA are perfectionists in a lot of ways, so I think many feel similarly.

Kathryn: Relief. After searching and searching for answers I finally had one. It had taken years of seeing different OBs and endos, and finally my RE at CCRM told me straight up: you're too skinny.

ReAnn: Frustrated, as nothing had changed in my habits, but all of a sudden at 30 after stopping birth control I was diagnosed with something that I'd probably had since I was 13.

Chrissy: I was very frustrated, as I was not an overexerciser and was not "underweight," but deep down I knew that I was never eating enough, and that the low BMI I was maintaining was likely not a healthy enough weight for me. But I was relieved that I was not totally broken, and I knew I WOULD be able to get pregnant!

Louise: I was pretty mad, actually, since I was still in a bigger than average body and had worked so hard already to lose 70 pounds. Didn't make sense or seem fair.

Kira: I was somewhat angry at myself for doing this to my body, since my body will probably always be more sensitive to calories and exercise. I also was thankful in a way that this is what motivated me to finally face my demons and mentally recover fully vs. the partial recovery/controlled prison I had been living in for years.

Leah: I had already diagnosed myself months ago, so was annoyed that I was still forced to go through all the extensive testing (although now that I work in a fertility clinic I know that's routine).

Julie B: I felt like a failure. And mad at myself and feeling like there was no way to have kids. Doctors told me that the only way to ovulate was drugs.

Deanna: I was upset that I wasn't diagnosed with HA by my doctor and actually resented him—but then I realized that I had diagnosed myself, made lifestyle changes and by the time I saw him I was no longer "HA" by any of the medical definitions ... my hormones were on the rise and I was getting Provera bleeds. So, while I wanted that diagnosis SO badly to validate everything I'd done and been working for, I thankfully never got it. If that makes sense. But it took me a while to come to terms with that

> and not hold the non-diagnosis against my doctor just because he didn't believe in the Recovery Plan that clearly was working.

It's not always easy to correctly diagnose HA. Some are lucky and receive the appropriate diagnosis early on. Others are told there is no explanation for their missing period or there is nothing to do besides go on birth control pills or hormone replacement to prevent bone loss and then use fertility medications when the time comes for pregnancy. In other cases, people are told they have PCOS and head off in the wrong direction (chapter 6). As you probably realize after reading this chapter, an accurate diagnosis takes time, and this period of limbo can be extremely frustrating when you have nowhere to turn for support or answers. In addition, outside the United States there seems to be much less awareness of HA and therefore folks are simply diagnosed with "unexplained amenorrhea" and given no further direction. We do not want this to be your experience. This chapter and the rest of the book are meant to arm you with knowledge so that you have a good idea of what to expect and how to conquer HA.

Additional Tests

There are some additional blood tests that your doctor might perform in your diagnostic workup that you might be curious about. We will discuss AMH further in chapter 20.

Additional hormones and expected results

Hormone	Purpose	Normal result	Abnormal result
Anti-Mullerian Hormone (AMH)	Secreted by small follicles in your ovaries	Normal to high*	Low-may indicate low egg reserve, suggests more aggressive fertility treatment.† High-indicates a large number of follicles; suggests caution with any fertility treatments to avoid OHSS.
Progesterone (P4)	Secreted after ovulation; helps maintain the uterine lining	<3 ng/mL unless ovulation has recently occurred	No levels considered abnormal

* The ranges for AMH are still under development and are dependent upon age. The laboratory should supply this information. However, normal is often considered a value from 1.5 to 4.0 ng/mL, high is above 4.0 ng/mL.

† Low AMH alone is NOT sufficient to diagnose diminished ovarian reserve, especially if your other hormones are low; AMH can be affected by FSH and LH levels. If a follicle scan early in your cycle shows the expected number of small follicles, the AMH is likely an aberration[9], especially if paired with a low or normal FSH (chapter 20). Diminished ovarian reserve is possible when your AMH and baseline (a.k.a. antral) follicle count are low and your FSH is elevated.

Summary

We described a number of tests that are commonly performed in order to determine the cause of your missing periods. The keys to diagnosing HA are:

- low to normal LH
- probably no bleed in response to Provera
- thin uterine lining when examined by ultrasound
- no large "dominant" follicles in your ovaries
- many small follicles

The good news, if you do in fact have HA, is that you absolutely *can* recover, as long as you are willing to put in the effort and time to make some changes to your habits and thinking.

> *Lisa*: OK, so nothing earth shattering here other than some rock solid instruction for specific tests to better confirm what you most likely already know or suspect. I sort of grin as I write this because I was in such denial when I was first told I had HA. I thought there was *no way* I have this—my eating was healthy and I wasn't training hours a day. I mean, really… I was a fitness coach proclaiming the word on good health and nutrition and most, if not all, of my female clients commented on the epitome of fitness I represented. (Ironically, my guy buddies regularly remarked that I could use a few more hamburgers and fries.) Though, if I hadn't been in such denial, not having a period along with my abnormal blood work results would have clearly raised a red flag. Could you too be in denial?

5
Hypothalama-WHAT??

ONCE YOUR DOCTOR tells you that you have hypothalamic amenorrhea (also referred to as hypogonadotropic hypogonadism), or you do some reading and determine for yourself that this is probably your diagnosis, your initial reaction might be, "What the heck does that mean?" You might have tried searching online to get an idea of what's going on and what you need to do, but still feel none the wiser as to what comes next. To get you started, this chapter will cover everything you need to know to understand HA: how menstrual cycles are supposed to work; how they're connected to what you eat, the stress you experience, and your exercise habits; and why your cycles are not doing what they're supposed to be doing right now.

If you are not so interested in the science and just want to know the bottom line, it's this: **the hypothalamus controls your reproductive system, and it tries to regulate how much you eat**[1]. If you're not eating enough (deliberately or otherwise) to fuel your daily activities, and/or exercise so much that you create an energy deficit, that information is quickly transmitted to your brain. Eventually, your hypothalamus responds by shutting down your reproductive system in an effort to conserve energy needed for other bodily functions such as breathing and blood circulation. These mechanisms are needed for survival, whereas reproduction is not. In essence, your brain ceases communication with your ovaries until conditions are optimal to sustain a healthy pregnancy (for you and baby).

We will go into more details in the next few sections. It is fascinating how our reproductive, feeding control, and stress response systems all work together for our own protection.

Don't get hung up on the technicalities, though. The key is to understand that the amount of food consumed, weight (and/or amount of body fat), exercise performed, stress experienced, and genetics all strongly affect the reproductive system. And no matter what our *conscious* minds think, if the hypothalamus senses an unfavorable nutrient balance or stress environment, it will shut down the ability to cycle and procreate.

> **Lisa**: *"No matter what our conscious minds think."* Did you catch that? In the midst of HA, most of us feel like Wonder Woman (start humming the theme song). Seriously, the only things missing would be the invisible airplane, bullet proof gold cuffs, and lasso of truth. Consciously, while deep in HA, we feel in control, have tons of energy (usually due to adrenaline or an exercise high), and appear to be lean mean fighting machines, but this is not the case. The hypothalamus, which takes no notice of our conscious thoughts senses the energy imbalance, increased stress, and decreased weight or body fat and says, "Hey Diana Prince, that spinny thing you do to turn into Wonder Woman ain't gonna work no more," and puts the kibosh on hormone output. Well, not exactly. What it actually does is attempt to reach homeostasis again by shutting or slowing down extraneous systems such as our menstrual cycles. So basically Wonder Woman doesn't have enough energy to even spin in a circle at this point.

Defining HA

The hypothalamus is a small area in your brain, about the size of an almond. It takes in information from the rest of your body, including different areas of your brain, nerves from other organs, and chemicals that are in your blood. It processes that information and then sends out a host of other hormones that control food intake, temperature, sleep, thirst, and the reproductive system[2].

We've already talked about amenorrhea; it's the technical term used to describe when you're not getting your menstrual period. In fact, it literally means "without menstrual flow": A (without)-men (menstrual)-o-rrhea (flow). As the hypothalamus is intricately involved in controlling the menstrual cycle, this leads us to the term "hypothalamic amenorrhea"—a lack of a period caused by improper signals from the hypothalamus. Be aware that not every case of amenorrhea is due to the hypothalamus, so your doctor should be involved in your care to rule out other causes (chapter 4).

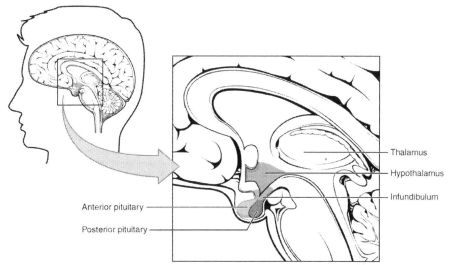

Control centers in the brain. The location of the hypothalamus (and pituitary gland, which will come into play soon) in your brain. Image reprinted under CC BY 3.0 license: "1806 The Hypothalamus-Pituitary Complex" by OpenStax College - Anatomy & Physiology[3].

How does this situation of improper hypothalamic signaling come about and result in the loss of your period? To answer this question, it is helpful to understand what goes on in a typical menstrual cycle, so we will go over that first, then briefly discuss how appetite is controlled, the effects of exercise and stress, and how the systems interact[4]. Lastly, we talk about what might be happening when someone has HA.

A Typical Menstrual Cycle

Many of us have been on some form of birth control since our teenage years. As a result, we have little experience with natural cycles. And middle school health class was way too long ago to remember anything that was covered—so we're going to go back there for a bit.

A regular menstrual cycle is driven by a network of hormonal signals, both positive and negative, which ultimately stimulate an egg to grow, mature, and be released. Simultaneously, the uterine lining is prepared so that an embryo can implant. If there's no implantation, the lining sheds and the whole process starts over again. The major hormonal players in this cycle are FSH, LH, progesterone, and estrogen. The changes through the cycle are inter-related; we'll go through what happens step by step.

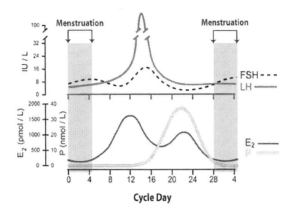

Reproductive hormone levels through the menstrual cycle. Levels of gonadotropins (*top*): follicle-stimulating hormone (FSH), which leads to egg growth and maturation, and luteinizing hormone (LH), which causes ovulation. Levels of hormones secreted by the ovaries (*bottom*): Estrogen is secreted by the maturing egg and affects levels of gonadotropins. Progesterone from the corpus luteum helps prepare the uterine lining for implantation of an embryo. Image reprinted under CC BY 3.0 license: "Figure 28 02 07" by OpenStax College - Anatomy & Physiology[5].

The first thing you need to know is that our cycles are divided into two parts:

- In the first half, an egg grows and matures in a sac-like structure called a follicle, inside your ovary. This is called the *follicular phase*.
- Around the middle of your cycle, the follicle bursts and releases the egg, which travels to your uterus. This release of the egg is termed ovulation.
- The second half of your cycle, after ovulation, is called the *luteal phase* (LP). During this stage, the former follicle (called a corpus luteum) secretes additional hormones like progesterone to prepare your uterine lining for an embryo to implant.
- If no pregnancy occurs, the corpus luteum breaks down and progesterone secretion stops, leading to shedding of the uterine lining (your period). Estradiol levels also drop, signaling the start of the next follicular growth phase, and the cycle starts over again.

Follicular Phase

Step 1: Your menstrual cycle officially begins on the first day of bleeding (not spotting), designated as cycle day 1 (CD 1). At this point, egg-containing follicles in the ovary produce a low level of a hormone called estradiol (E_2), which is a form of estrogen. The E_2 travels to the hypothalamus in the bloodstream and the relative amount controls the release of another protein called gonadotropin releasing hormone (GnRH), by the hypothalamus.

When E_2 is at its lowest, as in this early part of the cycle (CD 0–3, bottom panel), GnRH secreted by the hypothalamus is kept to a minimum, and it is released in slow pulses. These slow pulses cause the pituitary gland (another part of your brain) to release a small amount of follicle-stimulating hormone (FSH), which helps the egg (inside the follicle) grow and mature.

As the follicular phase continues, FSH increases to a small degree, causing further maturation of the egg, which produces more and more estradiol as it matures (CD 4–12).

Step 2: Once the egg is fully matured, around CD 12–13, the now high level of estradiol triggers an increase in the frequency of the GnRH pulses, leading the pituitary gland release a large amount of luteinizing hormone (LH) in addition to FSH. This surge in LH (measured by ovulation predictor kits (OPKs)) causes the follicle to burst and the egg to release about 36 hours later (CD 12–16, top panel). Now begins the second part of the menstrual cycle, the luteal phase (LP).

Luteal Phase

Step 3: After ovulation, the leftover follicle becomes the corpus luteum and begins pumping out progesterone, which has a role both in shutting down the LH production by slowing the GnRH pulses again, as well as preparing the uterus for potential implantation. Progesterone rises until about the middle of the LP (CD 21) and then gradually decreases again (unless an embryo implants). The corpus luteum also secretes additional estradiol.

Step 4: The drop in progesterone back to baseline at the end of the cycle (CD 28) initiates menstrual bleeding. The drop in estradiol leads to increased GnRH secretion from the hypothalamus, and the whole process starts all over again.

There are quite a few other hormones involved, such as inhibins A and B, but that goes beyond the scope of what you need to know to understand HA.

So to recap, in a normal cycle:

1) CD 1 is the first day of menses. At this time, FSH slowly increases, which encourages growth of an egg.

2) At about CD 12, the egg is fully mature and producing lots of estrogen, which in turn leads to the LH surge that causes ovulation around CD 14.

3) After ovulation, the follicle becomes a corpus luteum, which secretes progesterone to prepare the uterus for implantation and pregnancy, as well as estradiol to maintain the uterine lining.

4) If there is no pregnancy, progesterone drops leading to shedding of the lining. Estradiol also drops, causing the FSH increase that starts the cycle over again.

Appetite Control

What complicates matters is that the reproductive hormones are far from the only input to the hypothalamus[6]. In fact, the hypothalamus is a key control center for regulating hunger. It receives hormonal signals that indicate both how much and what is being consumed on a daily basis, as well as how much stored energy (body fat) you have. This information is processed by various nerve cells in your hypothalamus, which then attempts to encourage (or discourage) eating to balance energy needs with energy intake. The hypothalamus accomplishes appetite control by sending out hormonal signals that stimulate hunger when food is needed, as well as signaling when a sufficient amount has been eaten (by making you feel full). If there is no conscious override of these signals, they typically balance out to keep weight stable.

Appetite control hormones: ghrelin. After you eat a meal, there are hormones that are created by cells in your stomach and small and large intestines that signal to your brain how many calories you've just consumed, as well as whether they come from protein, fat, or carbohydrates. The hormone ghrelin (Ghr) increases to stimulate appetite when these calorie signals are low. The hypothalamus contains ghrelin receptors to sense when levels increase[7].

Appetite control hormones: CCK and PYY. The small and large intestines secrete additional hormones in response to each type of nutrient that has been consumed[8]. Cholecystokinin (CCK) increases in response to protein, while peptide YY (PYY) increases after ingestion of fats[9]. This is one reason it's important to eat a wide variety of foods in the recovery phase (chapter 9).

Appetite control hormones: insulin. Insulin is another important hormone. Made in the pancreas, this hormone is an indicator of what and how much you're eating[10]. Insulin levels increase after eating (particularly simple carbohydrates, those that are quickly digested) to help maintain the glucose level within a tight range. Insulin is also affected by how much body fat you have—increased body fat leads to increased insulin[11]. Just as with the other hormones we've mentioned so far, insulin travels through your blood to your brain, and the levels are sensed by the hypothalamus[12]. Interestingly, in people with chronically low insulin due to uncontrolled type 1 diabetes and in animal models of that disease, amenorrhea is common, showing that this one pathway alone can repress the hypothalamus[13].

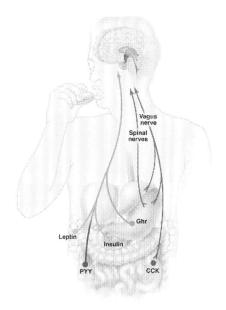

Hormones and hunger control. Hormones derived from many different organs are influencing your hypothalamus, and through it, how much you want to eat. There is ghrelin (Ghr) from your stomach, cholecystokinin (CCK) and peptide YY (PYY) from your intestines, insulin from your pancreas, and leptin from your fat tissue. Reprinted with permission from Marx 2008[14]. Illustration by Katharine Sutliff.

Appetite control hormones: leptin. There's one more hormone to mention—leptin. You may have come across information about an association between leptin and HA[15]. Leptin is secreted by fat cells, and signals to the hypothalamus how much fat is available in the form of fat stores[16]. If you have only a small amount of body fat, leptin levels will be low. If you lose weight, leptin levels also decrease. In both these cases, your hypothalamus will encourage you to eat more (by increasing hunger signals) because you need more energy. Some of you will be able to recognize when this happens because you feel hungry. Others, however, are still unable to recognize these physiological hunger cues as a result of long-term disordered eating.

Appetite control hormones: glucose. Finally, glucose, which is both a product of the breakdown of foods that you eat, and produced by your liver, is also sensed by your hypothalamus[17]. The nerve cells that respond to glucose levels are very sensitive to below-normal levels, and that sensitivity is also affected by the levels of insulin and leptin[18].

Appetite control hormones: summary. There are actually many more hormones and molecules that are involved in the regulation of eating and appetite, but we've described the major players. The function of each molecule is not important; **what you really need to understand is how closely the hypothalamus monitors what and how much you're eating. Each molecule and pathway can be targeted to encourage recovery** (chapters 8-9).

Stress and Exercise

Both psychological stress and physical stress (e.g., exercise) can also affect the hypothalamus. You've probably heard or read about the loss of menstrual periods in times of severe mental stress. Levels of a group of hormones we haven't yet discussed are increased during stressful times[19]. These hormones include corticotrophin releasing hormone (CRH), adrenocorticotropic hormone (ACTH), and cortisol. Just like the eating-related hormones, stress hormone are sensed by the hypothalamus[20], with pituitary involvement as well[21]. A number of studies have found that women with HA have elevated levels of cortisol in their blood[22] and also in spinal fluid[23]—indicative of a direct effect on the brain. We must note that those with HA don't always realize that they are stressed, but living up to self-imposed high expectations can cause a great deal of underlying anxiety[24].

In addition, exercise has been shown to increase cortisol in much the same way as mental stress[25]. In fact, one study found that exercise at 60% and 80% of maximal capacity (moderate and high intensity) raised cortisol by 40% and 83% respectively[26]. Many of us believe that exercise helps with stress relief[27], probably due to endorphins produced during strenuous physical activity[28], but in reality, cortisol levels rise and the brain senses additional stress.

You may be thinking: "Did I read that correctly?" Yes, you did—*exercise is actually a form of stress,* especially when you are undernourished. This is a challenging concept to wrap your mind around. You might be saying, "But...but...I exercise to reduce my stress!" We know. However, right now, any high-intensity exercise in which you engage is sending suppressive signals to your brain. So, although a person with regular cycles might be able to reap the stress-relieving benefits of exercise, with HA, exercise is yet another factor that keeps your reproductive system subdued.

> *Lisa*: Stress...it kills our reproductive systems. Two years before I went "all in," I made a bogus attempt "trying" to gain weight and stop exercising. What's a word for when you believe you are trying but you really aren't? I don't know either, but that's what happened. (Another form of denial?) I was pretty darn miserable attempting these changes and as a result sucked everyone who cared about me into my messy, unhappy mindset. It was what I now refer to as an "adult tantrum." After I wasted time and energy with that nonsense and was still not getting my period, I decided to do something different. I made the *choice* to change my stinkin' thinkin'. Instead of kicking and screaming, stressing myself out, I chose to be thankful for the opportunity to dig myself out of the deep hole I was in. This was a freeing time and there was a significant decrease in my stress levels, which I would have never thought possible without exercise or food control. Yup, there is stress reduction outside of training the heck out of your body and strict eating. It's called freedom of self!

Speaking of exercise and stress, it's been documented in multiple studies[29] that disordered menstrual cycles are present in 48% to 79% of women who exercise three hours a week or more*, even if they are menstruating. The disorders include no ovulation (anovulation) and LP defects—either a shortened LP (defined as less than 10 days), or one without adequate progesterone production. The lack of increase in estrogen and progesterone associated with anovulation, or lowered levels of progesterone with luteal phase defect mean our body is not getting the benefit of these hormones (see chapter 7). In addition, these conditions have been demonstrated to have a negative effect on the ability to get pregnant[30]. Are you thinking the same thing that we were? As little as three hours of exercise a week can impact cycles negatively? That's a day of training for some of us!

---

* The women in these studies were at a stable weight, however, caloric intake was not monitored so it is possible they were underfueling.

Putting It Together—Getting to HA

> *Steph*: Phew, this is a lot. For someone who trudged her way through science class, this chapter is hard for me. Nico does an amazing job explaining things, and after reading it a couple of times, I actually get it. But that does not mean my eyes don't glaze over... If you feel the same, give yourself a little break and come back to it. Or better yet, I urge you to press on to read these final paragraphs. It all comes together here. You don't want to miss this, I promise!

Now we get to the really remarkable part—the interaction between what you eat, exercise, stress, and your reproductive system. What we've told you so far is that:

- Your reproductive system is controlled by your hypothalamus, and it produces hormones that affect the hypothalamus. The interplay is cyclical, with each influencing the other.
- The same is true of what you eat. The hypothalamus controls the signals that cause you to feel hunger and fullness, and the act of eating produces additional hormones that also affect the hypothalamus.
- Cortisol and other related hormones increase with psychological stress *and exercise*.
- Finally, hormones are produced by fat cells, which indicate the amount of fat stores to the hypothalamus.

The links between these systems (reproduction, eating, stress, and fat stores) occur right in the hypothalamus. First, the GnRH nerve cells are directly controlled by some of these hormonal inputs[31]. Cortisol, which increases with stress and exercise[32], and glucose, leptin, and insulin—affected by what you eat[33]—all bind directly to the GnRH cells and affect the speed at which the nerve "fires," which in turn affects the production of FSH and LH[34].

In addition, these hormones bind to feeding-related nerve cells to control food intake but also communicate with and affect the reproductive nerve cells[35]. **Lowered body fat, decreased food intake, constant hunger, stress, and exercise can all result in decreased communication with the reproductive neurons.** These reduced signals keep the level of FSH at baseline so that egg maturation never begins—and voila, you have yourself HA[36]. Another method by which these nerve cells are controlled is that connections between cells (synapses) are constantly created and broken, in response to hormones like E_2[37] and leptin[38]. Finally, stress hormones can affect reproductive hormones in other ways, for example, cortisol directly inhibits secretion of LH by the pituitary[39].

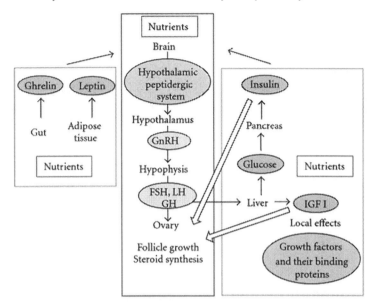

Interrelationship between nutrition and reproduction. The different ways that nutrients affect the hypothalamus are shown. "Hypothalamic peptidergic system" is another way of saying the signaling between nerve cells that are in the hypothalamus (through small proteins called peptides), and "hypophysis" is the pituitary gland. Image reprinted under CC BY 3.0 license from Garcia-Garcia RM (2012)[40].

Keep in mind that the levels of body fat, food intake, exercise and so on do not need to reach extreme lows or highs in order to affect the communication between the hormones and the hypothalamus. Because each of us is unique and has different sensitivities, any marked changes for an individual can have an impact on menstrual cycles.

Summary

A complex network of hormones communicates the status of the body to the hypothalamus. When food is plentiful, exercise is well-fueled, and psychological stress is reasonable, the cycle works just as described. However, each of the following conditions, perhaps with quick or significant weight loss in the past, can upset the hormonal balance, causing periods to cease:

- body fat is low/lowered

- insufficient calories are consumed to power daily functions
- exercise is undertaken, particularly high-intensity
- acute or chronic stress is experienced

Not only are hormone levels altered, but the connections between nerve cells change based on the inputs being received[41]. Ultimately **there are no signals to stimulate an egg to mature, and therefore no ovulation, and no menstrual cycle.** The key is that these processes are all controlled in the same place, which makes it easy to understand how the lack of adequate fuel and exercise or stress translate into the lack of a cycle. This is hypothalamic amenorrhea.

Honestly, it's not important that you remember or even understand all these details. What's important is this: these systems are intricately related. Therefore, what we eat, how much stress we experience, and how much we exercise have profound effects on our cycles.

> *Clover*: While reading I can't help but go back to that place where I did NOT want to accept the solution for HA. I continued on in rebellion but could no longer claim ignorance because I had been privy to the same information you have and probably more.
>
> No one can convince you to give up your current less-than-healthy coping mechanisms (overexercise) or your desire to be in control and comfortable (current weight and eating habits). But what we can do is share our experiences and the experiences of others. You see, for me, my desire to stay comfortable prevented me from having a period for a LONG time. Like some of you, I simply did not want to change. I loved being comfortably numb—running hard, restricting, isolating… I thought it was freedom, but now realize it was a type of self-imposed prison. I believed I was different and could escape the consequences of not getting a period. I deceived myself into believing that as soon as I gained some weight at a later date and was ready to have children, my body would snap back and do what I wanted it to. Why wouldn't it? I was "super fit" and those words were echoed many times among my friends and training partners. For so long my choices were about me, my stuff, my time, etc. I never thought about the ramifications of robbing my husband of a child and my parents of the opportunity to be grandparents, or the very real possibility of burdening my husband with the responsibility of an osteoporotic wife. All because I was comfortable, loved what I was doing, and was NOT willing to change.

6
The HA/PCOS Conundrum

WHEN WE TELL our doctors we're not getting our periods, there's a diagnostic path they follow to determine the cause (chapter 4, "Diagnosis"). This includes a verbal history, a physical exam, some hormonal assessments, and perhaps an ultrasound to look at our ovaries and uterus. Based on these findings, they propose a diagnosis. Often, that diagnosis is hypothalamic amenorrhea (HA). However, there is another condition, called polycystic ovarian syndrome (PCOS) that affects around 12% to 18% of the population[1] and manifests similarly to HA in some cases. So it is natural for this to be among the conditions suggested when we visit the doctor complaining of a missing period.

In this chapter, we talk about how to correctly diagnose PCOS and/or HA, as well as some treatments and long-term issues to think about if you do in fact have PCOS. If you're not interested in reading through all the research and just want the short version, here it is: it is common for doctors to diagnose PCOS based on the presence of amenorrhea and an ovarian ultrasound showing lots of small follicles (egg-containing structures called "cysts"). BUT, this information is not sufficient to diagnose PCOS **over** HA, especially when the risk factors for HA are present[2], as discussed in Part 1, "Hypothalamic Amenorrhea Nuts and Bolts." If you've been told you have PCOS, please ask some more questions and make sure that it is the correct diagnosis for you.

> *Kelli*: Where do I begin? Let me keep this to the point: you know yourself best. You know best what you have done to yourself, regardless of

> your diagnosis. Have you been restrictive with food? Have you overdone working out? Were you ever at a low weight or lost weight quickly by creating a severe calorie imbalance? The thing is, we HAers will be told many things. I have been diagnosed with PCOS by one doc, HA by two others, and with thyroid dysfunction by another. All reproductive endocrinologists. All correct to a degree. Yes, my ovaries are polycystic. WHY? Because the eggs I have are not getting released so they just hang around. Yes, my thyroid hormones are abnormal, but when I dig deeper into the results, I realize it is my T3 that is low—the marker of "illness" and "starvation"—so no, I don't have thyroid disease. I caused my hypothalamus to slow down my metabolism to keep me alive, and also to shut down reproduction. Could I believe I have PCOS, take fertility meds and metformin, which lowers sugar, and continue working out like a psycho and eating low carb? Yes, I could. I would love to believe that and continue in my destructive ways... but in the end I know the truth. I under-ate and worked out every day. I lost weight, was too lean for my body, and lost my periods.

What Is PCOS?

PCOS is a condition in which various hormone levels are not typical. There are a number of ways in which PCOS manifests, and any given person with PCOS can exhibit a different cluster of symptoms. Some issues that are common with PCOS, and the symptoms they elicit, include:

- An excess of "male" hormones like testosterone—leading to physical side effects like male pattern hairiness (hirsutism) and acne.
- Insulin resistance—the body does not respond appropriately when the hormone insulin is produced to help process sugar (glucose). This leads to more insulin being made to try and overcome this resistance. The continued overproduction can lead to diabetes over time if left untreated.
- Issues with ovulation—abnormal levels of androgens can work to prevent timely release of an egg and lead to issues with fertility.

PCOS is often thought of as a condition associated with being in a larger body because the hormonal imbalances can make it easy to gain and difficult to lose weight. But, about a third of PCOS cases are found in people with a BMI <25 [3]. This is sometimes called "lean" or "thin" PCOS, but it's not a different condition and the diagnostic procedures don't vary. The distinction is only based on body size which is a result of fatphobia in the medical field. A larger body size in someone with PCOS may be due to the degree of hormonal imbalance, in turn associated with the degree of long-term concerns; see the "Long-Term Concerns with PCOS" section.

Diagnosing PCOS

Over recent decades there have been a number of attempts to develop standardized criteria for diagnosing PCOS to include all the varied manifestations. The current gold standard was agreed to by the members of a consensus workshop held at the National Institutes of Health (NIH)[4], and originally put forth by a group of experts in the field[5]. They are often called the "Rotterdam" criteria because the workshop was held in Rotterdam, Netherlands. In order to be diagnosed with PCOS by these criteria, someone needs to exhibit two out of three of the following[6]:

1) Polycystic ovaries viewed on ultrasound (P)
2) Oligomenorrhea (long periods of time between menstruation) or amenorrhea (no menstruation) (O)
3) Hyperandrogenism (excess androgens) (H)

First, to diagnose polycystic ovaries, a transvaginal ultrasound should be performed. The machine needs to be able to scan at 6 MHz (megahertz) or greater in order to properly visualize the small follicles (2 mm to 9 mm) that need to be counted. Doctors who specialize in PCOS are clear that it is not sufficient to take a quick look at the ovaries, see a lot of follicles, and say they are polycystic[7]. The most recent criteria require more than 25 follicles between 2 mm and 9 mm to be present in each ovary, and/or the ovarian volume (three-dimensional area) must be greater than 10 mL[8]. In PCOS, the follicles are often lined up at the edge of the ovary with a "string of pearls" appearance, although this is not always the case and is not required for the diagnosis.

> **Steph**: When I went for my first ultrasound, the ultrasound technician told me I had polycystic ovaries. I immediately asked her if that meant I had PCOS. She said no, not at all. She told me, "Many women, about 30%, have the appearance of polycystic ovaries but that does not mean they have PCOS."

Second, diagnosing missing or infrequent periods is the easy part; that is just based on a verbal history from you. A missing period is obvious—you just don't bleed. With PCOS, periods can occasionally be normal, but more commonly cycles are either irregular (coming at varied intervals), and/or infrequent (more than 35 days in between periods). However, if it's a question of PCOS versus HA, you're obviously coming to the doctor with absent periods.

Finally, diagnosing hyperandrogenism. This gets a little trickier as not all androgens will necessarily be elevated when one has PCOS. Below, we show some of the hormones (including androgens) that might be tested, along with results that commonly point to PCOS. The more severe the PCOS, the more hormones are elevated, and to a higher degree.

Hormonal levels in PCOS

Hormone	Normal result*	Expected value with PCOS
FSH	3.0–20.0 IU/L	Low-normal to normal
LH	2.0–5.0 IU/L	Normal to high-normal (greater than FSH)
Estradiol (E_2)	20–150 pg/mL	Normal to high
Sex hormone binding globulin (SHBG)	40–120 nmol/L	Low to normal
Total testosterone	2–45 ng/dL	Normal to high
Free testosterone (T)	0.1–6.4 pg/mL	Normal to high
Free androgen index (FAI)	7–10	Normal to high
DHEAS	Age 20–29: 65–380 ug/dL Age 30–39: 45–270 ug/dL	Normal to high
Androstenedione	28–230 ng/dL	Normal to high
Anti-Mullerian Hormone (AMH)[9]	>4.2ng/mL (automated assay) >5.6 ng/mL (manual assay)	High

* We have listed standard ranges. You should ask for the reference ranges from the laboratory that performed your testing in order to compare your results.

There are also physical symptoms of hyperandrogenism that should be evaluated by your physician (next page).

The different criteria met will affect the ease of the diagnosis. If there is hyperandrogenism (H) along with oligo/amenorrhea (O) and/or polycystic ovaries (P), a diagnosis of PCOS can be made (assuming other similarly presenting conditions are excluded). It becomes a bit blurrier from our perspective when a patient presents with O + P only, as these are the same symptoms that someone with HA may exhibit[10]. In this case, the diagnostic criteria specifically state that HA must be excluded before making a diagnosis of PCOS[11].

Physical symptoms in PCOS

Symptom	Normal	PCOS	Frequency in PCOS
Hirsutism (FG Score)*	Score < 6	Score >= 6	21–76% [12]
Acne	Perhaps some facial acne	Facial and chest/upper back, not responsive to standard treatments	50-58% [13]
Androgenic alopecia (scalp hair loss)	Not present	Sometimes present	16% [14]
Acanthosis nigricans (skin darkening / texture changes)	Not present	Sometimes present	23% [15]

*Hirsutism can be quantitated through a "Ferriman-Gallwey (FG) score," in which the amount of hair on nine different areas of the body is graded on a scale of 0 to 5, and then the sum is taken[16]. The cutoffs for a "normal" score range from 5 to 8, depending on the investigator.

When PCOS Is Actually HA

As we just mentioned, the category of PCOS that consists of amenorrhea and polycystic ovaries (O + P) shares the same symptoms as HA. In fact, somewhere between 15% and 55% of those with HA have multi-follicular or polycystic ovaries[17], and obviously, missing periods. Doctors may diagnosis PCOS based on an ultrasound, along with amenorrhea, without understanding the precise requirements needed to qualify as polycystic ovaries (outlined earlier). In one recent study, if the PCOS diagnostic criteria were applied and HA not considered, 86% of those with HA would have been diagnosed with PCOS[19]. This makes it important to confirm a diagnosis of PCOS via methods other than ultrasound. The best way to do this is by looking at blood work and physical symptoms.

The next table compares blood work results if one has PCOS with what is expected in someone with HA. There are a couple of key differences between the two conditions hormonally. First, LH is almost always lower than normal with HA, although occasionally it is normal. In those with PCOS, LH will at least be normal and is often elevated to two to three times FSH[19]. Second, estradiol(E_2) is also often low in HA, but normal to high with PCOS. Finally, androgen levels will be normal with HA but are commonly elevated with PCOS, especially free testosterone (T) or free androgen index (FAI)[20]. If your blood work picture is HA-like and doesn't include any elevated androgens, it becomes much less likely that you have PCOS. Also, be aware that Anti-Mullerian Hormone (AMH) is being tested more frequently, with a high level thought to be associated with PCOS. However, people with HA often have similarly high levels so this can not be used to distinguish the two conditions[21]. Interestingly, HA can also be associated with quite low AMH values; see the HAers with low AMH table in Chapter 20, "When You Need a Jumpstart."

Hormonal levels in HA and PCOS

Hormone	Normal result*	Expected value in HA	Expected value in PCOS
FSH	3.0–20.0 IU/L	Low to normal (around 6 IU/mL)	Low-normal to normal
LH	2.0–15.0 IU/L	Low to normal, less than FSH	Normal to high-normal, greater than FSH
E_2	20–150 pg/mL	Low to normal	Normal to high
Total T	2–45 ng/dL	Low to normal	Normal to high
Free T	0.1–6.4 pg/mL	Low to normal	Normal to high
Free Androgen Index (FAI)	7–10	Low to normal	Normal to high
DHEAS	Age 20–29: 65–380 ug/dL Age 30–39: 45–270 ug/dL	Low to normal	Normal to high
androstenedione	28–230 ng/dL	Low to normal	Normal to high

* We have listed standard ranges. You should ask for the reference ranges from the laboratory that performed your testing in order to compare your results.

The next table compares the physical symptoms. Keep in mind that "hirsutism" does not mean a couple of extra stray hairs here or there (we all have those). The hirsutism associated with PCOS is a much greater degree of excess, "male pattern" hairiness. And "acne" does not mean a few pimples on your face; with PCOS, severe acne on both the face and other body parts, and often resistant to prescription treatments, is common. The presence of these symptoms may well suggest PCOS, but without them, again, HA is more likely the correct diagnosis.

Finally, lifestyle habits play a big part in correctly diagnosing HA over PCOS. If a number of the criteria below describe you and your habits, HA is much more likely than PCOS.

- being in a smaller than average body (although as we have discussed, HA does occur in those who are not "underweight")
- recent significant weight loss (>10 lb)
- a history of a larger weight loss (>10% of bodyweight)
- recent increase in exercise time or intensity, such as adding a few Zumba classes, or training for a race
- frequent high intensity exercise, e.g., more than one hour/day, multiple days of the week
- running
- low caloric intake on a regular basis (<14 kcal/lb/day)[22]
- a diet restricting certain food groups (e.g., low carb or low fat)

Physical symptoms in HA and PCOS

Symptom	HA	PCOS
Hirsutism (FG Score)	Score is 0–5	Score >= 6
Acne	Some facial; sometimes increased with weight gain	Facial and chest/upper back; often resistant to treatment
Androgenic alopecia (scalp hair loss)	Not present, although hair can be brittle	Sometimes present
Acanthosis nigricans (skin darkening/ texture changes)	Not present	Sometimes present

Among our survey respondents, 15% were diagnosed with PCOS by a doctor, and another 20% were told PCOS was a possibility. Unfortunately, we do not have sufficient data to make an assessment of whether these diagnoses met the criteria we are suggesting here. However, we can tell you that of those who reported blood work results, androgens were only tested in 45%, and elevated in less than half of those. This implies that in many instances the diagnosis of PCOS was based solely on lack of periods and the appearance of the ovaries on ultrasound examination, therefore HA was much more likely the correct call.

Among our survey respondents, those diagnosed with PCOS regained cycles at a similar frequency after following the Recovery Plan, with very similar weight gains compared with those not diagnosed with PCOS. This supports the argument that their amenorrhea was likely caused by HA.

> *Nadia*: I was diagnosed with PCOS. It was something I fought for over five years before I found a doctor who knew what HA was. She told me I likely never had PCOS and that it was possible that thinking I did (and changing the way I ate and exercised because I thought I did) made my HA worse. With my diet I had gone low carb: very limited starches, limited fruit, limited sugar, no gluten, and lower fat. I exercised daily for no less than 30 min, and often close to an hour. It was a lot of cardio (walking), but also weight training. *(Nadia's PCOS was subsequently confirmed by two different endocrinologists, but she was still able to conquer HA and regain her cycles by three months of consistent, "all in" work toward recovery.)*

While it is true that many who are told they have "lean" PCOS probably have HA instead, it is also possible for an individual to have both PCOS and HA. The PCOS hormonal imbalances are not hypothalamus-derived, so they can be present at the same time the hypothalamus is shutting down the reproductive system because of underfueling, stress, or overexercising. In general it seems HA trumps PCOS; that is, if both are present, the hormonal and physical picture will be more HA-like. Once an individual is recovering or recovered from HA, more PCOS-like symptoms may become apparent[23], both biochemical (e.g., blood work) and physical. Although in many cases the appearance of PCOS-like symptoms after HA recovery is only temporary, so we encourage waiting at least a year after HA recovery before confirming a PCOS diagnosis[24].

To reiterate, if all your blood work is normal, and your doctor just noted there were "a lot" of follicles in your ovaries (possibly without counting them), PCOS may not be the correct diagnosis.

Does It Matter If I Have PCOS or HA?

As far as getting pregnant goes, there aren't huge differences in recommended methods for HA versus PCOS; one can usually try naturally (perhaps with additional supplements that will be discussed in the "I definitely have PCOS" section) if cycles are restored, or use oral medications, injectables, or IVF. The biggest concern with multifollicular or polycystic ovaries is that the more follicles one has, the greater likelihood there is for ovarian hyperstimulation syndrome (OHSS) if injectables or IVF are used. OHSS is a complication of fertility treatments in which your ovaries become very swollen, and in severe cases leads to fluid buildup in your abdomen and chest, sometimes requiring hospitalization. Doctors should be mindful of the possibility of OHSS when choosing dosages for these treatments in women with high numbers of follicles. For more discussion on the possible ovulation induction methods and avoiding OHSS, read chapters 20 through 23. Much of what we discuss in those chapters is applicable to both HA and PCOS.

Where the diagnosis matters most is in recommendations for lifestyle modifications. Typically, those with PCOS are told to exercise more and eat less, which has been found in some cases to reduce the hormonal effects of PCOS[25] (although long-term compliance is a serious issue with these recommendations, and many "Health At Every Size" dietitians now work with people to reduce symptoms without specifically working toward weight loss.). However, exercising more and eating less is the exact opposite of what one needs to do to recover from HA, so receiving the correct diagnosis is important.

> *Jessica O*: After a year of unsuccessfully trying to conceive (TTC), my doctor ran a bunch of tests and did an ultrasound. Everything was normal, except that the ultrasound showed ovarian cysts. So, they diagnosed me with PCOS and put me on metformin. I actually ended up getting pregnant the very next month. I don't know if the metformin helped, or if it was just the fact that it was over the holidays, so I was eating more and exercising less than usual. At any rate, I lost the pregnancy fairly early on. After that, I decided to get serious about treating my supposed PCOS, so I went on a low carb diet, lost some weight, and became obsessed with getting my daily workouts in. Surprise, surprise; at that point, I developed full-blown HA. My doctors continued to assume that my problems were caused by PCOS and no one knew why things were getting worse rather than better. It was an incredibly frustrating experience. I was never actually diagnosed with HA, but when I found Nico's blog and the Board, it all started to make sense. I gained weight, cut back on exercise, and regained my cycle.
>
> *Katherine*: Don't get sucked into the "maybe I have PCOS and can exercise as much as I want" trap. Been there, doesn't work.

HA and PCOS??

There is a small group who have both HA and PCOS, as we described earlier[26]. When HA is active, they exhibit the classical symptoms of HA—low LH and E_2, often along with the physical issues like being cold all the time, low libido, night sweats, brittle hair and nails, etc. Once they recover from HA by eating more and exercising less, their hormonal profile swings to be more PCOS-like, with perhaps an LH level that is higher than FSH, and a higher E_2, along with increased androgens and possibly physical manifestations of PCOS[27]. The latent PCOS may prevent cycles from returning to normal even after recovery from the HA component. Amenorrhea may persist, or cycles can continue to be lengthy and/or irregular. So, treatment may still be needed to induce ovulation for pregnancy, despite HA recovery. It is worth noting that in some folks LH increases to more than FSH with no other symptoms of PCOS. In these cases we suggest waiting a few months and retesting, as the increased LH may simply be a consequence of the hypothalamus overshooting and speeding up too much[28] (http://noperiod.info/HAvsPCOS2).

> *Grace*: I was diagnosed with both PCOS and HA. My doctor did extensive testing to confirm that I had both. I did all of the ultrasounds and hormone testing, but he also had me completely cut out exercise for a while and then add it back in to see how my hormone profiles adjusted. When I cut out exercise, the labs showed more of a PCOS profile, but when I added it back, all levels were low, an HA profile. I also have the cystic ovaries and abnormal hair growth.

If it turns out that you do have PCOS in addition to HA, it can be a discouraging realization, especially if you have already worked to recover from HA. You may question everything you've done—did you make things worse by gaining weight and not exercising as much? You might feel like the only thing you've accomplished is to go from one problem to another.

That is not the case! If you have PCOS masked by HA, you have two issues to overcome—first the HA, then the PCOS. Once you recover from HA, the first and overriding issue, your likelihood of ovulating on your own is higher. If you aren't able to ovulate on your own and need help from treatment, your chances of responding are significantly better when you are not trying to work around both an energy deficit and the issues caused by PCOS.

Liz: I cycled regularly for two years (age 13–15). Then my periods started to become slightly irregular and I got some PCOS symptoms without any dietary changes. Then I started restricting, and boom, my period was nowhere to be seen. I definitely have PCOS-like symptoms now, but I started cycling for the first time in forever when I started eating a normal amount of calories for the amount of energy I expend (and being more intuitive and not restricting). I also take some herbs and vitamins, but I did this throughout the years, and until I completely stopped restricting and gained weight I did not have a period. My thinking I had PCOS absolutely contributed to my restriction. Even after I got my eating disorder under control, I was obsessed with maintaining a certain weight and never letting myself gain, even if it meant eating very little, thinking I was controlling my PCOS when actually I was preventing myself from cycling. (*After many years of visits to endocrinologists, a 17-OH-progesterone test showed that Liz has late-onset congenital adrenal hyperplasia, a condition that manifests similarly to PCOS.*)

Shayla: I was diagnosed with HA in July 2011 and didn't commit to making true, significant changes until the end of the year. Between July and December, I would throw in an intense spin class or exercise a couple days harder than I should have. December is when I got real with myself and realized that I needed to commit to a lessened exercise routine in order to see results (four to five days per week, 40 minutes max, walking or easy elliptical). From July 2011 to January 2012, I got my weight up to a place where my body was happy. And while I haven't gotten a natural period because I have hormonal PCOS, I know I recovered from HA since I tried Provera a couple weeks ago and got a significant, heavy bleed from it—marked improvement since I had failed it in July 2011. So all in all, with significant changes made around December and my weight to a better place for me by January, now I'm responding to treatment. I'd say it took me about three to four months. And to be honest, what every single person has said here is absolutely true. For a while last year, I was in denial about it all, but if you really commit to gaining, eating fats, and lowering your exercise, you WILL respond to treatment or get your period naturally. (*Shayla got pregnant with her son on her second round of Femara. Her second child, a daughter, was naturally conceived*)

I Definitely Have PCOS

If you have PCOS and not HA masquerading as PCOS, the obvious next question is, now what? There are two areas of concern: 1) management of the syndrome (perhaps with future pregnancy in mind), and 2) longer-term health issues associated with PCOS. We are far from experts on PCOS, but recent research we discuss below suggests some avenues for you to consider and explore.

Lifestyle modifications, medications, and nutritional supplements can potentially help manage PCOS by:

- lowering androgen levels
- improving insulin resistance
- promoting ovulation (if cycles were absent or irregular), which can lead to pregnancy
- perhaps improving ovarian morphology

Discussing all the possible alternatives to help with these symptoms is beyond the scope of this book. We will discuss a few options here; we recommend having a conversation with your doctor about what treatment plan is most appropriate for you. You may want to visit the website "SoulCysters: Women with PCOS Speak from the Heart" (www.soulcysters.com) to learn more.

First, lifestyle modifications. As mentioned, weight loss and exercise are commonly recommended to manage complications such as insulin resistance that seem to respond to such interventions (although long term benefits are unclear[29], and many "Health at Every Size" dietitians are working with patients to manage symptoms without focusing on weight.) In those without insulin resistance, or who have experienced HA, weight loss is not encouraged, although exercise in moderation can be beneficial. If you have an HA/PCOS combo, keep in mind that reduced exercise is needed in the short term for recovery from HA (chapter 12, "The HA Recovery Plan: Exercise Changes"); it can be added (slowly!) in the longer term as your HA recovery stabilizes. After you work on recovery and achieve a natural cycle, we encourage you to continue with your new, improved lifestyle for at least three months before you consider making any changes, like changing eating patterns or increasing exercise. That way, you allow your body to trust that you are not going to return to an energy deficit. Those who have immediately added exercise or cut calories once regaining their cycles have been much less regular than those who waited for at least the recommended three months. Once you've got a few natural cycles under your belt and you decide to make changes, incorporate them slowly and pay attention to your cycles to note any effects (chapter 16, "Recovering Natural Cycles").

A different lifestyle approach that has showed improvements in PCOS symptoms involves changing the timing of meals. Women with PCOS were put on a meal plan in which they consumed 54% of their calories at breakfast, between 6:00 and 9:00 a.m., 35% at lunch (noon to 3:00 p.m.), and only 11% at dinner (6:00 to 9:00 p.m.)[30]. Their diets were also high in protein, at 0.64g/lb, which reportedly helped them to feel full and satisfied throughout the day. After three months, hormones were normalized (androgens and insulin decreased, sex hormone-binding globulin increased) to the same extent as when the medication metformin (a standard PCOS treatment) was used (see table on p. 68). In addition, more frequent ovulations were observed, commencing between one and three months after dietary changes were implemented. The more frequent ovulations are clearly helpful when one is trying to conceive. There are no long-term follow-up studies, but there are few concerns with side effects from a dietary change like this.

It may feel overwhelming to consider making breakfast your biggest meal of the day, especially if you had/have to modify your eating patterns significantly in order to recover from HA. So if this is something that interests you, perhaps you could start by adding more protein to your breakfast and making that a higher calorie meal, without going as far as making it more than half of your calories for the day.

A second option for managing symptoms of PCOS is medication. Metformin is a standard treatment for PCOS that reduces the amount of glucose produced by the liver. As a side effect, it also improves some of the other hormonal and physical symptoms of PCOS (see table). However, metformin can cause gastrointestinal discomfort and weight loss, which is not recommended for those who have or had HA.

A third solution to ameliorate PCOS symptoms is nutritional supplementation, including d-chiro-inositol and/or myo-inositol[31]. These dietary supplements are readily available at health food stores. The table on the next page includes data on reductions in androgens and insulin sensitivity in individuals taking a 40:1 combination of myo and d-chiro-inositol.

Recent research has found that both myo- and d-chiro-inositol can help normalize insulin response and hormones by acting on different tissues[32]. Myo-insoitol plays a role in glucose uptake, and is active in ovarian tissue, also affecting FSH/LH ratios. D-chiro-inositol affects glycogen synthesis and is active in tissue outside the ovary, mediating insulin-related androgen production.

A study that compared different ratios of myo- to d-chiro-inositol found strong support for a 40:1 ratio[33]. This ratio has also been found to be optimal in other research[34], and is therefore our suggestion as a supplement to take to potentially help reduce PCOS symptoms (once again with a reminder to discuss with your personal physician).

Effects of PCOS treatment options on hormones and ovulation.

Treatment	50% of calories at breakfast [35]	Metformin [36]	D-chiro-inositol [37]
Study Duration	3 months*	6 months*	6–8 weeks*
Free Testosterone	−50%	−67%	−73%
DHEAS	−35%	−23%	−49%
Androstenedione	−34%	NR	−27%
SHBG†	116%	−13%	138%
Fasting insulin	−53%	−61%	−36%
	% ovulating in test group (% in control group)		
First month	0% (0%)	0% (0%)	60% (0%)
Second month	28% (7.6%)	10% (0%)	NA (20%)
Third month	50% (20%)	50% (5%)	NA
Months 4-6	NA	95%	NA

* Note: Negative numbers indicate decreases in listed hormones
† Sex hormone-binding globulin, used in calculation of free androgen index (FAI); an increase yields a lower, improved FAI. (FAI = 100 * Total T / SHBG)
NR = Not reported
NA = Not applicable (e.g., study too short)

Long-term Concerns With PCOS

When you are diagnosed with PCOS, you probably also hear about the potential long-term complications: diabetes, heart disease, and cancer. By now you may feel weary—yet more health issues to worry about, on top of the issues from HA. Let's take these long-term issues one by one. First, the criteria for a diagnosis of metabolic syndrome (MetS), which is thought to be the precursor to diabetes and heart disease, are three out of five of the following[38]:
- high waist circumference (> 35 inches)
- triglycerides > 150 mg/dL
- high-density lipoprotein-C (HDL-C) < 50 mg/dL

- blood pressure > 130/85
- a fasting and 2-hour glucose reading from a glucose tolerance test > 110mg/dL and > 140mg / dL respectively

Although studies have suggested a link between PCOS and cardiovascular disease based on blood work (e.g., high cholesterol), the clinical research to date does not support a strong association[39]. The cardiovascular risk is based on insulin resistance being associated with greater susceptibility to the disease, as well as abnormal processing of cholesterol and other lipids. Additionally, the two factors most correlated with risk of cardiovascular disease are an abdominal waist measurement greater than 35 inches and an above normal non-HDL cholesterol. Your doctor should gauge your risks by assessing your psychosocial stress, blood pressure, glucose, lipid profile (cholesterol, triglycerides, HDL, LDL, and non-HDL cholesterol), waist circumference, physical activity, nutrition, and smoking[40]. If the results suggest an increased risk, you can work together to develop a plan for the future. Note that both metformin and the inositols reduce insulin resistance and can therefore help mitigate some of these other issues as well, however most studies performed to date have been short term (12 weeks to 12 months), so the longer term effect of these treatments is yet to be determined[41].

The final potential long-term consequence of PCOS that has been suggested is endometrial cancer (cancer in the lining of the uterus). Many studies have been performed through the years with conflicting results; a recent analysis of multiple studies found a possibly three-fold increased risk in those with PCOS[42] (9% versus 2-3% in the overall population). However, the criteria used for PCOS diagnosis were not high quality in all studies. Theories attribute the increased risk to[43]:

- uterine lining buildup because of high estrogen, with irregular shedding due to oligomenorrhea or amenorrhea
- increased levels of LH (and receptors for LH in the cancerous cells)
- increased levels of insulin (and receptors for insulin in uterine lining), increased levels of leptin, and decreased levels of adiponectin, all associated with fat mass
- increased estrogen due to high insulin levels

If you do *not* have increased LH, estrogen, or insulin[44], your risk of endometrial cancer is unlikely to be higher. Most hormonally-driven endometrial carcinomas seem to derive from long-term higher estrogen exposure without progesterone in opposition. With the estrogen level of <20 to 30 typically seen with HA the uterine lining remains thin and therefore not of concern. If your estrogen levels are higher and your uterine lining does build up without a regular bleed, you could talk to your doctor about using progesterone pills or cream to shed the lining from time to time[45]. Regardless, PCOS-related endometrial cancer is slow to develop and often found at an early stage due to abnormal (mid-cycle or post-menopausal) bleeding in middle-aged or older people, so if you and your doctor are aware of your potential risk and maintain vigilance, you should be able to catch it early and treat it.

Again, these side effects do not occur in everyone with PCOS, and if they do manifest, the symptoms are usually mild in those who formerly had HA.

In Summary: PCOS or HA?

We know many who were given a diagnosis of PCOS because they were not getting their periods and had "polycystic-looking ovaries." With no other symptoms or corroborating blood work, and especially with other HA risk factors in play, PCOS is almost certainly not the correct diagnosis. Instead, it is much more likely you have HA. Many healthcare professionals seem to be unaware that research shows a high proportion of those with HA exhibit polycystic-like ovaries. It is also possible to have both HA and PCOS. In this case, one needs to work to overcome HA first and then potentially (and slowly) make dietary and exercise changes to help manage PCOS symptoms. Do not let a possible PCOS diagnosis lure you into thinking that restrictive eating and excessive exercise habits are a wise choice. If what we have described in earlier chapters rings true for you, please give the HA Recovery Plan in part 2 ("The Recovery Plan—Changing Your Habits and Your Life") a try and see what happens.

> **Lisa**: I know... the possibility of PCOS on top of having HA adds to the confusion and concern, and certainly doesn't make your decisions any easier. These frustrations among those with HA/PCOS have been echoed repeatedly, so know you are not alone. With that being said, what we *don't* want to see happen is for you to start waving the "I have PCOS, not HA" flag, derailing you off the track for HA recovery. (Can you tell we have heard that?) I only caution you because I can assure you that if I had a possible diagnosis of PCOS, you can bet your bottom dollar that I would not have decreased exercise and gained weight in order to

recover. Heck no! And on top of that, I am certain doctors would have recommended not gaining weight because of my "average" BMI. Only you know deep down if there is a possibility that restrictive eating and/or exercise are contributing factors to your HA, muddying the waters of a PCOS diagnosis. There is only one way to find out and, again, it's temporary and totally within your control.

So at this point you have possibly begun to consider that you might have both PCOS and HA and have chosen to press on with the HA solution; or you are concerned that you might have only PCOS and not HA and sure don't want to risk lifestyle changes for "what ifs." No one can tell you which path to take, but what we can do is give you a few things to think about.

1) If you press on with HA recovery and do indeed have both HA and PCOS, you will then only be dealing with PCOS, as opposed to both, and get all the benefits from option 2 below.
2) If you press on with HA recovery and do not have PCOS but only HA, then YAY! You will recover, your bones will likely increase in density, your brain and heart will be in tiptop shape, you will cycle regularly, and if you decide to make babies you will now have that option.
3) If you press on with HA recovery and don't actually have HA but do have PCOS then you should play the lottery because I doubt that will happen. Yet let's just say it's a possibility. (And based on the work of Health At Every Size dietitians like Julie Duffy Dillon, nourishing your body well, similar to "all in," is a good way to manage PCOS symptoms, possibly with the addition of some insulin sensitizers as discussed earlier in this chapter.)

7
Brittle Bones and Other Health Consequences of HA

WHILE MANY WANT to conquer HA to get pregnant, the reality is that there is much more to HA/REDS than the impact it has on fertility. Not getting your period can have serious potential health consequences both in the near term and even more so as you age. It may seem like your post-menopausal years are eons away, so who cares, right? But think about what you see yourself doing in 20, 30, 40 years.

> *Nico:* I imagine myself playing ice hockey well into my sixties, and playing golf for many years after that. I see myself running after grandchildren, having lucid conversations with them, and telling stories about their parents back when they were small kids. I don't envision having had a heart attack, being hunchbacked or breaking my bones because I have early osteoporosis, or living in a long-term care facility because my brain has degenerated. I'm guessing you don't either.

The negative health effects we will describe in this chapter are realistic consequences of not having a period, and are compelling reasons to do your best to get your cycles back soon, fertility motives aside. You've probably heard that not getting your period can mean that your bones are not as strong as they should be for your age. There is also evidence that HA can lead to an increased risk of heart disease down the line (despite the fact that exercise is usually thought to be good for your ticker). Finally, there are studies that suggest that low lifetime estrogen exposure is linked to a higher risk of dementia, Parkinson's disease, and Alzheimer's disease. Much of this is based on extrapolation from effects of low estrogen seen after menopause, which is not an unreasonable comparison. With HA, our estrogen and progesterone hormones are low and not increasing throughout the month as they should be, similar to the hormonal profile post-menopause.

We don't throw around claims without backing them up, so the rest of this chapter will examine the evidence in each of these three areas. If you'd rather have the short version, it's this:

- Not having a period is strongly correlated with below normal bone density. Birth control pills (or other hormone replacement) may help prevent further loss *but likely do not help replace lost bone. The best way to do that is to regain your cycles.*
- As for heart function, changes implicated in future heart disease have been found in concert with HA, particularly atherosclerosis (narrowing of the arteries that feed your heart). Recovery from HA reverses the changes.
- Estrogen appears to be highly protective of your brain cells; if they are not getting that protection in pre-menopausal years, there may be an earlier onset of neurodegeneration. Recovery from HA restores the protective effect.

The bone effects of HA are undeniable. The evidence for heart and brain effects is more circumstantial, but that doesn't mean you should ignore the possibility that your current lifestyle may have these repercussions down the line.

Your doctor may be aware of the link between amenorrhea and these health risks, so you may have been offered birth control pills or hormone replacement therapy "to protect your bones." The artificial hormones may be better than nothing, but the best thing to do is to restore your own system to its proper working condition rather than to continue masking the issue. There also haven't been studies to determine whether the artificial hormones can protect your heart or your brain in the long term. *Ultimately, the best course of action for your overall health now and in the future is to follow our* HA *Recovery Plan (part 2) and get your system back in its natural balance.*

Brittle Bones

The negative effects of a missing period have been unequivocally demonstrated in the area of bone loss. Bone density and amenorrhea are linked tightly because bone cells contain estrogen receptors, and are also dependent on other proteins whose synthesis is driven by estrogen levels[1]. High estrogen levels (such as those found close to and after ovulation) increase the rate of bone formation in three major ways:

- Preventing formation of groups of cells that dissolve and reform bone.
- Promoting creation and slowing breakdown of bone forming cells (osteoblasts).
- Hindering creation and encouraging dissolution of bone breakdown cells (osteoclasts).

High progesterone levels, e.g., between ovulation and when your period starts, increase osteoblast maturation and differentiation, increasing bone density[2].

The net result at high estrogen and progesterone levels is increased bone formation. On the other hand, low estrogen levels lead to bone breakdown (resorption). Within three weeks of stopping estrogen supplementation in post-menopausal women, significant increases in markers of bone breakdown and decreases in a maker of bone formation were seen[3]. Essentially, bones are always being broken down to provide calcium—estrogen is needed to slow that breakdown and encourage formation instead.

This connection between estrogen and bone evolved to provide a calcium source for a breastfeeding infant[4]. A baby has massive calcium needs during the first few years as it triples in size. Estrogen decreases markedly during breastfeeding, increasing bone breakdown and releasing the stored calcium to breast milk. Breastfeeding has been shown to decrease maternal bone density by about 3% to 8% over six months[5]. Fortunately, the loss of bone during lactation is in most cases completely reversible; weaning, with the associated return of menstrual cycles and higher estrogen levels, leads to increases in bone formation[6].

When we are amenorrheic, our estrogen levels are low, just as when we are breastfeeding, and don't increase throughout the month as they should. This leads to increased bone breakdown as we have just described. Multiple studies[7] have shown significant decreases in average bone density (the amount of bone in a given area) in young women with amenorrhea. The same is true in our survey respondents.

Survey respondents' bone density results (67 participants)

Bone density category	Expected percentage (normal population)	Survey respondents' percentage
Normal	85%	50%
Osteopenia	15%	37%
Osteoporosis	<1%	7%
Don't Remember	NA	6%

As we've mentioned, the hormonal profiles of HA are similar to those of post-menopausal years (in terms of estrogen and progesterone levels). The rate of bone loss (a decrease of about 2.5% per year[8]) is comparable between the two states. These numbers sound scary—*but the good news is that there are things you can do to reverse this loss!*

The Basics of Bones

In case you don't know much about the bones in your body, here are some basics:

1) There are two types of bone: the hard outer shell is called cortical bone; the inside, which is less dense and spongier, is trabecular bone. When estrogen binds to and activates its receptors within the bone, bone formation increases as detailed on the previous page. Alpha-type receptors in cortical bone (compact bone) respond to low levels of estrogen. A mixture of alpha and beta receptors in trabecular bone require a much higher level of estrogen for activation. Therefore, chronically low estrogen as is seen with HA causes a larger decrease in areas such as the spine that are more trabecular. This is why spinal bone density is often lower than the hip, which contains a mix of cortical and trabecular bone.

2) Bone mass in girls increases approximately 2.5-fold from age 6 to 16 (3-fold in boys) due to increases both in bone size and density[10]. There is some debate as to the age at which peak bone mass is attained; estimates range anywhere from age 16 to 30 depending on the type of measurement and study[11]. After that, cortical bone density remains relatively constant until menopause. Trabecular density decreases slowly throughout adulthood as estrogen levels decline, then more rapidly upon menopause[12]. The post-menopausal decreases are largely due to the low estrogen (and other menstrual hormones) that occurs when periods stop; taking hormone replacement therapy after menopause significantly reduces bone loss[13]. Bone loss is typically not an issue in those with PCOS as estrogen tends to be higher overall, even if no menstrual cycles are occurring.

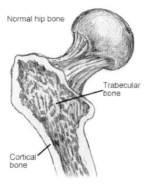

Types of bone. The location and architecture of cortical and trabecular bone. Reprinted with permission from Medscape Drugs & Diseases http://emedicine.medscape.com/, 2015[9]

3) Bones are a work in progress, with a balance between being dissolved to access minerals, a process called "resorption," and being formed again. The balance is skewed in favor of bone breakdown when estrogen and other reproductive hormones are low[14]. An ongoing energy deficit also decreases formation of new bone[15].

4) Bone density is related to bone health and strength. The risk of bone fracture increases as bone density decreases[16]. Bone density can be measured in a few different ways: currently the standard is a dual-energy x-ray absorptiometry (DXA or DEXA) scan. Results are often reported as a T-score, which relates the measured density to the distribution of bone densities seen in 30-year-olds, or a Z-score, which is similar but relates the measured density to an age-matched population. Osteopenia is when the T-score is between -1.0 and -2.5 (15.1% of 30-year-olds); osteoporosis is diagnosed when the T-score is -2.5 or less, which is found in approximately 0.6% of 30-year-olds (remember that in our survey respondents, 7% were diagnosed with osteoporosis). A Z-score of less than -2 warrants followup. Blood tests that measure markers of bone turnover are becoming more common and may replace the DXA testing in the future (this is not standard practice in 2023, however).

Bone Density and Energy Intake

Doctors Loucks and Thuma performed an experiment in which the energy intake and output of women was completely controlled for five days at one of four different levels, and effects on hormones, including markers of bone turnover, were measured[17]. On the next page, changes in bone markers at different energy levels (given as energy per unit of lean body mass, LBM, which is every part of you excluding body fat) are shown. At lower than optimal daily intake, markers of bone formation decreased. In addition, at the lowest energy intake of approximately 500 calories a day, bone breakdown markers increased. This study provides excellent evidence that ongoing energy deficiency contributes to bone loss. **It also suggests that weight gain and continued adequate caloric intake are important for bone rehabilitation.**

Change in bone markers at different energy levels[18]

Energy intake level	Daily energy intake	US equivalent	Bone breakdown markers	Bone formation markers
Sufficient	45 cal/kg LBM	20.45 cal/lb LBM	Normal	Normal
Minimum	30 cal/kg LBM	13.64 cal/lb LBM	Normal	-10% (PICP and OC)
Deficient	20 cal/kg LBM	9.09 cal/lb LBM	Normal	-20% (PICP), -30% (OC)
Severely deficient	10 cal/kg LBM	4.54 cal/lb LBM	+34%	-30% (PICP and OC)

Note: To convert from cal/kg to cal/lb, divide by 2.2 (the conversion factor from kg to lb).

When bone is dissolved, proteins called cross-linked collagen N-telopeptides (NTx) are released. In the study we just described[19], when the researchers examined these markers at the different energy levels, they found that bone dissolution stays at a normal level unless a severe caloric deficit is attained, when dissolution intensifies as indicated by the marked increase in bone breakdown markers (row for 10 cal/kg LBM). On the other hand, when bone is formed, levels of procollagen type-I C-terminal peptide (PICP) and osteocalcin (OC) are increased[20]. *The researchers found that bone formation was reduced by minor caloric deficits, and continued to slow down as fewer calories were consumed.* A severe caloric deficit leads to rapid bone loss, as there is both an increase in the breakdown of bones and a decrease in formation[21]. This study shows a clear relationship between not eating enough for your activity level and changes that can decrease bone density, or conversely, suggests that eating more will increase bone formation.

Hormone Replacement for Low Bone Density?

In many cases when someone goes to their doctor with amenorrhea and isn't interested in conceiving, doctors will prescribe birth control pills (BCP) or hormone replacement therapy (HRT) "to protect your bones." HRT consists of a combination of an estrogen pill or patch with the addition of a progesterone pill for some part of the month, and possibly testosterone.

However, the evidence for a positive effect of either treatment on bone density is underwhelming. Studies are split fairly evenly between showing no change (although this is better than the loss that can occur with continued amenorrhea) and small increases in bone density over varied lengths of time from one to four years[22]. *Further reductions in bone density can be seen even while on BCP or HRT when a caloric deficit is large enough to lead to additional weight loss*[23].

Birth control pills have been shown to decrease the rate of bone breakdown, but they also reduce bone formation[24]. This explains why those on BCP don't lose additional bone mass, but nor do they gain (much, if any). It also sheds light on why there can be further bone loss with weight loss while on BCP—the effects of the BCP are outweighed by those caused by an ongoing energy deficit. The upshot is birth control pills and hormone replacement therapy probably do not truly "protect your bones." (http://noperiod.info/bcp) They may be better than nothing, but are far from the optimal solution (see the next section). Newer evidence suggests HRT is superior to BCP, as the pills suppress insulin-like growth factor-1 (IGF-1)[25], which is involved in bone density increases. Going on hormone replacement therapy for a few months to prevent additional bone loss while you work toward recovery is a reasonable course of action.

Recovery of Lost Bone Mass

What seems to be more uniformly true is that weight gain and return of the menstrual cycle are associated with bone density increases. In a study in which bone density was measured in runners of various ages and hormonal statuses[26], the findings were:

- Runners under the age of 40 *with ongoing normal menstrual cycles* tended to have a higher bone density than average due to the positive effects of exercise (positive T-score).

- Those with amenorrhea had markedly lower T-scores (average <-1 in the spine, average approximately -0.5 in the hip).
- Runners over 40 years old who had been amenorrheic at one point but had since regained their cycles, had an average T-score around zero. This was not as good as the runners who had never lost their cycles, but still indicated a bone density similar to the average 30-year-old.

Comparing the bone densities of runners who had regained cycles with that of the currently amenorrheic runners suggests there can be a reasonable recovery of bone density with resumption of menses.

Other studies have addressed the issue of improving bone density upon recovery from restrictive eating/overexercising. A two-year study in anorexic women undergoing treatment highlighted the importance of both weight gain and resumption of menses in optimal bone health[27]. Three groups were compared. First, subjects who both gained weight and regained cycles showed a healthy 3.1% annual increase in spinal bone density and a 1.8% increase in the hip. The second group consisted of those who gained weight but did not resume cycling, and gained bone density in the hip only (0.6%). The third comprised those who did not gain weight, but resumed cycles (note that this can take years, and there are no guarantees), with bone density increases in the spine only (% change not reported)[28]. The difference between groups 2 and 3 can be explained by the more estrogen dependent nature of the trabecular bone that is a larger component of the spine[29]. Similar correlations between weight gain, periods, and bone density increases were shown in two other studies, one in which anorexics were followed for a year through recovery[30], and another where former anorexics were restudied three to nine years after recovery[31].

A series of case studies shows similarly promising correlations between weight, menses, and bone density:

- A 12-year study in an anorexic runner with a starting BMI of 16.4 showed that she continued to lose bone density as she lost weight (low BMI 14.7), *even though she was on BCP*. She then regained 12.1% (from her lowest point) of spinal bone density through the use of HRT, and increased her hip density by 19% (from the lowest point) due to weight gain[32]. Her final bone density in both areas was 1% to 2% higher at age 37 than at 25.
- An individual with a starting BMI of 15.8 had a spinal T-score of -2.5 and a hip T-score of -1.5. No changes were observed over the next two years with ongoing BCP and maintenance of weight. From age 25

to 31, BMI increased to 21.3, menses were restored, and bone density increased 26% in spine and 20% in hip to within normal values[33].
- A third runner (21 y.o.) had starting Z-scores* of -2.2 (spine) and -0.5 (hip). In the initial two years she increased training and showed negligible changes in bone density. However, marked improvements were seen over the next four years with reduced training and further increase in weight, including resumption of menstrual cycles, pregnancy and breastfeeding. Her final measured Z-scores were -0.6 (spine, 18.4% increase), and -0.1 (hip, 5.7% increase)[34].

The bottom line is even if your bone density is currently low, it can be improved over the coming years by weight gain and return of menstrual cycles, well into your thirties and perhaps even beyond. *It is not too late to change your habits and change your future health.*

There are other things you can do to improve your bone density in addition to regaining your cycles—*but not before*! Exercise that provides high or "odd" impact, as in quick changes in direction, can help increase bone density[35] and strength[36]. These types of exercise include many team sports like volleyball, softball, soccer, lacrosse, rugby, and basketball, as well as individual sports like gymnastics, tennis, sprinting, and jumping. Exercise with repetitive or low impact such as distance running, swimming, cycling, and walking, while beneficial, does not lead to the same increases as the higher impact sports. Particularly encouraging was a randomized control study in which 89 women aged 35 to 45 participated in three one-hour exercise sessions each week for 18 months that incorporated 20 minutes of jumping and step aerobics. These women saw a 2.8% to 3.8% increase in bone strength over that time—significant compared to the controls. The gains were maintained for the next 3.5 years[37]. This study highlights that gains in bone strength are possible even into one's fifth decade.

> *Ami*: I just had a DXA that shows I have osteopenia in my spine. Even though I knew I had to have something due to the amount of damage I have done for sooooo many years, it was good to know. I want to reverse what I have done! The scan was painless and easy. I did have a little breakdown on the way home beating myself up for giving myself osteopenia at such a young age but all these life lessons I am learning are just shaping me into a better version of myself. They will do the same for you. Do not get down if you have bone loss, you CAN and WILL reverse it!

---

* A Z-score is similar to a T-score, but corrected for age, gender, weight, and race. A Z-score less than -2 suggests bone density loss not due to aging.

Clover: My DXA scans (see next page) from 2002 (32 y.o.) to 2011 (41 y.o.) provided evidence for a slow and steady decline in bone health. In 2011 my DXA was at its worst, and it was during that same year in September when I finally went all in. Six months later, March 6, 2012, my periods returned. After cycling regularly for two consecutive years, I anxiously went for a follow-up DXA in 2014, praying and hoping that in spite of my age I might see some sort of improvement. I have good news. Our bodies are machines! At 44 years of age my body has shown some bone restoration.

Now, while I am still in the osteopenia/osteoporosis category, I have almost reversed the damage of the last eight years. The increase in density since I started cycling is pretty significant, which should give you full confidence that if you are in your twenties or thirties your bones can and will recover. My density has increased by almost 8% in just the last two years!

Yes, I know … this will pretty much want to make you run out and get a DXA. Not a bad idea!

Clover's DXA results 2006-2014 (recovery March 2012)

Body area	Year	Bone density (g/m^2)	T-Score	Difference from previous scan
Spine	2014	0.823	−3.0	+7.2%
	2011	0.768	−3.4	−1.4%
	2009	0.779	−3.4	−8.5%
	2006	0.851	−2.8	NA
Femur neck—left*	2014	0.782	−1.8	+8.2%
	2011	0.723	−2.3	−4.5%
	2009	0.757	−2.0	NA
Total femur—left*	2014	0.806	−1.6	+4.0%
	2011	0.775	−1.8	−1.6%
	2009	0.788	−1.7	−2.2%
	2006	0.806	−1.6	NA

* Results are similar on the right.

Recommendations

The clear consensus among the doctors who specialize in this area is that the optimal solution for bone density improvement is to gain weight and restore menstrual cycles (see part 2). The hormone changes that occur with adequate nutrition along with the resumption of menstrual cycles lead to a net increase in bone density by increasing bone formation and slowing down bone dissolution. Your bones may not get to where they would have been if you had not had amenorrhea[38], but there will almost certainly be improvements, even well into your thirties and perhaps forties.

If a decision is made *not* to gain weight, resulting in continued amenorrhea, it is certainly better to have some form of hormonal supplementation like birth control pills or estrogen plus progesterone (and possibly testosterone) to at least stabilize bone density where it is. Without weight gain and cycling, or hormonal supplementation, further decreases in bone density on the order of 2% to 3% a year are seen[39].

In addition to the diet and lifestyle changes that will be described in detail in part 2, various vitamins and/or supplements are known to improve bone health and are strongly recommended for those who exercise more than a few times a week[40]:

- Consuming adequate calcium, from a combination of food and supplements (~1200 mg/day, not more than 1400 mg/day[41]).
- Calcium is better absorbed from food than supplements, so adding calcium rich foods is beneficial.
  - Green leafy vegetables, sesame seeds, and black-eyed peas are good sources of calcium that are also high in magnesium which is necessary for proper absorption.
  - Other good sources of calcium are eggs, raisins, and artichoke.
- Consuming prunes may be beneficial for bone density[42]. The recommended amount is 100g/day (9-10 prunes).
- Boron (3mg/day)[43].
- Vitamin D (800 IU/day, or more if deficient).
- Vitamin K (60–90 ug/day).
- Protein (0.54–0.73 g/lb/day [equivalent to 1.2–1.6 g/kg/day]).

> *Amy S*: I just wanted to say something about the bone loss issue. I did in fact have significant bone loss when I had my bone scan about a year ago. I actually had osteoporosis in my spine, and mild osteopenia in the hip and femur areas. Needless to say I was both shocked and terrified when I found out. My RE was expecting some amount of bone loss since I'd had HA for about 8 months at that point, and also had HA at other earlier times in my life. But I was not expecting it. I thought I was being so healthy by exercising and maintaining a low weight.
>
> After I got those results I was terrified of what further deprivation of estrogen would do to my body. So I made up my mind to gain as much weight as I needed to in order to get my body cycling again—my RE was convinced that weight gain would get me going again. I am only five feet

> tall, and I gained 22 pounds (and believe me I am not mostly muscle; far from it at this point since I also stopped all exercise except walking while I was waiting to cycle). I got my period back within four to five months of the weight gain and reduction in exercise. My RE said she'd put me on Fosamax right away, or a different drug for bone loss, but it's not a good idea to do that if you are going to be pregnant in the near future. Apparently the medication stays in your bones for up to 10 years and can go across the placenta.
>
> Nonetheless, it is scary stuff. And I will likely have to take some kind of medication to improve my bone density at some point. In the meantime, I'm pregnant with twins! Yay! And I take a ton of calcium/vitamin D/magnesium combo supplements, and I get a lot of calcium from milk and cheese and yogurt. I make sure to get A LOT every day since the babies now need it too and will take it from my bones if they aren't getting enough.
>
> Finding out how bad my bones were really shocked and scared me. And it still does. But, at least you can do something about it now to get your cycles and estrogen back.
>
> Bone Density for Amy:
> 2008—spine T-score: −3.2
> 2009—twins born, exclusively breastfed for 13 months
> Late 2009—spine T-score: −3.4
> Dec 2011—spine T-score: −2.6
> Dec 2013—spine T-score: −2.2 (out of osteoporosis range)
> Nov 2015—spine T-score: −2.0
>
> This equates to a 22.3% improvement in spinal bone density over the last six years, with the last scan at age 39.

Heart

There haven't been any studies linking HA directly to cardiovascular disease (CVD), probably because of the long time frame and large numbers such a study would require. Therefore, suggestions of a possible connection between HA and CVD are based on the commonality of low estrogen. With that, there's enough evidence to demonstrate that CVD is a realistic long-term concern in those with HA:

- First, there is a marked increase in incidence of heart disease after menopause[44].

- Second, in a study of women who underwent surgical menopause by having both ovaries removed, the risk of death from heart disease was increased by 85%[45]. If estrogen replacement was used immediately following the surgery, there was no increase in risk.
- Third, in pre-menopausal women, cardiac events that require hospitalization are much more likely to occur in the first half of the menstrual cycle when estrogen is low[46].
- Fourth, other studies have examined estrogen levels in women with CVD and found them to be significantly lower than in controls[47].
- Finally, cardiac issues have been well documented in anorexia, where estrogen is extremely low[48], including abnormal heart rhythms, reduction in heart mass, bradycardia (heart rate < 50 bpm), and systemic vascular resistance, which makes the heart work harder to pump blood.

Based on these studies it is reasonable to conclude that low estrogen, as is experienced with HA, is potentially associated with an increased risk of heart disease.

Signs of Future Heart Disease in HA

We mentioned "systemic vascular resistance" in the previous section as a common issue in those with anorexia, where the heart has to work harder to pump blood. This vascular resistance has also been demonstrated with HA[49]. A test called "flow mediated dilation" (FMD) can expose some of the early changes that lead to CVD. It measures artery elasticity; how easily arteries can expand to accommodate increased blood flow. Think about it as the difference between blowing up a normal balloon versus the small balloons for making balloon animals; the latter can turn your face red and make you feel like you just can't get the air out. That's what your heart feels like when you have reduced FMD. Athletes with HA have an FMD about 60% to 75% lower than in normally cycling peers[50], and about 50% lower than sedentary controls[51]. Do you need to rush out, see a cardiologist, and get your FMD checked? Probably not. Our recommendations (see below) would be the same regardless of the results.

Like bone density, FMD is correlated with estrogen levels. Estrogen drives the formation of hormones like nitric oxide (NO) that are vasodilators (help with expanding the arteries when necessary) and keeps levels of vasoconstrictors (which constrict the arteries) low[52]. Restoration of normal estrogen through return of menses or supplementation with BCP (or hormone replacement), led to normalization of FMD[53]. Along with reduced

FMD, high cholesterol is also associated with an increased risk of heart disease. A finding of increased total cholesterol or low-density-lipoprotein (LDL) is common in those with "athletic amenorrhea"[54]. In our experience, cholesterol levels generally normalize upon recovery.

Once again, low estrogen as seen in HA, appears to be a catalyst for negative health effects; however, restoring the monthly estrogen fluctuations allows for repairs and normalization.

> *Lauren*: I first found the Board in February. Then, pretending I didn't read what I read, I tried to forget about it, made like 10% to 20% changes in my diet and exercise, and wasted a solid seven months being amenorrheic until I decided: besides the threat of infertility, I'm tired of the acne, the brittle nails, the shedding hair, the extreme thirst, and the low libido. Then I got my cholesterol tested and it was high (an effect of low E_2)! I laughed in the woman's face because I told her there was literally nothing better I could do in terms of eating and exercise to lower cholesterol. I then read that low estrogen puts us at an increased risk for heart attacks and osteoporosis. I said, "I've had it." It was killing me emotionally knowing that my body was literally deteriorating, and although I knew I could do something about it, I did nothing. I couldn't deal with the inner conflict any more. (*Lauren's cycles came back two months after going all in. Eight months later she and her husband conceived their baby girl on their very first try.*)

Recommendations

Evidence in this area suggests that hormone replacement can restore cardiac parameters to close to normal[55]. However, the artificial estrogen and progesterone do not mimic all the effects of weight gain and restoration of normal cycles, so artificial hormone supplementation is likely to be a Band-Aid rather than a long-term fix. Once again, the best course of action is regaining your cycles. Otherwise, BCP or HRT should be considered.

Brain

The final area of concern in those with HA, particularly in the long term, is the possibility of an increased risk of neurodegenerative disease like dementia, Parkinson's disease, or Alzheimer's disease. While there is no direct evidence of a correlation between HA and future risk of neurodegenerative disease, this caution is again based on studies that included women who have undergone either surgical or normal menopause, studies in animal models, or studies on individual cells.

As we discussed regarding the heart, estrogen promotes vasodilation, i.e., elasticity in your arteries (remember the normal balloon versus the difficult-to-blow-up balloon animals?), which makes it easier for the heart to pump blood. This elasticity also leads to a better blood supply to the brain[56]. There is evidence that estrogen enhances the building of new nerve connections and prevents nerve cell death[57]. In addition, new evidence suggests that many neurodegenerative diseases are due to long-term, low-level inflammation in the brain, caused by a type of cell called "microglia cells." Microglia are turned off by estrogen and progesterone, reducing inflammation[58].

The evidence suggesting a link between low estrogen and neurodegenerative disease comes from two sources, one being the long-term follow-up of patients after surgical menopause. There is a clearly demonstrated 1.5- to 2-fold increased risk of dementia[59] in these women with chronically low estrogen, as well as an increased risk of death from neurological disease[60]. The risk was highest in women who had the surgery younger than 45 years old and did not use HRT, which may be a good model for what may occur with long-term HA. Studies in animal models have shown similar effects[61].

The second way of looking at the issue is to determine approximately how much estrogen someone has been exposed to in their lifetime and see if that has an effect on cognitive outcomes. One group collected information from subjects such as:

- when the person's first period started
- how many pregnancies and live births they experienced
- whether babies were breastfed and for how long
- the age at which menopause occurred
- when hormone therapy started (if it was used)

A "lifetime estrogen exposure" score was calculated using the information. A higher score indicated more estrogen exposure and was correlated with better performance on memory tests[62]. When the components of the measure were examined individually, the strongest association was that longer breastfeeding predicted lower scores[63]. This may be a good proxy for HA, as breastfeeding keeps estrogen low and prevents menstrual cycles (we're not saying *not* to breastfeed—there are a myriad other reasons that it's a good idea). Other groups used bone density as a surrogate for estrogen exposure and likewise found that high bone density, which equates to high estrogen exposure, was associated with better performance on memory tests[64].

Recommendations

Long-term effects of estrogen depletion on the brain during reproductive years are not well defined, although the suggestion of negative effects is not unreasonable. Although there haven't been studies on whether the standard hormonal treatments are helpful, estrogen and progesterone supplementation following surgical menopause does show decreases in the risks of some neurodegenerative disease. This suggests that the same recommendations hold true as in the case of bones and hearts; the best course of action is to work toward restoring your menstrual cycle, most likely in concert with gaining some weight. In the absence of recovery, it is probably advisable to use some form of hormonal supplementation.

Overall Recommendations

As we have discussed, it is clear that in the case of bone density, the optimal course of action is gaining weight and restoring natural menstrual cycles. The same is presumably true for protecting heart and brain as our hormonal systems are complex and much more than just the estrogen and progesterone that are provided by hormonal supplements. We will spend lots of time discussing how to work toward restoring your cycles in part 2.

- Trying to get pregnant?
    - o If you follow the HA Recovery Plan (part 2) and do not resume cycles in a timeframe acceptable to you, fertility treatments can help you ovulate and hopefully get pregnant. Our systems often reset after pregnancy if we are careful not to fall back into restrictive eating and under-fueled exercise habits; you may very well start menstruating after pregnancy (see part 4).
- NOT trying to get pregnant?
    - o If you are not able to resume natural cycles within a year or so after following the Recovery Plan (part 2), we would suggest going on hormonal replacement, perhaps with a break of a few months every year to determine whether you cycle naturally. Other options are discussed in chapter 18.

If you choose not to follow the Recovery Plan right now, it is likely better to use hormone replacement in some form than to do nothing.

> *Clover*: Good grief ... do not, I repeat, do NOT follow in my footsteps by ignoring the fact that you aren't getting a period, especially if you've already been diagnosed with osteopenia and/or osteoporosis.
>
> You would think I'd have had some sort of concern after being diagnosed with osteoporosis in my spine and osteopenia in my hips. It didn't scare me, though; I chalked it up to my small build (even though I didn't naturally have a small build... denial), bad luck, and genetics. This was pure folly. Then I rationalized it even further—there was no way I could have osteoporosis because I spent years lifting heavy, doing Olympic lifts which surely built my bones, right? I was really into my running sport, worked hard at staying fit, and ate meticulously. Obviously NONE of that matters when you aren't getting a period. No period means you most likely have low estrogen, and if you have little estrogen you are probably losing bone mass. Now is the time to be steadily increasing bone density, not losing or simply maintaining. The preservation of bone is for later, when your body goes through menopause.
>
> I'll share with you a little word picture. I am currently caring for my 72-year-old osteoporotic mother. Within the past two years she fractured a hip (then had a replacement), then fractured her sacrum, two months later her tib/fib (this is beginning to sound like a horror flick), and then a week later her pelvis. Ouch! Ouch! Ouch! If I had a dollar for every friend that asked how she keeps falling... The irony is that she was not falling but simply engaging in everyday life—carrying groceries, doing laundry, stepping off a curb to cross the street, etc. Osteoporosis does indeed live up to its name as the "silent killer," having no symptoms leading up to the fractures. Thankfully our bodies are designed in such a way that we can directly impact our bone health by making lifestyle changes now!
>
> Pay now or pay later because we all pay one way or another. This might be a great reason to get uncomfortable NOW with the Recovery Plan (part 2) rather than getting uncomfortable later with osteoporosis... or dementia... or cardiovascular disease.

Part 2:
The Recovery Plan—Changing Your Habits and Your Life

Nico: As I've mentioned, when I was trying to recover from HA I had to figure out my own recovery plan. Eventually, after a bunch of diagnostic tests, my doctor told me I should probably eat a little more and reduce my exercise, but with no guidance as to what that actually meant. Even though I had come to the same conclusion myself, putting that into practice was a struggle. I enjoyed my exercise, thought I looked fantastic after my recent weight loss, and it seemed really unfair that I had to undo all my hard work when others around me were getting pregnant at the drop of a hat. (Like a party I went to with FOUR "oops" pregnant women who proceeded to tell me that all I needed to do to get pregnant was to *not* want to be. Gee, thanks! But I digress.) With no information as to what I really needed to do to recover, I didn't go far enough in my changes. Even after seeing a nutritionist I don't think I was eating enough, and I was almost certainly exercising too much. I finally got my period back when I went on a three-week vacation, ate whatever, and did no exercise other than walking.

Steph: I fought recovery kicking and screaming. I was *not* running too much, I *was* eating enough, why was this happening to me? It seemed so unfair! I had done my time. I had been through eating disorder treatment, I was recovered! How could there be more?! My doctor told me exactly what I needed to do, the Board provided story after story that confirmed her recommendations, but I liked my life and didn't want to have to change yet again. The whole plan seemed pretty preposterous. Yet when I finally did go all in, I reaped the benefits—happiness, health, and pregnancy!

In this section we will outline our recommendations on how much to eat, what to eat, and how much to exercise. We know that these changes are incredibly hard to make and keep up, so we include chapters with tips and tricks that we and others have used to cope with these challenges.

8
You Want Me to Eat WHAT??
The HA Recovery Plan

DID YOU SKIP AHEAD to get to this chapter? We probably would have too. It's what we all want to know— "What do I have to do?" But before we get to that (sorry for the tease!), it's important for you to know that the Recovery Plan detailed throughout the next few chapters works. When all was said and done, 98% of our survey respondents resumed natural cycles.

You might be tempted to think that your weight and eating habits are just fine because you aren't "underweight," and this section does not apply to you. That's not true, because no matter what your current size, you can be underfueling *for your body*. This is particularly likely if your LH is on the low side of the normal range (below about 5 IU/L). Among our survey respondents, there was no difference in recovery rate based on starting body size. It's evident that if you are missing your period, and your lifestyle is as we have described, when you apply the Recovery Plan you too will benefit from the changes.

What Does Recovery Mean?

First, the fundamental goal is recovery of your health and fertility (and for many, to get pregnant). To get to that point, you need to supply yourself with energy not just for your current day to day needs, but also to replenish your body after months or years of underfueling.

It is important to address the restrictive eating and food habits, and the mindset that goes along with those behaviors that for many are a fundamental tenet of HA. Irrespective of your current level of food restriction, the eventual goals for your eating habits include:

- To enjoy and fully participate in work and family gatherings that involve meals.
- To spend your free time thinking about work, family, friends, kids, anything—but NOT about what or how much you're going to eat.
- To let food be something that provides nutrition and pleasure; no more, no less.
- To never count calories again (unless you need to occasionally to confirm you are eating enough).
- To eat when you are hungry and stop when you are full.
- To eat all foods (aside from allergies and religious or ethical choices) in moderation, while realizing that occasional indulgences are part of a happy, healthy outlook and nothing to feel guilty about.

> Lisa: A couple of things came to my mind upon reading these goals. If you can't relate with anything I am about to share, well then, good for you! <smirky smile>
>
> - *"Never count calories"*??? Oh gosh... are you kidding? I have never been a huge calorie counter but did tend to glance at the package to make sure there wasn't over X amount of calories. After recovery I remember talking to a friend on the Board about a protein bar. I asked, "Aren't those bars good? They are low in sugar too!" She replied, "Oh! I didn't even notice. <laughing> I don't ever look at calories, fats, carbs, or anything anymore." Huh???? This is a true story. I know it sounds completely far-fetched, but it's not. As time passes and women recover, similar healthy changes are experienced. True freedom!
> - *"Eat when you are hungry and stop when you are full"*...whoa...so at this point for some of you, eating an extra carrot stick might push you over the edge, let alone a single-scoop ice cream cone (it did for me—the ice cream, not the carrot stick). That is because hunger and fullness signals are off kilter from the ongoing caloric restriction. The only antidote is to eat more. So, for now, you will experience sitting with the uncomfortable in order to reach the long-term goal of "sensing when full," and then you can make a choice to stop (or not). That being said, it's important to note that many of our non-disordered eating peers eat beyond fullness from time to time without going into panic mode, which could be another goal to strive for.
> - *"Eat all foods."* Yup, anything. Eventually those mysterious allergies you developed over the years (that no one else in your family has—lactose intolerance, sugar, gluten... no, not all of you have true gluten

> allergies) will miraculously disappear. I think I ate so strictly and was underfueled for so long that my body couldn't digest properly—as if it was losing the necessary enzymes. I was lactose intolerant (great excuse to not eat anything out of my comfort zone); oh, and I even developed a mysterious beef allergy that landed me in the hospital three times for anaphylactic shock! I don't make this stuff up, folks. And the coolest part about these mysterious allergies is that along with recovery I can now eat a burger and chocolate shake with the best of them with NO allergic reaction. The body is amazing when properly fueled.
>
> I could keep going but you get the point. And besides, there is NO convincing to be done. Just sharing some truth.

Does living your life that way sound appealing to you? Our survey respondents felt and acted very differently after recovery than when they had HA.

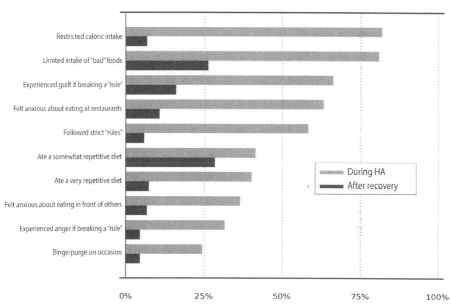

Subclinical eating disorder symptoms during HA and after recovery. The percentage of survey respondents (326 participants) exhibiting each behavior during the time they had HA (light gray) compared to after recovery (dark gray). You can see that there are still some with issues even after recovery, but overall symptoms are *much* improved.

> **Shayla**: I used to live in such full-fledged anxiety over eating anything that wasn't part of my "scheduled" eats… God forbid I had an extra carrot or a piece of candy. Yes, I was that crazy about every.single.calorie. Or heaven forbid I got in 58 minutes of cardio instead of 60, or burned 550 calories instead of my usual 600. I'm not saying that's where you are now,

> but it's easy for our minds to get back to that place. Now that I'm free from that prison, I want you to be free from all the demons as well...not only for *your* health, but to portray a healthy, positive example to our precious children (present or future in whatever way kids may be in your life). I *know* you can do this and I *know* you can free yourself from it all. You deserve absolutely nothing but the best in this precious, short life we have.

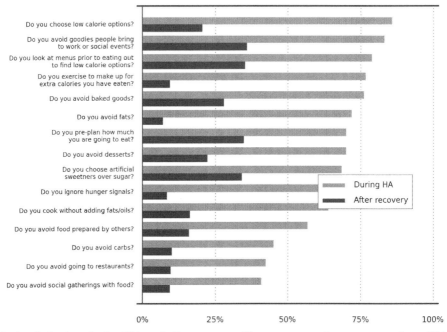

Eating behaviors during HA and after recovery. The percentage of survey respondents (284 participants) selecting that they "always" or "often" exhibited each eating behavior, during HA (light gray) and while gaining/recovering (dark gray).

The Recovery Plan: Are You Ready?

You may have gathered from what you've read that the Recovery Plan will entail eating more and gaining some weight. You're right. You will probably have to eat quite a bit more—in amount as well as variety. And yes, eating more will probably lead to some degree of weight gain.

Is the idea of eating more and/or gaining weight scary to you? That's not unusual—it was for us! As we've discussed, our appearances and abilities to control food and exercise often become a large part of our identities. Considering any changes to those integral parts of us can be frightening.

It often takes a complete mental shift in how we think about food, eating, and our bodies. Hopefully it helps to know that thousands before you have accepted this challenge and found themselves better off afterward both mentally and physically.

If you are ready to jump in and begin to follow the HA Recovery Plan, you will find that the very common feelings of concern over food (what, when, why, and how) will decrease in intensity and frequency over time, while your feelings of freedom and relief increase overall. If contemplating these changes makes you anxious, gather the information found in this book, then you can choose whether or not to put our recommendations into practice. If you decide not to follow our suggestions right now, keep them in the back of your mind because you may feel differently in the future.

> *Deanna*: I thank my lucky stars every single day for this process. I love that I am free, can eat what I want and live how I want, and that I am no longer tied to my old body and ways. I know I will be a better mommy and person for it. I know this weight will help me get pregnant. I do not for any minute of any day regret going through this. I will never revert to my old habits of restricting, losing friends and sleep over exercise, and living in a self-made prison—I will continue to live free now and in the future after baby. *(Deanna got pregnant seven months after going all in, using Femara, with three subsequent natural pregnancies.)*

> *Chassta*: Skinny is not the ultimate achievement. These bodies are ours, but for a moment in time. Even if I don't get pregnant, I will one day be a mother and I WILL NOT pass this horrible distorted view of unattainable perfection to my children. Even though some of us "reached" our so-called ideal body, what did we have to sacrifice in return? Our bodies and minds were not created for such consuming anxieties and stress. So now, in order to regain the things long thought lost—shiny, thick hair; glowing skin; deep sleep; sexual appetite; feminine curves; clear thinking; strong bones; fertility; positive attitudes; compassion and non-judgmental attitudes toward others and ourselves—we have to sacrifice our "skinny" bodies. Which one is really more of a sacrifice? *(Chassta recovered her cycles after three months all in and got pregnant five cycles later.)*

The hardest part of getting ready to take the plunge to change eating thoughts and habits, for many, is the unknown. Most of us are excellent planners and will do whatever it takes to make our plans happen. But this? There is no way to know exactly what is going to make your body happy (i.e., recover), or how long it will take. It is a leap of faith to go forward with making these changes without knowing for sure they will work for you or when. Yet, it is not a blind leap of faith; weight gain, rest, decreased stress, and time equal a restored reproductive system.

So let's say you take that leap. What comes next? Probably some disbelief, denial, doubt, and fear. Maybe some anger. But also excitement, relief, and joy. You will probably experience each and every one of these emotions during the roller coaster ride you are about to take. Ready?

I Have to Eat How Much?!

And finally, we get to the question you've been waiting for: how much do you have to eat? We're providing these caloric targets as guidelines to give you an idea of how much you really need to be eating to fully fuel your system and recover. But as we've said, the eventual goal is to stop counting and eat the food your body needs. As time passes you will learn what you should be eating in a day and be able to eat intuitively, without that calculator in your mind (or on your phone) keeping track. It's important too that if you feel hungry, even though you're already increasing your caloric intake, you feed that hunger and eat even more!

> *Megan*: I agree that calorie counting can be a trigger, even if it is counting in the opposite direction. I'm sure most of us are aware of the ballpark amount of calories in the foods we eat. If you know you were eating 1500 before, it shouldn't be too difficult to figure out what 1000 more would be.

> *Jessica*: I used to get angry with my body when it got hungry before I thought it should. I used to think "I just fed you, why are you hungry already? Can't you give me a break?" Now, I find myself thinking "OK, body. I hear you. I am not sure why you are so hungry today, but I will get you food." It is a crazy shift but I think it is a freeing one. I feel like I have shifted from relying totally on my brain and pretty much ignoring my body to trying to rely mostly on my body (e.g., I am feeling hungry, better grab a snack) and only a little on my brain (e.g., I haven't had much protein today, maybe I'll include that in my snack).

Keeping the eventual goal to stop counting calories in mind, as a general rule you should be eating a minimum of about 2500 calories a day. Yes, you read that correctly. Twenty-five hundred calories a day. That probably sounds like a huge amount. In truth, you may even need to eat more than this—certainly if you're having hunger pangs you should continue to eat! The recommendation of 2500 calories is not an upper limit, it's a minimum. To help you understand where this number comes from we will go over the rationale and calculations below.

You may have concerns that if you eat that many calories you will immediately pile on the pounds, becoming "unhealthy" (never mind that you are not healthy right now . . .). Contrary to what many believe our physiology doesn't work like that. In fact, some noticed that the weight gain was slower than expected. This is because the body first uses the extra energy toward repairing and restoring the systems that were slowed and shut down. Others have experienced a rapid initial gain as the body stores fat in case starvation is coming again, then works on systems repair after that. No matter what, weight gain levels off over time, as we will discuss later. And many markers of "health" improve with giving our bodies necessary fuel. (For example, many find cholesterol levels actually decrease.)

> Liz: I gained about 20 lb in six months or so and then my weight stabilized (based on how my clothes fit; I rarely weigh myself). I didn't cut back on what I ate and continued eating freely. My weight has been about the same since that initial quick jump.
>
> Devon P: At first, the weight I gained was "lean weight": muscle and water that had been depleted during my years of restriction. Side note—I saw a doctor when I'd made an attempt to recover about 10 years earlier. She tested my resting metabolism and found it was crazy low because my body was trying to conserve as much energy as possible, to the point where I had started metabolizing muscle and hair protein to make up the deficit. Anyway, after that lean mass was restored I piled on weight (fat and more water) really quickly. But after seven months, I stopped gaining despite the exact same (zero) exercise and (plentiful) eating regime.

Prove It!

If you're thinking that we are nuts and there is no way a person your size needs that many calories (some small adjustments are provided on the next page), we will describe two different methods of calculating energy requirements that show how we arrived at this number. We will also discuss some additional clinical studies in which weight gain (from added calories) was important in recovering from HA. But if you'd like the quick and simple version, here's a summary:

- Equations from the Institute of Medicine (IOM) lead us to compute that a 5'6", *weight stable*, active woman at a fertile BMI of 22 burns about 2450 calories each and every day. The stable weight indicates consumption of the same amount, which means that for a fully functioning metabolism, that's how much a woman of similar size should be taking in each day[1].
- Various research groups studied the relationship between lean body mass (e.g., heart, muscles, lungs, bones ... the parts of you that use energy) and caloric intake and derived equations to calculate the energy levels at which optimal metabolism is achieved. For an active woman at a fertile BMI with 20% body fat this is a daily intake of 2533 calories for a fully functioning (menstruating) metabolism[2].
- Four additional research studies have found a strong correlation between weight gain and resumption of menstrual cycles.

Energy requirement calculation: method 1. The first method for determining the recommendations used formulas calculated by researchers at IOM who measured metabolism of safe radioactively labeled water to accurately determine energy expenditure[3]. These formulas include other variables so you can adjust your intake slightly depending on your age and height.

Recommended daily caloric intake[4]*

Height	Recommended calories if you are active†	Recommended calories if you are sedentary
< 5'0"	2250	2000
5'0" – 5'4"	2350	2100
5'4" – 5'8"	2450	2200
5'8" – 6'0"	2550	2300
> 6'0"	2650	2400

* If you're 19 or younger, you should add an additional 100 calories because you're still growing and your body needs even more!

† "Active" is defined as the equivalent of walking five to seven miles per day. Most HAers fall into this category.

Energy measurements were performed while the study participants' weight was stable[5], indicating that caloric intake equaled output. So, on average, participants were burning *and consuming* 2450 calories per day (although from here on out we're just going to say 2500 as a ballpark figure—eating an extra 50 cal per day will be good for you as you work toward recovery, and again, you shouldn't be counting going forward!). This is the answer to how much *you* should be eating (taking into account your height as shown) in order to have a fully functional metabolism and restore your missing periods, because your basic metabolic needs are just the same as everyone else's. Your heart beats, blood pumps, hair, nails, and bones grow, immune system fights infections, and so on. As you consume the additional energy, a large proportion will go to repairing, restoring, and revving up your metabolism. And if you eat more than our recommendations? Well, that will just get your body back to where it desperately wants to be that much faster.

One other thing to mention is that if you're in a sedentary job and not active at all (e.g., not walking or performing any other exercise whatsoever), you can subtract 250 calories from the daily minimums. Conversely, if you continue with an exercise program that is high intensity (not recommended, see chapter 12), you should add additional calories to account for your exercise on a given day.

You may be wondering how this jibes with the recommendation that you see to eat 2000 calories to maintain[6], or 1500–1800 (or shockingly, less) to lose weight. Those recommendations are outdated. They are based on the same idea, that 2000 is the number of calories one needs in order to be weight stable—but that amount is based on self-reports of caloric intake rather than any actual measurements[7]. The majority of people tend to underestimate the number of calories they are consuming[8], which leads to the recommendations being lower than what is actually required. This is probably fine for the average person who is likewise underestimating what they're eating—but for those of us who are in the opposite camp, more likely overestimating our daily intake, we need an accurate target!

Energy requirement calculation: method 2. A different yet equally accurate method used to measure the energy expenditure of hundreds of people involves a room specially designed to track daily activities, including sleeping, preparing food and eating, working, and exercising[9]. The researchers found that the energy expended going about normal daily activities is proportional to "lean body mass" (LBM), which is every part of you excluding body fat. This makes sense because muscles, bones, brain, heart, circulatory system, lungs, etc., carry out the work of running your body. For example, your heart uses up energy every time it beats to send blood to your lungs and through your veins.

It turns out that 20.45 calories per pound of lean body mass[10] is the amount of energy you expend each and every day going about your normal activities*. *This does not include any purposeful exercise.*

Lo and behold, if you assume 20% body fat, the calorie requirement for a 5'6" woman at a fertile BMI of 22.5 is 2283, which is remarkably close to what you would calculate from the IOM equations for a sedentary woman (2450-250 = 2200). If your body fat is lower (for example, the average among our survey respondents was 14%), you need MORE calories than that, as your LBM will be higher! Then you also have to add in extra calories for those burned performing daily physical movement and exercise (yes, walking counts!), which gets you to approximately 2500 calories per day.

If your BMI is currently below 22.5, you may think that you don't need to eat this amount because you weigh less. Not true! There are three important reasons: 1) if your low/lowered body mass is because of lower body fat, your bones, muscles, and organs are doing the same work as someone at a higher BMI and therefore need the same amount of fuel; 2) if your lean body mass is in fact lower, your body needs at least this amount of energy to rebuild muscle and organs that were used for energy while underfueling; and 3) the lower your current weight-for-height, the more complete the shutdown of your systems tends to be, so the same amount of energy (if not more) is needed for repairs and to turn everything back on again.

Is Eating More Really Going to Work?

Do you want even more evidence? Although you're probably convinced by now, when it comes down to being purposeful in putting on weight (especially in our current society in which this is rarely encouraged), there is never too much information. The next table shows the weight gain in women whose cycles returned while participating in clinical studies. *As you can see, most of those with returning cycles made a willful decision to gain weight; those with ongoing amenorrhea did not.* It's your choice. Our survey population is by far the largest group in which this question has been assessed, and there was a significant difference in weight gain between those who resumed periods and those who did not (an increase of 2.25 BMI units in those who recovered versus 1.35 BMI units in those who did not, $p < 1 \times 10^{-4}$). Particularly if you're currently under a BMI of 22, weight gain is going to be important,

---

* The concept of metabolic rate being correlated with lean body mass has been corroborated in many studies[11].

much as you may not want it to be. Note that in the other studies, just as with our survey respondents, the weight gain tended to bring people to a BMI of 22 to 23 or more, which we call the "fertile zone." The study by Falsetti *et al.*[12] was particularly interesting as they calculated the likelihood of returning menstrual cycles; for every one unit increase in BMI, they calculated a 34% increase in the odds of recovering.

Resumption of menstrual cycles and weight changes

Study	Number in study	% Regaining cycles	Time to recovery	BMI change in recovered women	BMI change in non-recovered women
Sykes (Rinaldi) (survey respondents)	302	52%*	Median 6 months	+2.25	+1.35 ($p < 1\times10^{-4}$)
Falsetti[13]	92	71%	NR	+2.4 (33 women) or remained at 21.8 (32 women)	-1.5 (4 women) or remained at 19.0 (19 women)
Arends**[14]	51	18%	Average 16 months	+1.9	+0.5
Misra[15]	34	41%	< 12 months	+3.1	+0.8
Berga[16]	16	88% (CBT† group), 13% (control group)	20 weeks	NR, estimated at +0.5 (starting BMI 23.2)	NR, estimated at +0.0 (starting BMI 21.2)

NR – Not Reported, estimated from information provided.
* The remainder used fertility treatments to achieve pregnancy.
** The Arends *et al.* study was performed in college-age athletes, for whom recovery was likely not a high priority.
†Cognitive Behavioral Therapy

> **Kira:** Soooo... just thought I'd fill y'all in: I have kicked "intuitive eating" to the curb and am back to stuffing my face (3000+ cals) and am going to be more *regular* about it as opposed to in the past where I'd eat anywhere from 1800 to 3500 calories/day (but usually around the 2000 to 2200 mark). I spoke to a very knowledgeable registered dietitian yesterday who was so encouraging about it and I think that's what I needed—a professional telling me things would be OK, the weight gain would eventually stop, and I might end up tapering down once my metabolism is back to functioning optimally. She has worked with clients with amenorrhea

> and they all got their periods back within three weeks to three months! So here's to hoping the same for me. I ate the biggest breakfast I think of my life this morning and rolled all the way to work, but I'm ready to push past any discomfort and negative thoughts that get in the way. I'm running this race (without *actually* running of course) all the way to the finish line and am going to be victorious and win! I'm going where I've never been before and it's daunting, but when I feel down (which I already have today and it's only day 1), I will remind myself to have faith in a greater plan and that I am made for so much more than my weight and appearance. I won't be able to be the best version of me until I conquer all demons. (*Kira got her period back after six weeks of focusing on recovery, and has been cycling regularly ever since.*)

How Long Will It Take?

What determines how long it will take to recover? There is no magic formula or crystal ball that will tell you. What we can tell you is that there is a high probability it will happen. The time frame seems to vary greatly, between one month and a few years. There are many variables that impact the recovery time frame, such as your age, how quickly you gain weight, your exercise activity, how much stress you are under, and things you have absolutely no control over like genetics and how sensitive your system is to your energy balance. One factor that does not impact time to recovery is the length of time for which your period was missing, in those who took our survey there was no correlation between time without a period and time to recovery (http://noperiod.info/time).

Factors in Recovery: Going "All In"

Of the factors we mention, the biggest one you can control is how quickly you make changes and go "all in," which does affect how soon you will recover. What we mean by "all in" is

1) Following our eating plan every day.
2) Cutting all high intensity exercise (chapter 12).
3) Reducing stress and making time to relax.

Let's be clear, we do not mean just eating a few extra handfuls of nuts and gaining a couple of pounds. Sure, you can try that if you like, but in our experience it will just prolong the time to recovery.

> *Devon P*: When I first realized I needed to get real—cut exercise and eat more—I thought I could get away with some minor changes. I cut my exercise back from 45 minute cardio workouts (usually elliptical) to 20 after an RE said "there was no way" 20 minutes a day would cause HA. Maybe so but he didn't realize I'd exercised three or four times that much for years! I also was a little more generous with food and gained couple of pounds. After a few weeks of nothing, I quit all cardio and just did weights, rationalizing that it was good for my bones. Upped my food intake a little more. Still nothing. After about another month of these watered-down efforts I got frustrated and finally committed. I was wasting time; gaining weight maybe but not getting closer to my goal, and it was making me *more* anxious. I wondered if I was slowing progress down by exercising; if all I was doing was pushing my goal of getting a period further and further away. That anxiety was getting almost as strong as my anxiety about gaining weight. So I decided to go all in. Eat at least 2,500 calories (probably twice what I was taking in before) and do no exercise other than slow walks and gentle yoga. After three difficult, soul-searching, questioning months, I got my period!!! The very next month I was pregnant. To those in my situation, I say don't dither! Quit working out, the sooner the better. It's only slowing you down and your bones aren't getting the full benefit of weight-bearing exercise (I know that excuse) without estrogen coursing through your blood. Your body needs REST. You've gotten in this situation because you've been majorly stressing yourself and you need a break. You need it and you need to build up those energy stores to carry that baby. You can go back to working out, it'll be there, but if you have HA, your workouts aren't healthy, they're anything but.

Factors in Recovery: Time

The second factor you control is the length of time you spend on the Recovery Plan before moving to other options. Are you trying to get your period back for overall health reasons, or do you want to do so in order to get pregnant? Are you preparing for pregnancy a year or two down the line, or did you only find out about your missing period when you were ready for a baby? Depending on which category you're in, you will probably have a different time frame for which you are willing to wait to see changes and resume your cycles. In a perfect world we'd love to see you put in at least a solid six months of recovery effort. Why six months? On average it seems that those who spend at least six months all in feel more at peace with the total weight gain and exercise reduction, and *have a more complete recovery*.

This might have something to do with the willingness to sit with the uncomfortable and unknown for so long, leading to developing new healthy coping skills. With that said, please realize we are not saying recovery can't happen in a shorter time because it can (and does), but we do feel a responsibility to share what we have seen work best overall. Among our survey respondents who regained natural cycles, 24% did so within three months of starting lifestyle changes, 34% within four months, and 57% within six months. Of those who did not regain natural cycles prior to their first pregnancy, 63% started fertility treatments before completing six months of recovery efforts.

> *Claire*: I really think a lot of this is about patience. Several months ago, I was feeling very impatient. I was debating meds, obsessing about cervical mucus and temps, etc. Then I decided that I was going crazy and was unhealthily focused on getting pregnant. So, I decided to concentrate on the rest of my life, while still continuing to take the steps necessary to allow my body to heal from HA. So far, it's working (both from a physical and mental health standpoint).
>
> There is more to life than getting pregnant tomorrow. If I get pregnant a year from now, or even two, it will still be OK, so I'm willing to try to be patient while my body does its healing work.
>
> Who knows, maybe my husband will have a horrible sperm count, or we'll miscarry, etc. Maybe we'll end up adopting regardless. Either way, for the health of my bones, mind, and family, I need to heal this HA thing. I'm taking steps to get there, and in the meantime, I'm living the rest of my life.
>
> Patience... time, food, rest, weight. It really will work; your body is created to create. (*Claire conceived her first three weeks later, then got pregnant with her second two years later, within a few weeks of weaning.*)

If you choose not to put in the time, there are certainly treatments you can use to help you ovulate to get pregnant (part 3). We will caution you, however, that jumping to those treatments without having made any strides toward recovery can lead to thousands of wasted dollars and dealing with the emotional stress of failed cycles. Not to mention the reality of having the same unhealthy mindset with food and/or exercise that landed you here in the first place. Fertility treatments do work for some with HA, but there are many others who are not successful until they have made lifestyle changes. There is also the fact that pregnancy is much easier to deal with mentally and physically when you're on your way to recovery.

> *Joy*: I unfortunately did go ahead with treatments that did not work (at least not the three failed IVFs before my current totally natural pregnancy—which came after I found the Board and gained weight, as my RE did not tell me I needed to gain weight to get pregnant). *(Joy's RE told her to use donor eggs to get pregnant. Instead, she worked on recovery for three months and commenced cycling; she got pregnant on her seventh natural cycle. Her third and fourth children were conceived naturally as well.)*
>
> *Ami*: I wasted soooo many months thinking I was doing enough to recover and when I failed to ovulate on Femara twice, I was like, "That's it, I will gain 300 pounds before I go through life without a baby!" My advice for ladies reading this is to DO IT NOW! Don't wait. I thought I might be the exception—that I wouldn't have to give up all my behaviors and would still get pregnant. WRONG! The faster you make the changes, the easier this process is. *(Ami gained some more and stopped all exercise except walking. She got pregnant on her next Femara cycle!)*

If you don't resume natural cycles before getting pregnant, chances are *excellent* that you will get them back postpartum, assuming you don't go crazy with weight loss and exercise after you have your baby. Overall, 83% of our survey respondents resumed cycles in between pregnancies, and 98% after their final pregnancy. The possibility of regaining cycles is a great carrot… or cupcake! (See chapter 27 for more info on the postpartum period.)

Coping With the Changes

Changing your thoughts and feelings about food can take time and a lot of mental energy. It helps to continually remind yourself of why you are doing this. In fact, why don't you quickly jot down five reasons why you need/want to recover from HA. Is it for physical heath? The opportunity to have a baby? Tired of being a lackey to yourself? Bone health? Why?

This is hard. But so are many other things that you have striven for and achieved. Look at this as another project you have chosen to tackle. Actually, it's probably the most important project you will ever take on for yourself and your future family. Many of us with HA are driven, perfectionist overachievers. Take that energy and use it toward building a new, healthier body for the rest of your life—a five-star baby hotel instead of a run-down, tired, overused side-of-the-road motel.

> *Ami*: I've said this before but the *biggest* part of this is letting go of the thoughts, restrictive behavior, exercise, and negative body image. The

> weight gain is secondary because if your mind isn't right, you will either spiral back after you have a baby or you won't ever get to the point where your body trusts you enough to allow you to get pregnant. You CAN do this!

How do you get from where you are to what we're suggesting? It's different for every person. Each journey is unique. Some can jump in feet first and never look back, while others dip in a toe and take it out, and have to make a few attempts before they can wade in. Then there are lots of people who fall somewhere in between.

Are you ready to begin?

Summary

The first component of the plan to recover from HA is to fuel your body by eating more. Not just a little bit more, most likely a lot more; a minimum of ~2500 calories each and every day. And if you feel hungry, don't let that number limit you—give your body the energy it is crying out for. That energy goes to fix everything that has been neglected or shut down while you've been underfueling and then keeps all your systems in optimal working condition! You've read about the freedom that many have experienced after they've followed our path; now it's your turn.

Recommendations:

- Eat a minimum of 2450 calories a day (*and then stop counting!*)
    - Subtract 100 if you're less than 5'4", add 100 if you're taller than 5'8".
    - Subtract 250 if you're totally inactive; add more if you are continuing to exercise.
- Aim for our "fertile zone"—a BMI of 22 or more.
- Remember that you can have HA no matter your current body size, especially if you are underfueling your body as we have described. Following our suggested caloric targets and gaining some weight can potentially help. See more on this topic in chapter 10.
- Some of our survey respondents (13%) find that their fertile weight is higher than a BMI of 23.
- See chapter 9 for more discussion on what to eat and how to add all these extra calories.

Lisa: So, not to beat a dead horse over the "six-month challenge," but I would like to reiterate that although half a year seems like a long time, in actuality it's a small investment that will pay dividends for the rest of your life. Setting small short-term goals may help if this is the path you choose. Initially, I went in with the thought process of applying these changes for two months. I remember telling myself that as miserable as I might be, two months was doable. Heck, I could stand on my head for two months if I had to. Then when the two-month mark hit, although I was still uncomfortable at times, I was getting used to my new normal and chose to continue for another month. After four months had passed I was becoming concerned, wondering if getting my period back would even happen for me. I thought, "Now I have a darn muffin top, hail damage on my butt, and feel very deconditioned." Comments from neighbors wondering what was wrong with me because they didn't see me running added insult to injury. I was ready to throw in the towel and return to my comfort zone. My husband recognized this and asked, "What do you have to lose giving it a few more months? Besides, you are much more fun now, look healthier, and are not so rigid about EVERYTHING." This was true. Ha! So I gave it another month, but was still not confident about getting my period back (because I was "different" from others with HA ... sound familiar?). At the end of that fifth month (the following description is not for the squeamish) I was in the bathroom doing my thing and noticed blood in the toilet. I immediately panicked, "What now??? I have a hemorrhoid!?" I frantically grabbed a mirror to figure out if I was going to have to go to the emergency room from bleeding so much. And it was in that incredible moment I discovered ... I HAD MY PERIOD!!! Can you say, OVERJOYED?!?! You too will experience this indescribable feeling (I am certain). In hindsight, I realized that two weeks prior I was having tons of EWCM (egg white cervical mucus; chapter 17), was bloated like a tick, and my breasts even hurt. But I was still totally clueless and caught off guard with my period of the century!

OK ... all this is to further encourage you that six months is a small investment that will impact your physical and mental health for the rest of your life in a positive way.

9
Putting Recovery Into Practice

IF YOU'RE STILL THINKING, "This is nuts, there is no way I can do this," remember that where there is a will, there is a way. The key is increasing your total intake and eating from all food groups (except for those limited by legitimate allergies or morals—and no, you cannot be morally opposed to carbs or fats!).

Many of you have become comfortable with eating healthy, eating whole foods, and eating "clean." The problem with this type of eating is that it tends to fill you up without providing many calories and is another way to restrict and control your intake. Now you need calories along with a balance between healthy, nutritious foods and what you might currently see as "unhealthy" or "junk" foods. Rather than make a black and white distinction between "good" foods and "bad," recognize that *all foods provide nutrients and energy your body needs*. There is no such thing as a bad food; right now, it's ALL recovery/fertility food. If you've been restricting your overall calories, let go and eat more. If you haven't been allowing yourself any fat, add some. Lots. If you're following a Zone, Keto, or Paleo type diet, add in some of the forbidden carbohydrates (carbs). If you're only eating carbs, include more proteins and fats.

> *Steph*: I was not in any way happy when my doctor told me to eat more. I was scared. Scared of gaining weight, scared of being judged, scared of losing control. I cried. I was angry. You name it, I felt it. It was not easy, and it did not feel comfortable, but I began the process of re-examining my eating plan. Nancy (the registered dietitian mentioned in chapter 1)

> and I looked more closely and added more to my diet in both variety and quantity. My morning granola bar became two or three tablespoons of peanut butter on graham crackers. My mid-morning granola bar became a hefty serving of almonds and cashews. I really listened to my body. If I was a tad bit hungry, I ate. If I was not hungry, I still ate: yogurt, peanut butter, avocado, eggs, ice cream, French fries, potato chips, hamburgers, and so on.
>
> *Alaina*: I encourage you to think of fats as healthy for people like us (HAers) since that is what we need in order to get our periods back. Obviously, our bodies are not in good health since they are struggling to provide energy and hormones to allow us to cycle, and thus won't support a pregnancy. With all that said, enjoy this time of indulgence and realize that we will begin to get used to our changing, more womanly bodies. When I feel my flabby belly now, I think 'this belly is getting ready to have a baby'—it helps.

To get the energy you need, aim for less filling, calorie-dense options: handfuls of nuts or seeds; avocados; full fat dairy (like ice cream); olive, coconut, or canola oil when you cook; spoonfuls of nut butters; fatty fish like salmon; full fat salad dressing; and smoothies with added protein. Toss the low-fat and nonfat out of your fridge and out of your life. Seriously. The full-fat versions are soooo much tastier, and much better for your body[1]. Cut out the "diet" foods and drinks altogether. No more "sugar-free" sodas; enjoy caloric beverages instead, like orange juice, lemonade, and milkshakes (YUM!). No more chewing low-calorie gum to help curb your hunger. When you're hungry, eat. If you're eating huge salads or similar low-calorie yet bulky foods to fill yourself up without getting many calories, you may need to shrink those portion sizes in order to make room for what you're trying to add. Let other selections make their way into your daily fare too. Foods like pizza, burgers, chocolate, donuts, and chips can all have a place in your diet—especially when working toward restoring your endocrine system.

Each HAer (among those with restrictive eating habits) limits her eating in different ways. However, it is important to understand that each of the food groups we mentioned above provides an additional signal to your hypothalamus. Ingesting a larger variety of foods will activate many different pathways to restart your hypothalamus. For example, in 2010's it is common to follow a diet in which simple carbs are reduced or eliminated. But researchers have found that high concentrations of glucose in the body (which occur after you consume simple carbs like bread, pasta, or sugary treats) cause your GnRH nerve cells to fire at a faster rate, which, as we discussed in chapter 5, leads to an increased production of FSH and LH *and more growing eggs*[2]. Insulin plays a part as well, and more glucose equals more insulin, which also leads to cycle resumption[3].

If you've forgotten what all these hormones do, no matter—the point is that for now, healthy is added calories and variety. Listen to your cravings. Even so-called "bad" or "unhealthy" foods can help get your system going again; think of them as recovery or fertility foods instead of feeling guilty for indulging. Also, recognize that we are not suggesting you eat like this forever. Right now the goal is to do whatever it takes to refuel, rest, and replenish your body until it has recovered; then over time you can tweak what you're eating to include more wholesome choices (without reducing calories by much), while still enjoying your fair share of indulgent "fertility foods."

> *Lisa*: While the majority from the Board embrace the idea that adding "forbidden" sugars and processed foods would be beneficial during HA recovery, both mentally and physically, there have been a few naysayers along the way (understandably so since sugar has been vilified in our society). Because of the skepticism, I decided to take a community poll. My hope is that the results inspire you to be more confident in making necessary changes.
>
> The following question was asked in a private Facebook group among those who had recovered from HA:
>
> "Hi friends, please comment on this post to let me know if during HA recovery you went "all in," eating whatever you wanted, i.e., simple carbs like cake, cookies, ice cream) to help weight gain, and to get cycles back and/or get pregnant—or did you continue to avoid certain food groups?"
>
> The results? A whopping 96% (64/67) ate some "bad/forbidden" foods in order to recover from HA. These folks also increased proteins and healthy fats. The remaining 4% increased their complex carb load along with proteins and fats, but did not add simple carbs.
>
> Adding different foods and decreasing food type restriction and control is an integral part of recovery, both mentally and physically. You too will experience a true sense of liberation when you let go and realize that you don't suddenly increase your morbidity rate or never stop eating. Instead, you will gain freedom, flexibility, and a lot more joy.
>
> One of the reasons I felt this was important to share is that *many of us waste time trying everything but the simple stuff.* We overlook the obvious—that our bodies need more calories *of all types,* now.

> Here are a few responses from those who took part in the poll (with key points italicized):
>
> **Kaysie**: My goal was to get to a fertile BMI as quickly as possible, so my diet was generally healthy, just more of it. AND the fun part: a daily pint of Ben and Jerry's ice cream—full-fat and full of simple sugars! I also ate more liberally at restaurants. *I looked for what I actually wanted to eat instead of the healthiest thing on the menu.* I think if you only eat clean you're going to miss out on not only the speed of the weight gain but also the fun of it!
>
> **Candace**: I tried the "clean eating" approach to gaining weight, but could not eat the volume of food I needed to take in the calories my body required. Eating "unhealthy" fats was the healthiest thing I did for myself because that led to weight gain and a functioning reproductive system! *Same thing with simple carbs... less filling and more easily digested so I could eat more.*
>
> **Vicky**: I did attempt only increasing healthy fats but didn't see much movement on the scales. It was when I increased portion sizes, added healthy fats, AND consumed lots of cakes, biscuits, and chocolate that I really saw a difference. The other thing I would suggest is throwing all calorie counting and attempts to follow a "diet" out the window, *because all the time you do this you are still practicing restriction of some sort.* I'm sure there are many different approaches we have all taken that work; this was mine. But I do believe for everybody, letting go of any type of restriction is key.
>
> **Nadia**: Initially I ate a very specific way—I was still counting calories and managing my macros (protein, fat, carbs). *I realized that I was still hanging on to disordered eating by doing that,* so I stopped and just ate whatever whenever.
>
> **Meg**: I mostly avoid refined grains, but I do think that allowing a little sugar and white bread was absolutely critical in getting my cycles back. Refined grains were the last things that I added before my body started waking up. *I really wanted a high-calorie clean diet to work, but it just didn't for me.*

Now that we have shared the importance of adding simple carbs to your diet, let's talk about other ways to consume more fuel. Full-fat dairy is a great way to get additional calories and fat. In fact, recent studies have suggested that folks who eat at least one serving of full-fat dairy a day (ice cream, yogurt, or a glass of whole milk, for example), while keeping caloric intake constant, are less likely to have ovulatory disorders (i.e., no ovulation and/or no period) than those who consume low- or nonfat dairy products[4]. Estrogen dissolves in fat and therefore is present in full-fat dairy. Androgens (the "male" hormones like testosterone) dissolve in water; so when you remove the fat to get low-fat or skim milk, you're taking out the estrogen but leaving the androgens, which can throw your system out of balance[5]. These androgens have been demonstrated to negatively impact ovulation and fertility and cause an increase in acne[6]. You might find it hard to make an immediate switch from skim to whole milk; the latter can seem too creamy when you're not used to it. Instead, if you're used to nonfat you could start by transitioning to low fat, then move to full fat in a few days or weeks. Or (*and*) you could start a nightly tradition of a bowl of ice cream with a friend or partner... and don't make it a paltry half-scoop "no thank you" helping of ice cream. Go for at least one full serving—the more the better!

> **Steph**: There is an unspoken rule between Nico and me that came about while we were writing this book. Since we are lucky enough to live only 15 minutes away from each other, we get together every so often to work. And that means it's ice cream night. Not just any run of the mill ice cream, but delicious, homemade, full-fat ice cream from a local ice cream stand. Whoever is traveling picks up a "large" (the equivalent of more than a pint) of a wide variety of flavors ranging from Milky Way to apple pie to peppermint stick to coffee Oreo. And, of course, we add sprinkles. The ice cream is all gone by the time we're done!

Aside from adding new foods into your daily fare, you can increase the amounts you're eating. Add some extra snacks through the day. Make larger portions or eat a few more bites before deciding you're done with your meal. Instead of only eating half when you go to a restaurant, eat three quarters or, heaven forbid, the entire meal! If you can't stand the full or over-full feeling you get from larger portions, eat more frequently throughout the day. Make a pact with yourself to never (except while sleeping) go more than two hours without eating something. These are all strategies that have worked for people as they try to reach the 2500 daily calorie range.

This includes eating fairly soon after you get up in the morning - no more waking up, going out for a run/walk, getting ready for work, heading in, and then eating a few hours later. An analysis was performed in 25 high level athletes in Sweden[7], all of whom were eating the same amount (~3500 calories a day), and doing the same amount of exercise (~1000 cal). Ten women continued to have regular ovulatory menstrual cycles, another 15 had no period. The researchers found the difference between the two groups was those without a period were in an energy deficit for approximately four hours longer per day. So loss or recovery of your period is not just about how much you eat, but also how that food is spread through the day (http://noperiod.info/energy-balance).

Another common restrictive habit is to eat less throughout the day if we know we're going out for a meal; or if we "overeat" one day, to eat less the following. This is counterproductive. Even just a short span of restriction can negatively affect your hormones. In an experiment in which energy intake was restricted for only five days, there were significant changes in hormones like LH, insulin, glucose, and cortisol[8]. Each day is a new day. How much you eat doesn't depend on how much you had yesterday or how much you're going to have tomorrow. Or even what you're going to have later in the day. For now, you need to keep eating to keep your hormone levels heading toward their optimal levels, and do it like it's your job. Think of the days when you're eating at a restaurant as estrogen building days. Eat just as you have been during the day, and then enjoy your meal at the restaurant. No reducing or restricting the next day; just keep on going.

> *Nico*: When I was trying to dig my way out from HA, my ob-gyn suggested that I see a nutritionist. Initially I balked; my eating was just fine, thank you very much. I am very independent, and very good at whatever I put my mind to, so I thought I could deal with it myself. But I realized in short order I didn't really know how much I should be eating, or how to get there.
>
> Off to the nutritionist I went. She told me I should be getting around 2100 to 2200 calories, which I now know was a severe underestimate based on how much I was exercising. I probably needed even more than the 2500 calories we are recommending to you. The 2100 to 2200 recommendation likely still had me at a deficit of 500 to 600 calories a day, which may not seem like much, but certainly is enough to delay recovery, and it did—I didn't cycle again until I went on vacation and cut my exercise completely. At the same time, she did have some excellent tips on how to accomplish increasing my intake. First of all, switching the milk I drank from skim to 2%. Knowing what I know now, I'd have switched to whole instead, although that would have been H-A-R-D! Why had I not thought of that myself? Then she suggested handfuls of nuts or trail mix as snacks, and cooking with OIL; even adding it to pasta sauces and soups to increase fat. Gasp. I had gotten so used to trying to get everything as low fat as possible that was practically anathema to me. But I knew she was right. (In fact, when he was alive, my dad and I used to have arguments all the time on this; he would argue that olive oil was good for you, and I would say, "Yeah, but it's still *fat*." Guess he had the last laugh on that one.) She also suggested whole wheat toast with peanut butter for

> breakfast instead of a granola bar; more fiber, protein, fat, and calories, all of which I needed.
>
> I walked away from the appointment with lots of great ideas and good intentions. But when it came down to it, I had to fight hard against my ingrained tendencies and thoughts. Over time, I went from carefully measuring each almond snack and making sure I stuck to my 2100 to 2200 calories a day to just grabbing a big old handful and enjoying them. I started enjoying the creamier taste of milk, drinking two big full glasses a day. I *did* use oil while cooking. I stopped counting calories altogether and just *ate*. And it all led me to exactly where I wanted to go.

If you need to slowly work up to our recommended caloric intake, that's fine. It can be challenging to break out of your thought patterns around food and eating, but you can do it. How about if you take a baby step *today*? Baby steps can get you to the same place in the end. Eat one thing today that makes you feel uncomfortable. You'll notice later that you are doing all right. Maybe even feeling pretty good. Have an extra snack even if you don't feel hungry (and especially if you do!). Buy something at the grocery store that you would "never" buy—a bag of nuts, or a candy bar—and then eat it. If there's a candy jar at work or someone brings in donuts, don't just walk by; stop and have a bite or two, or heck, the whole thing. It's a start. If your friends invite you to coffee or dinner, say yes and don't check the menu beforehand. Go and eat or drink what you want without worrying about how many calories it contains. Choose what actually sounds good to you instead of looking for the menu items that have the low-calorie symbol next to them. If you make your lunch, make it a little bigger. If you're buying, don't split the meal in half as usual, eat the whole thing. Or get some French fries.

> **Laura:** I joined the Board with a BMI on the low side of "normal". When I read that I needed to gain up to a BMI of 22 to 23, I said, "No way, not me... I don't need to do that, I'm just fine and healthy." Honestly, it scared the pants off me. But once I got more involved, I realized that people who seriously gained the weight did in fact get pregnant or get their period back. From there, I gave up my crazy running schedule, ate LOTS more (especially fat), and started gaining. It really helped me to make gaining goals for myself... I would first say that I needed to gain to a BMI of 20. Once I reached this goal, I would make another for 21... and so on. This really helped me take it one step at a time (baby steps!), as I found myself getting too scared to even think about getting to a BMI of 22 to 23 all at once. Anyway, I am now free of my obsession with exercise

> and fear of fats, and... I'm loving life (and my pregnancy). (*Laura gained weight over the course of nine months. She started fertility treatments after three months, getting pregnant on her third cycle.*)
>
> **Samantha**: So I took a test this morning and it was... Positive!! I can't even believe I just typed that and I'm starting to cry *again* as I write because there's no way I'd be here right now if it weren't for the Board and all of you. I can't even begin to express my gratitude. Here's one more success story, one more person who has given up herself completely to the Recovery Plan and had it work. For anyone who is hesitant about going all in or wants to try and do it gradually, if you're trying to get pregnant, it will happen MUCH quicker if you dive right in, no regrets, no holding back. Quit the gym and eat with a vengeance. Pack away the skinny jeans and buy a lot of yoga pants. Ditch the scale if needed; don't let the weight gain and what you see in the mirror stop you. There's an end game, an ultimate goal, and after that positive test, you won't care how much weight you've gained or how many sizes you've gone up. It just doesn't matter anymore. I gained 25 lb and went from a size Small/4 to a size Large/10-12 in two months. I don't think I've ever had so much jiggle on my body, but I don't care, and you won't either, I PROMISE. I am 100% convinced it was all due to this Board, there's no way I could have done it without this support group. (*Samantha got her first period 11 weeks after going all in, then conceived on her next ovulation.*)

Coping With Eating More

You might find yourself struggling with feeling full. Or over-full. We mentioned that one of the goals of our Recovery Plan is getting to a point where you stop eating when you're full. For the time being, though, you cannot trust those signals. Part of the recovery process involves eating even though your stomach is telling you it's had enough. Your body has been trained to expect small portions so when you go beyond that, even though it's what your body needs, your stomach isn't on the same page yet, which might result in feeling uncomfortable. This will improve with time. If you're having trouble with eating larger portions you can try eating small, frequent meals throughout the day. Breakfast, second breakfast, snack, lunch, second lunch, snack, dinner, maybe even second dinner! Don't worry about eating late at night; in a way that helps because your body can use those calories for repair without having to provide energy for moving around as well. Eating frequently like this may seem like you never stop eating, but keep in mind that this is temporary; your body will adapt. Also, remind yourself you are providing the fuel that your body needs to be fertile!

Some of these "sensations" may also be psychological. Allowing yourself more food may be uncomfortable mentally, leading to the manifestation of physical symptoms, or the belief that they are there even when they are not. While you are working on dealing with the initial discomfort of recovery, keep your mantras and distraction skills close as explained in chapter 11.

At some point you may question if you are eating too much or possibly bingeing. This is a common and natural feeling! For example, you decide to have some chips or cookies or whatever you are allowing yourself, and all of a sudden you've eaten the whole container or more. You might feel ill or may even feel a need or want to throw up. Stop. Take a deep breath. Realize that this is a normal response to finally allowing yourself to have the calories (and treats!) your body desperately wants. As you continue with your recovery, you will feel less and less of a need to eat the entire package. Call on your support team—your partner, a friend, your therapist—to help you get through these feelings. Find an online support group, or start a blog, and write them out instead of acting on them. Check out chapter 11 for more tips on distracting and forgiving yourself. Afterward, keep going just like you have been. Do not be angry with yourself; accept that your body needed that food, and keep providing it with more. Restricting is no longer an option!

> *Kelli*: So, the bingeing. Is it really bingeing? You need to ask yourself this and be honest. Years ago, I was anorexic. I was only bones and some muscle. I remember the day the bingeing started. I was at the supermarket food shopping, which was so hard to do but very pleasurable in a twisted way. I don't know what happened, but the next thing I know, I am behind the deli counter which was closed at the time, eating frosted cupcakes that came in a six pack container... I didn't know what I was doing. I felt out of control and I just remember feeling like I was out of my body watching myself do this. That was the first time... the behavior continued and got worse—more food, more frequent, and always like I was in a trance and out of touch. I think my unconscious mind saved me from dying by making me do this. I continued to work out (even more) to compensate. This went on for years. Restricting as much as possible, working out as much as possible, then bingeing on obscene amounts of food. A few times I even fell asleep chewing the pile of food in front of me. That is

> bingeing. I think what you are doing IS recovering. You lifted the brakes on restricting food, you are allowing yourself to eat food, and your body and your unconscious mind are taking what they can before you freak out and stop yourself. I get that it is scary. When recovering this time around, I went through this phase too. I was worried I would start bingeing like before. What I realized is that I am not bingeing. I am just recovering and I am hungry. As I worked out less and gained some pounds, I wanted less junk, and found myself more full after meals. It will get better, and it will pass. If eating healthier will make you more comfortable, then do that, but also allow yourself some other stuff. If you keep certain foods taboo, you will keep wanting to eat tons of it when you are around it. It happened to me many, many, many times before I got to the point where I could take a handful of chips and be content rather than finishing the whole bag. It takes time! I've been at this for six months and every day I learn something new.

Summary

Strategies for eating more:

- Add nutrient rich calories and snacks: avocados, nuts/nut butters, fatty fish such as salmon, sweet potatoes, full-fat dairy; add oil or butter when you cook; add coconut oil and protein to smoothies.
- Add fat to your diet; aim for at least 30% of your calories to come from it!
- Full-fat dairy may have additional properties that help restore cycles (hello, estrogen), beyond just the added fat and calories.
- Simple carbohydrates are more easily broken down to glucose and can aid in recovery by increasing signaling in your brain.
- Eat what you crave, even if it isn't "healthy." Your body knows better than your brain what it needs in terms of types of food. It needs the fat, sugar, and quick energy that you get from recovery/fertility foods.

> *Lisa:* When I started my climb out of HA, I remember feeling awful due to the addition of all those extra calories; the *full feeling* was totally pushing me over the edge in the discomfort department. Although I wanted and needed this extra fuel, I did not want to feel like I had just swallowed an extra-large pizza and tub of ice cream when I had only consumed an average-sized meal. Do I need to mention the accompanying obsessive thoughts until the stuffed feeling subsided? At that point, I made a decision to temporarily cut out most of my fruits and vegetables in exchange

for calorically dense foods. It seemed so upside-down and counterintuitive, but in reality, I wasn't healthy in spite of my super strict diet and needed calories to regain my health no matter the form. With these changes decreasing the fullness, I was able to consume more protein, sweet potatoes, olive oil, avocados, nut butters, pizza, ice cream—really calorically dense foods—without feeling uncomfortably full. It was as if I was *sneaking* in the calories. An additional benefit to this strategy was that I immediately noticed a decrease in bloating and constipation. How crazy is that—less fiber resulting in less constipation? This idea of temporarily decreasing fruits and vegetables has been shared with a number of people who have also found this dietary change useful during the transition to increasing food variety and calories while crushing HA.

Fuel that hypothalamus and you will reap the rewards in many ways. Health, performance, and if you so choose, babies.

10
What to Expect...

> EVA: I AM NOT trying to conceive, but I am engaged and want to have a baby right after we get married in April 2014. I resisted and resisted and fought myself on weight gain the past eight months. I was convinced my lack of a period could *not* be a weight issue. Well, finally I really started eating, as in gaining weight relatively quickly (like six pounds in a week) and BAM, this morning, my period arrived! I was shocked, but now it makes sense. I've always been that "healthy" eater but lately, all I've wanted is junk—ice cream and cupcakes. I never have a sweet tooth but I couldn't get enough of *real* ice cream and sugary frosting. Gaining some weight, eating more treats, and cutting down cardio *will work*. I didn't believe it would but *here I am*!! Truly nothing feels as good as being fertile feels. Honestly.

There are dozens of reasons to go ahead and put the Recovery Plan into practice, but we're not going to lie; it's not all going to be sunshine, rainbows, and butterflies. However—and we really cannot stress this enough—the end result of a healthy, functioning, feminine (pregnant!) body is so worth any temporary not so wonderful bumps along the road. What are the bumps? Well, you might feel some physical discomfort as you start eating more, and you will almost certainly have to deal with mental discomfort as you rewire your brain from your old destructive thought patterns to new healthier ones. You are probably going to gain some weight, and that will most likely cause you even more distress, given our societal obsession with being as small as we possibly can. But the weight gain will not be unlimited, and the physical discomforts you may initially feel will subside over time. The mental distress will also diminish, especially with each of the positive changes and signs that you notice. When you get your period, or see the longed-for positive pregnancy test, that is just the icing on the cake (which you are now allowed—no, required—to eat!).

Before we discuss some of the discomforts you might experience, we do want to reinforce the positive reasons to go "all in" and eat like your life depends on it—which, in many ways, it does. The extra calories you consume will allow your body to restart and stimulate the systems that have been slowed or shut down. This means that over the next few weeks, yes, you will be eating more, but your body will make good use of that extra energy. After just a few days to weeks, you'll notice the effects of your metabolism revving up—you will most likely feel warmer, be less constipated, and sleep better at night. Down the road you'll notice healthier nail and hair growth, better vaginal lubrication, and increased libido. You might notice some low abdominal cramping and/or sore, fuller breasts. And then, hopefully, you'll get your period. Finally, your weight gain and restored menstrual cycle will lead to improved bone density over the long term[1].

To put some numbers and hard data around this, two women were studied intensively as they went through the process of recovering from HA[2]. Their resting metabolism was measured when they had HA, and again after recovery. The difference was *300 calories a day*! That means their bodies were able, with the added food intake, to expend 300 more calories each and every day toward their basic needs, *including reproductive cycles*. This doesn't mean, however, that you just need 300 extra calories—you need to fully fuel *all* your body's activities and allow for repairs to the systems that have been neglected, and then the extra energy can go toward the processes that need more fuel.

> **Kelli**: My boobs are fuller, my temps don't dip below 97 (I was getting 95's), my husband thinks I'm sexy, and people are more attracted to me these days and they can't figure out why. I think it's because when we are healthier we give off more positive vibes and look more attractive. I smile more, I sleep better, I don't wake up in the middle of the night doing a beeline for the fridge. I don't think about food 24/7, I have more time with my husband, and I see friends I haven't seen in years because I was too afraid food would be a problem or that I would miss the gym. I am more myself in that I make jokes and laugh... just more social. I had a great personality once; people just loved to be in my presence, and I see that person in me coming back out. My hair doesn't fall out and it is

growing. My nails are growing too, and they don't break easily anymore. What else? Oh—I used to be in so much pain going up the stairs at work (used to work out every day); my legs were always sore, my feet were always puffy, and I had a mean case of plantar fasciitis ... no more. What a relief. SEX!!! Much better LOL. Pizza! Pizza, pizza, pizza, pizza, like every day. You know how Scarlett said, "I will never go hungry again"? I will never be without pizza again ever. Never. My God, so many things have changed for the better.

Rainbows and Butterflies

With an increased metabolism you get a slew of positive effects. Some changes you will notice immediately, while others may take a bit longer. In chapter 1, we listed common symptoms that people feel in concert with a missing period. Now we show how much those symptoms improved with added calories and increased metabolism. Notice that the level of discomfort after recovery (represented by the dark gray lines) is reduced significantly.

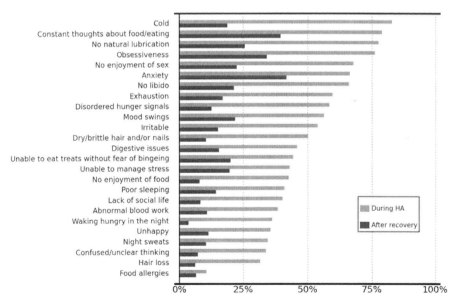

Physical symptoms during HA and after recovery. The percentage of survey respondents (276 participants) who "always" or "often" experienced each listed symptom while having HA (light gray), and after working toward recovery (dark gray). The differences between rankings during and after HA are highly significant in all cases ($p < 1 \times 10^{-4}$) because the changes for every person occurred in the same direction, indicating improvements in overall health and quality of life after recovery.

> *Chassta*: Still no period, but I am creeping toward the "fertile" zone, with LOTS of rest (hardly any workouts) and TONS of food! Loving it! I definitely am in awe of my body right now. Sure, there are jiggly bits here and there that are not so comfortable, but who cares? I have BOOBS (still A, but bigger than a training bra—LOL!), and baby got her "back" back! I know that I have gained a belly in the process, but I am happier that I have gained joy, freedom, and peace! I went to my chiropractor (whom I have known for many years) and he said he barely recognized me. We talked about the HA Recovery Plan and he told me that I was glowing and looked beautiful. I laughed and I felt like I could kiss him.
>
> I am the "heaviest" I have been since 2009, but the "lightest" I have been in my whole life. That burden was WAY heavier than ANY amount of "fertility butt" and "baby house" that I will acquire. And just to make it known to myself and others, even if the healing doesn't come for my womb (still believing, though!), it has been and will be worth EVERY moment of this journey toward complete surrender! (*Chassta did in fact get pregnant on a natural cycle. That pregnancy unfortunately resulted in a miscarriage, but five cycles later she conceived again; her daughter was born December 2015.*)

A Bit of Discomfort

Now that we've talked about the upside of extra calories, we will tell you about the not-so-fun physical feelings that some encounter. Each person experiences a different range of these symptoms, from none to quite a few. Hopefully you will fall in the former category, but if you don't, keep in mind that these symptoms improve with time.

In the first few days of your new eating plan, you might find that you feel overwhelming hunger, despite eating more. Because you are finally following your body's signals asking for food, the hunger hormones increase further and make you feel hungrier in an attempt to get more of calories needed for repairs while the going is good. Another common concern is feeling bloated and gaining more weight than is possible for the number of calories eaten. This is almost certainly water weight. What happens is that the body will initially hold on to water to help with the cellular repairs it is now able to undertake[3]. *This is normal*, and is the start to recovery! Eating a lower sodium diet may help to some degree, but if not, the water retention will decrease over the first weeks to month. The bloating is probably not obvious to anyone but you, but if you feel like it is, simple flowing tops, stretchy pants, and skirts can do wonders in both covering the bloat and making you feel more comfortable. It seems completely counterintuitive, but many find these symptoms improve if they reduce the amount of vegetables they eat for the time being. It's worth a try…

You might also experience some other digestive discomfort such as gas or indigestion. Or, if you've been diagnosed with irritable bowel syndrome (IBS), you might feel like you're getting a flare-up. Gastro complaints are not uncommon and usually go away in a few days to weeks as your body gets used to actually having energy to support its daily functions. On the other hand, you might find that IBS-like symptoms you used to experience diminish as you eat more.

> *Melli*: I tend to be a volume eater when I'm in my "healthy" phases, which means stuffing myself with veggies galore. Whenever people say you can't possibly overdo it on fresh produce, I guffaw. I can—and do—habitually. I've had many a salad binge that ended in extreme discomfort, and contributed to the lovely IBS-type symptoms we've all commiserated over. Well, lately, I'm piling lots of heavy things on top of my usual farmer's market buffet, and I've had a few episodes of awful indigestion actually waking me up. Last night was the worst—I actually ended up spending half the night on the bathroom floor, getting sick, and shivering all over. It's funny; my first instinct is always to blame myself, so I laid there thinking about how I should not have had that apple AND cookie after dinner… only secondarily did it occur to me that I might have gotten an actual bug or food poisoning, because I was clearly feverish and out of sorts. Whatever it was, it was gone by morning. But it was a good thing ultimately because I had a lot of time laying on cold tile and feeling miserable to decide that I needed to go "all in" on the food, too—to just start eating like a normal person, and not like a barnyard animal strapped to a feedbag of carrots and hay. And I did!

Sleep might be the only thing you want to do aside from eating since your body wants to use the extra calories you're feeding it for repair. Repairs happen as you sleep, which is why rest—and decreased exercise as we'll discuss in chapter 12—is so important during the recovery phase. You may find that you feel more tired during the day as well. In the evening, when you sleep, you might experience night sweats, while during the day there is the possibility of hot flashes. Low thyroid hormones are often associated with HA; as you start eating more your thyroid can overshoot and become hyperactive, causing these symptoms. They should disappear within one to two weeks. On the other hand, you may find that you are staying up later because you have more energy, that you sleep through the night because you are satiated, and you are less constipated because your body has all of the nutrients it needs to function properly.

As you continue eating more, and gain some more weight, you might notice that the added weight is going mostly to your stomach, your rear end, and thighs. Right now your body is holding onto the extra calories by packing some fat around your abdominal organs to protect them in case you decide to go back to your old restrictive ways. This, too, is normal. And as time passes, with weight restoration maintained, your body fat will redistribute more evenly[4].

> *Phoebe*: Oh my god, those are THINGS?!? Like all the weight going to my stomach and the bloating so I look pregnant and it makes it even more depressing is a THING??? It happens to other people?? It might go away?? Oh, thank GOD! Lol.
>
> *Jodie*: I thought you all would get a kick out of this: I just popped a button on my pants when I went to the restroom! The weight gain sneaks up on you. What places on your body have you gained weight? Mine is my tummy (mid-section), boobs and butt.
>
> *Lisa*: When I was on my weight gain endeavor I TOTALLY gained weight around my midsection... I even saw little ripples of cellulite on my stomach, which freaked me out. But then I would calm myself, recognizing the overwhelmingness of it was temporary. My body did eventually redistribute the body fat just as I was told. I also went from an almost A to a full A, smaller waist, with fat in my butt and thighs. Dang proud of it too! My body is finally perfect again, i.e., *cycling*.

We've described the most commonly reported physical symptoms; you might experience others such as headaches or a racing pulse for example. We encourage you to check in with your doctor for symptoms such as these to confirm there is nothing else going on. You might, on the other hand, be lucky and continue to feel better from the get-go.

Mentally you might struggle with gaining, your identity changing, believing this lifestyle is unhealthy, feeling anxious, and/or out of control. These thoughts are often particularly bad in the first few days. Getting over the mental discomfort is by far the hardest part of this journey, and also the most important. Teaching yourself to appreciate and possibly love your body when it is in a healthy state, able to create new life, will provide you with a sense of peace as far as your appearance is concerned. Being content with your size, whatever it ends up being, will also help you impart your healthier body image and eating habits to your children and others in your life.

> *Katherine*: I thought I'd share a good body image day since I am often looking for support on the crisis days. My weight gain has led to much nicer curves. I think my body's "happy weight" actually looks like Scarlett Johansson's shape, just a bit taller. I had forgotten the hourglass shape I used to have before starving and exercising myself to muscle and bone. It's actually kind of nice.

Dealing With Weight Gain

For most, if not all of us, the idea and reality of gaining weight are big sources of mental discomfort and fear. As discussed, we have been indoctrinated for years to believe being "fat" is unhealthy and everyone should strive to lose weight or stay "thin." Yet here we are, telling you the exact opposite—that you need and probably are going to gain some weight in order to be healthy. The rest of this chapter will address some of the fears that lead to this angst, and hopefully convince you that it is worthwhile to continue pressing on. Trust that you can and will get through this.

One sticking point with this whole "eat more" plan is that no one can tell you exactly how much weight you will need to gain to regain your health. For some, the weight gain is significant before cycles resume, while for others much less is required. The amount you might gain depends on your body's set point range[5], and where your current size is in relation to that range. There are a number of models that describe this idea of a size or size range that bodies will defend, called the "set point regulation model," "settling point regulation model," "general model of intake regulation," and the "dual intervention point model."[6] There are nuanced differences between the models, but the general idea suggests our bodies have a natural weight range at which they prefer to operate. This range is determined through a combination of genetics (about 65-70%), environmental, psychological, and societal influences. The tools our bodies use to keep us within the desired range include adjusting our metabolism (exactly as has been done to cause HA, shutting down reproductive function in order to conserve energy), adjusting hunger and fullness cues, and adjusting our unconscious activity levels.

This has been shown clearly in experiments involving animals. In a study where mice were under or overfed[7], the underfed mice lost weight, and the overfed mice (given a high-fat diet) gained. No surprise. But once the mice were given a normal diet and allowed to eat as much as desired, the underweight mice returned to about their pre-weight-loss weight, and the overweight mice lost to around their starting weight.

If you have been chronically undereating and/or over-exercising to the point where you have lost your period, you are almost certainly not within your body's set point range, much as you might like your current size. Remember that we have been encouraged by the "diet culture" we live in, to embrace a thin, muscular look as "healthy" by those who will gain financially from us feeling less than perfect, without regard to actual health. With that said, we encourage you to trust that your body knows the right place for you as an individual. It is at those set point ranges (often at the higher end or a little above, http://noperiod.info/activate) where we see bodies thrive, becoming healthier and recreating fertile environments.

> **Sarah B**: I was reflecting on my HA recovery journey and wanted to share all of the reasons I am thankful that I had to go through this process. Thought maybe it could inspire those who are just beginning. I know in the beginning I was mad at myself, scared of gaining weight, scared of giving up the gym and my control over food but it was the best thing that could have happened to me. I learned to slow down and enjoy quiet mornings that don't involve the gym. I learned to enjoy meals with friends and family without fear. I learned to stop criticizing my body because it is truly just a vehicle for my inner being. I learned that my identity is not tied to my weight. I rediscovered who I am as a person without fitness. I honestly am not in a rush to return to fitness and don't think I ever will to the degree that I was before. I know that my life from this point forward will be different and that it is for the best. I wish everyone luck on their journey!!

You probably want to know, "How do I figure out my body's set point range?" As with just about everything else in this process, the answer is "it depends." Before we discuss, however, we want to encourage you to do your best to let go of the need to know, because it is derived from a place of wanting control, and so much of the process of recovery is about letting go of controlling our bodies. When you instead trust that your body knows what it needs and communicates that to you through hunger and fullness cues, you can just eat. Food becomes much less of a focus of your thoughts and energy, giving you time and space for other way more interesting and fulfilling pursuits. Your body is deserving of your trust. When you listen to and honor its cues, it will make sure your nutritional needs are met in the long term (short term you may want a lot of previously forbidden foods; that's normal and okay, it will balance out over time). Another issue to consider as far as having a specific recovery weight target in mind is what if your body needs more than that to get things restarted? If you reach that goal and nothing happens, then what? It is not a time to give up or stop: your ultimate size has to be your body's "decision," not your mind's.

Back to the set point range:

- If there was a time in your adult life when you were eating freely and exercising moderately, and at a stable weight, that is likely to be within your set point range. If you lost weight from there after discovering "clean eating" or starting a new, more intense training regimen, your pre-loss size or a bit more is probably a place where you could expect cycles to return (http://noperiod.info/activate).
- Another possible scenario is you have been restricting your eating and/or using exercise to control your body's size for most or all your adult life, so you never have been in a place where you might discover your set point range. In this case, you could look to close family members to get a rough idea of where your body might prefer to be. Of course, this approach assumes that you have family members who are eating freely and not stuck in the diet/exercise mentality themselves.
- As a very general rule of thumb, natural, fertile set points tend to be at a **minimum** BMI of 22-23. This absolute number depends on a lot of factors such as ethnicity, how much muscle you have, and bone structure—but if you are currently in a body that is smaller than that, it is a reasonable minimum to aim for. This also in no way means that being in a larger body means you do not need to gain. Your set point range is likely higher. Bodies come in all shapes and sizes and they are ALL worthy vehicles for us
- A third possibility is if you were in a much larger body at some time in the past then lost a significant amount of weight and have been maintaining that too-small-for-you size; chances are your set point range is somewhere in between.
- Alternately, if your body size didn't change much when you lost your cycles, removing all food restrictions and rules (which may or may not lead to weight gain), stopping high intensity exercise, and reducing stress may be more important factors for you. Although if you have more muscle now, you may still need to gain weight in order to increase body fat levels. Importantly, if that size is smaller than a BMI

of around 22, pushing to gain weight to aid in recovery and long-term health is only going to be helpful.

As you think about this, it's crucial to keep body composition in mind. If you are more muscular than in the past, your set point range might be higher than before muscle-building, because muscle is more dense than fat. It is likely that our bodies not only have a set point range in terms of overall size, but also in terms of either the amount of fat (which remember is actually a hormone producing organ) or the ratio of fat to "lean mass." Recall that leptin is one molecule that signals the size of our fat stores to our hypothalamus.

We still haven't given you a firm answer, have we? It's because the weight you end up at is really up to your body. You have an idea you're in the right place when you find that you don't have to work to maintain your size. You follow your hunger cues and do the exercises you enjoy without having to be obsessive, without having to work the rest of your life around either the food or the activity. Your metabolism, appetite, and digestion are all functioning well without micromanagement. Coming to terms with this uncertainty about what the number will be, and letting your body determine the weight at which it feels replenished, is part of the mental recovery we are talking about. Trust your body and its ability to perform as intended when nourished and rested.

> *Jade:* I had a comforting thought . . . Usually I hate, and to some degree feel sorry for myself, that I have amenorrhea, and have to be barely training, eating, and gaining weight. But I now see it as more of a blessing . . . as a result of the recovery process I feel I have broken the chains of exercise addiction and can enjoy eating food of all kinds with loved ones without feeling 'bad' . . . if I never lost my period and maintained my previous lifestyle I don't think I'd be enjoying life as much as I am right now. Don't get me wrong, the road is long and I am yet to get my period back-but I can say I am grateful to my body for making me reassess my lifestyle, see a new type of happiness, and sort my priorities.

> *Rebecca*: Hi everyone, dropping in to share some inspiration for those questioning the process. I consider myself recovered. I recently got my 4th all natural recovery period. I just got a full blood test workup done. After 6-7 months of no exercise, eating all the simple carbs, dairy, desserts, following ZERO restrictive food rules, and gaining LOTS of weight, I am literally the healthiest I have ever been. All my reproductive hormones were well within normal range for the luteal phase, which I was in at time

of blood being taken. My T4 was on the high end of normal and my TSH on the low end of normal (this indicates healthier thyroid function if you've been hypothyroid previously) and my T3 was in normal range for the first time EVER. I am still taking thyroid meds, but this is the first time they seem to be working properly. My cholesterol was perfect. Even though I am not happy at all about how I look, and I hate my clothing options, these results reinforce my decision to go all in for my HEALTH. Not babies, but true health. I feel like, for the first time, my body is doing what it's supposed to do.

Clover: What does it mean if you gain weight? I mean, what if you even went over your estimated BMI goal? Does it mean your friends won't like you? (They will like you more—mine love me now that I am not so consumed with myself, my food, and my body.) Will it mean that you are less intelligent? (Gosh, no... you will actually have clarity. I mean, really—I could have been a doctor if I had the brain back then that I do now. OK, exaggerating a bit on that one.) Does it mean your hair will be luxurious? Yup, mine sure is. (Totally kidding... it's a bit old like me, but I do have a hot mess and am getting ready to chop it and then donate it.) Does it mean you will *feel* uncomfortable and out of control with weight gain? Well, initially yes, but like ALL *feelings,* they change. I have seen that switch among HAers and experienced it myself. Stick with the yucko and it goes away. Also, keep in mind that society has totally warped our view of what healthy is. Sorry if I am rambling... just trying to help you wrap your head around gaining weight. Though I totally realize that my purpose is not to convince (which would never work) but to provide truth. The ball is in your court and ultimately you have to decide what your health is worth, *no matter what*. I simply have a hard time sitting back and watching anyone follow in my footsteps (no baby/osteoporosis) without a fight!

As we've said, regardless of your current body size, you should increase your intake to 2500 calories (modified as appropriate, chapter 8, and if you currently are at a very low weight due to an eating disorder, significantly more than that). Over time, as your systems repair, you will learn to follow your hunger cues. This means eating what you want when hungry and stopping when satiated—these cues are the way your body stays in your set point range. Recall that we discussed many of the hormones involved in the process of appetite control in chapter 5—if we leave our conscious thoughts out of it and let our bodies be the guide, they get it right. Following hunger cues also means eating if you find yourself hungry in the middle of the day or wanting a snack late at night—not overriding those signals because of diet culture messaging. You need to recognize that when you feel hungry, your body is telling you it needs energy to do its work, and you should feed it.

It is also essential, if you are recovering from an extremely low weight, that you do not take getting your period back as a sign that you are totally healed. It is possible to get your period while still at a low weight, with your body not fully restored. If you are below our fertile minimum, we encourage continued fueling and weight gain—you probably have not rebuilt your organs or muscles to their optimal sizes, and there are likely other systems that remain underfueled. Recall our discussion in chapter 8 of how the 2500 calorie recommendation was arrived at; the amount needed to provide our bodies the full amount of energy they need. Keep eating at that level for the long term even after getting your period back to allow your body to return to it's natural, optimal size (and health).

> *Marta L.S.*: I would say: forget about the kcal or food that you are eating, or how much your body is changing: just eat, rest and try to chill and embrace your "growing" momentum. Follow what your body is telling you, not your thin/fit self. This is the body of someone that loves herself so much that it's trying to have a healthier body. This is the body of a warrior that has to recover. Some battles are won not by fighting, but by letting yourself go.

Parting Words

We've noticed through our years posting on the Board that there are two versions of recovery: true recovery and pseudo-recovery. True recovery occurs when people gain the weight their body deems appropriate, learn to be content with their new shape and possibly even love it, and eat intuitively enough to avoid a recurrence of HA and associated symptoms. They learn to cope with stressors through means other than exercise and food control. Sure, every now and then thoughts of restriction pop up, but they are passing thoughts and not acted upon. Then there is pseudo-recovery: begrudgingly gaining a few pounds without allowing yourself to get bigger than a size X; making a halfhearted attempt at reducing exercise; then skipping over to fertility treatments to get pregnant (usually injections because the recovery has not been sufficient for the gentler oral medication routes to work). This leads to pregnancy eventually, maybe with adequate weight gain and maybe without… afterward, the pregnancy weight is lost as quickly as possible, and it's right back to square one—a life constrained. We hope that you can feel the joy and acceptance that exude from the words of those who have truly recovered and follow that road. Treat this time of working to conquer HA as a path to a new future, rather than a temporary detour to achieve a baby, only to get right back onto the same treadmill. Do it for yourself, your family, and your friends.

> **Deanna**: I want to tell you all that the BEST thing you can do is just let your body do the thinking for you. To really surrender yourself to the process, let go and dive in feet first is truly the best way to go about healing and overcoming HA.
>
> There is so much more to having hypothalamic amenorrhea than just being thin or having low body fat. There are deep ties to our mind and attitudes as well that affect our recovery simultaneously. Really freeing yourself from the chains and ties of restrictive eating, obsessive exercise, self-loathing, and the stress of it all (whichever category you may fit into, one or all) is the best thing you will ever do for yourself. Whether you want to be a mommy now, years in the future, or never, recovering fully from this is so much more, and gaining your fertility back is only one of the major benefits. You will also gain your life back, and more importantly, discover things about yourself and learn so many lessons that will make you a stronger individual, a stronger mother (should you so choose that path), a stronger wife, and a stronger lover.
>
> Modern medicine has come so incredibly far, so yes, perhaps a small percentage of those who don't want to gain weight and can't get past that hurdle will go on and get pregnant with the help of injections or IVF without making lifestyle changes, but sadly those people will be missing out on the incredible benefits and advantages of really truly recovering. It isn't easy; in fact, it is likely the hardest thing I've ever done, but it is so worth every ounce of pain, every day of struggle, and every tear I've cried.
>
> For the past six months I've been at a BMI over 25, and every day I struggle with my appearance, my ill-fitting clothing, and my extra padding, but every day I am also reminded of my freedom, of the beautiful, fun-loving person I've become, and of the wonderful mother I'll someday be. This journey has taught me patience (oh my, has patience been a virtue forced upon me), kindness, faith in the impossible, and a love for life that cannot be stifled or put out. I know in my soul had I never made these lifestyle changes, had I skipped gaining weight and gone straight to the heavy guns of fertility medicine, and had I remained the hollow

version of myself I once was—my life would not be as remarkable or enjoyable for me nor for those who share it with me. And likely those heavy guns would have failed and cost me large sums of money, time, emotional turmoil, and angst.

If there's one thing I want you all to know, it's that there is more to this process and more to recovery than just getting pregnant. There are so many joys in life that we miss out on and take for granted when we are absorbed in our own weight, size, looks, and fitness. Giving a piece of yourself up for the sake of others (your family, friends, partner, and future children) is something worth taking a risk for. If you can improve the quality of life of those around you, and trust me, people will notice that you are more fun, more carefree, a better lover, and a humbled person, then it is undeniably apparent that you should at least give it a try.

I wouldn't take back one second of this journey, not for anything. Not to be thin again, not to be fit, and not to feel sexy, because the sexiest, most beautiful version of me is who I am today and who I've become with the love and support of all the wonderful women from the Board. I try hard to tell myself I am beautiful (self-love is NOT overrated!). Do I cry about it a lot? Heck yes, but then I move on. It takes a ton of commitment—but is oh, so worth it. *(Seven months after going all in, Deanna used Femara to get pregnant. Her second was naturally conceived while still nursing her six-month-old son full time.)*

11
Expanding... Mentally and Physically

IT IS EASY to fall prey to the idea that being a certain size is all anyone ever needs; that being "thin" equates to acceptance, happiness, health, and success. Society has influenced us to believe anything else is unhealthy, unattractive, slovenly... the list of negatives goes on and on. The best way to be happy, loved, and successful, according to the media, is to be thin and toned. But what if society is wrong?

In chapter 8, we explained that one of the most important parts of beating HA is eating more to fully fuel our systems, which may lead to some weight gain. This idea is simple in theory, but for HAers, it is high on the list of seemingly impossible feats—for some, our worst nightmare. This chapter will offer tips and support to help you battle the negative thoughts that make the journey toward recovery challenging.

We are going to start by sharing some points that will hopefully ease your concerns.

- Gaining weight does not mean you will be unattractive (and honestly, we are so much more than our physical appearance!)
- Gaining weight does not mean you have lost control and let yourself go.
- Gaining weight does not mean you will be unhealthy or a failure.

Rather:

- Gaining weight means you will be more healthy-looking, attractive, and sexy (physically and mentally) than you were before.

- Gaining weight means you are making a choice to improve your health and taking back control.
- Gaining weight means you will be nourishing your body to allow it to menstruate (and have a baby if you so desire).

> *Lisa*: I'd like to take the previous statements a few steps further. As shared, gaining weight doesn't make you ugly, unhealthy, or a failure, but you may believe each and every one at different times. *These are fallacies and feelings, not facts!* With a little effort in avoiding stinkin' thinkin' (this is where "expanding mentally" comes in) the thoughts will pass.
>
> Let me add that gaining weight doesn't mean you're losing control but rather that you have faced reality, made a decision, and are learning how to cope in a new way, actually gaining control. *This decision to gain weight is conscious and purposeful*, not a mindless, out-of-control experience!
>
> Gaining weight does not mean you have let yourself go; rather that you've trusted your body enough to watch it change into the functional system it was intended to be.
>
> Gaining weight does not mean you have lost your discipline. In fact, in my opinion it takes much more self-control to be mindful, eat purposefully, gain weight, rest, and battle negative thoughts than hardcore training and food restriction ever did.

We have provided the solution to recovering your cycles: kick back, eat more, and gain some weight. But if this plan is so simple and easy, why do we have support groups full of people working each day to recover? What makes it so hard to just eat a little extra food each day, take in some more fats or carbs or whatever you have been denying yourself, and gain weight? To an outsider this is all common sense. Steph used to tell people, "I know what I have to do. I just have to get up off the couch, go to the fridge, take out some food, and eat it. But I never can get myself off the couch." Do you feel the same? You know logically what you need to do, but when the time comes to take action, you just, well, can't! The reason for this inability (unwillingness?) to change your habits may be personal to you, but we all struggle with various concerns that make it difficult to get off the couch. We worry, for example, about getting larger, seeing the number on the scale rise, clothes not fitting, and that others might think we've let ourselves go.

There are also deeper inner struggles, sometimes associated with eating disorders that can come into play. For instance, do you use food, exercise, and weight management as a way of coping with difficult emotions and/or stress? We hope to provide tips to help you learn to cope in other ways. However, we do suggest seeking professional help if you find yourself struggling with making changes toward recovery, and the support we offer here or that you find online isn't cutting it. Steph sees her counselor regularly and would be lost without her. Finally, if you need help combating a current eating disorder, we strongly encourage you to speak with a psychologist, psychiatrist, or social worker.

> **Karen**: Last December after another failed IVF cycle I decided to look at my struggle with HA, which I had tried to override with modern medicine again and again. In January and February, I eased up on my food controls, and with equal effort began to look at some of the psychological issues I had with pregnancy and having children. I talked to a counselor about some of my personal and sexual inhibitions. Turns out I had some inner conflicts with the idea of pregnancy, in particular with the idea of having children with my then-husband (whom I still love but he's not meant to be the father of my children). Long story short, I got my period in February 2013 for the first time in 16 years.

> **Maxine**: I tried cognitive behavioral therapy (CBT) last summer and found it really helpful. My husband and I decided to start trying to get pregnant in February/March 2008. Then in February 2009, my brother told us that his girlfriend was pregnant (by accident, no less). In May 2009, my sister told me she was pregnant too, after only three months trying. I'm super close to both of them, so I was feeling quite anxious about how I was going to cope with the unpleasant feelings I knew would arise (e.g., jealousy, feeling left behind). Meanwhile, I'd recently quit exercising and had gained weight, so I was also dealing with identity and body image stuff. I was feeling overwhelmed with emotions and found it so helpful to talk to someone outside the situation—I didn't exactly feel comfortable complaining to my mum or sister about how unfair I thought it all was. It was great to vent without judgment (the Board is great for that too). Anyhow, I saw my therapist seven or eight times between May and August and got my first natural period (after 18 months) in September. So I wonder whether the CBT helped me cope with the stress of my emotions, which in turn certainly didn't hurt the hormone situation.

> **Melli**: I feel like I'm making great strides with my therapist. She's amazing at helping me to re-frame the narrative of my life, which I never realized was so deterministic and fatalistic. I interpret every minor slip as complete failure, and let it catapult me into a downward spiral that I need to repeatedly drag myself out of. In some ways, I had just convinced myself that I would always be vulnerable to this cycle, this (as she put it) "bulimorexic" pattern of restricting and binge/purging. Now I'm starting to see

> my "slips" as "unskilled" moments—just little setbacks in a long, messy, but fertile (no pun intended) process of becoming who I really want and NEED to be. No more letting my "script" and my past failures define and control me. Somehow, just shifting my thinking in that way has been transformative. I can forgive myself for an "unskilled" moment, and get right back on the horse. I've also started to explore why I have this need to be a tiny, little, child-like person (I'm 5'0" and look high school aged, which doesn't help!). Lots of childhood stuff there to unpack, and I'm doing it, slowly and miraculously. And realizing that despite everything—being married, owning a house, and getting tenure in a job I adore—I still haven't acknowledged myself as a woman. So that's what I'm working on. I actually looked down at my little soft belly in yoga the other day, and for the first time ever, thought, "Oh, that's cute." We really do have the power to surprise ourselves, and that's been one of the best revelations so far in this journey

Dialectical/cognitive behavioral therapy teaches us that negative thoughts lead to negative feelings and in turn negative actions. With HA, thoughts like *"the weight gain will never stop," "others will think I've let myself go,"* and *"I feel fat,"* lead to the fear of gaining weight, along with, perhaps, anxiety, depression, or anger. These emotions can quickly cause destructive actions like restrictive eating or hitting the gym. We can counter this cycle by recognizing those negative thoughts, stopping them in their tracks, and turning them into positive thoughts instead.

> **Lisa**: You know what we're talking about here, right? Changing that stinkin' thinkin'! What you believe about yourself, what you say to yourself, and what you think about yourself has such a heavy influence on the choices you make. It's a reaction, if you will. Think about it for a minute. These negative thoughts can be the equivalent of quicksand. If I keep thinking and telling myself that I am *"gaining too much," lazy,* and *average* (gosh, that's sucking the life out of me simply writing that), then I probably won't have much gumption to try, let alone try hard. Instead, I take those negative thoughts captive and recognize how invalid they are. I then reflect on these truths: This *fat* is restoring my health. The *lazy* feeling is acknowledged as rest and allowing my body time to repair. Oh, and the average comment—that was just an example because I am far from *average* and you are too. Each of us is unique in a very special way (wink, wink). Can you feel the wind coming back into your sails?

So how do we transform negative thinking to positive belief? There are a number of strategies to help accomplish this, and different approaches work for each of us. Do not feel discouraged if one does not work; try another, and another!

Tips for Transforming Your Thinking

Positive self-talk. Ever find yourself in front of the mirror (or anywhere for that matter) and you start to criticize your body? We want to stop that right now because it is a method of thinking that will just make this whole process harder. In the moment the criticism strikes, imagine that you're looking at your best friend instead. How would you talk to them? Would you call them ugly or hideous? Would you look at their arms and say, "Wow, those look like sausages," or call their legs "tree trunks"? No. You would find something about them that looks great (because they do), and focus on that! You'd compliment their haircut, smile, jewelry, or outfit. Or even better, compliment something other than physical appearance! Show yourself the same care. When you find yourself worrying about gaining weight and having to eat more, reframe those thoughts. Instead, think about what you do love about your body. If you are not ready for that, try out "faking it until you make it". Pick something, anything, about yourself and give yourself a compliment. "I have beautiful eyes." "I'm a loyal friend/partner." "I'm a great karaoke singer." Even if you can't believe your positive thought right now, as you repeat it over time, you will. Words are powerful.

> *Jaclyn*: Feeling lazy and yucky and uncomfortable in your clothes means you are doing absolutely the right thing. If you feel that way, you are making progress because if you didn't feel uncomfortable and wish for thinner days, then I would think you weren't actually doing the hard work and gaining weight/eating more. I actually had to fake it to myself that I liked my body better and all of that. It does help to fake it, I find, because you train your mind to feel that way somewhat. As soon as those self-defeating thoughts start up, recognize them and switch them to something better, as in, "Doing this is allowing me to have a child. My body is a five-star baby hotel!" I also get feeling full and wanting to skip breakfast, but don't do it. It sets up the cycle! I am actually super full this morning from a big steak dinner followed by my spoon in the peanut butter jar, but I am still going out for my weekly Sunday brunch with my friends. Anyway, whenever you feel crappy, remind yourself that is how you are supposed to feel right now and if you didn't or don't feel that way, you aren't really

> working toward recovery as much as you should be. That's the way I like to look at it anyway.

Affirmations. We really like affirmations—encouraging statements that keep you focused on your goals—as a tool for recovery. Affirmations are pithy, powerful, and positive, bringing you back to the moment to remind you of the truth, especially when you're feeling down. Choosing affirmations that speak to you, spending time making them into attractive collages if you enjoy artsy activities, and decorating your house with them, can be therapeutic. Even if you're not one to typically try crafting, taking the time with crayons, paper, scissors, fabric, or whatever else you come up with can increase your mindfulness and help you to really think about what you're writing down and telling yourself. And there is something to be said for a warm, decorated affirmation instead of a sterile black and white printed quotation. Place your declarations, however they look, everywhere: your closet, pockets, kitchen, bathroom mirror. That way you come across positivity throughout your day, including times that might be challenging— for example, when convincing yourself to eat that extra scoop of ice cream, putting on a pair of jeans that used to be looser, or evaluating yourself in the mirror. Memorize your favorite affirmations and repeat them over and over again.

Here are a few suggestions from those on the Board—spend some time to find more that really speak to *you*. Inspirational blog posts, websites, and books are everywhere.

- My body has been designed perfectly and will recover with fuel and rest.
- I am PHAT—Pretty Hot and Tempting. Or FAT—Fertile and Thankful.
- I am a warrior. I can be a healthy, fertile, emotional warrior!
- Extra curves = estrogen!
- I am more than my appearance.
- Recovery is: Realizing you have a problem and not wanting to live that way anymore; allowing yourself food which is necessary to live and shouldn't be restricted; allowing yourself to relax and get better.
- I am confident in my need to keep eating and resting, even when I feel doubt.
- Food challenges are *non-negotiable* (e.g., you're having butter this week, non-negotiable).

Remember your goal. When the going gets tough, it is easy to lose sight of why you are doing this and yearn to go back to your old ways. It is at this exact moment that you need to remember your ultimate goal. Whether you are doing this for your health, in order to get pregnant, for your future family's health, or a desire to be free from the food/exercise compulsions, your end goal is as worthwhile as they get. What you are doing now will take you there. If you had to choose, would you rather be thin or pregnant? Have a slim-for-you physique with brittle bones, or be healthy with strong bones to carry you in your later years?

> *Jessica W*: Today when I looked in the mirror and realized I wasn't as skinny as I used to be, I just thought, "Yes, I'm totally getting there!" Like I viewed it with a little competitive spirit and felt like I was winning. So if you're a competitor/goal setter too (I'm sure you are, aren't we all?), try that out! Focus on winning the battle!

Reality check. Many of us, HA or not, have negative thoughts about our bodies from time to time. This is where "reality checks" are useful. While you are critiquing every little flaw in your body as you start to recover, others see you as a whole. They see a friend, partner, or sibling who is less consumed with themselves and probably a lot more flexible. They love you for what is inside and they notice how much more vibrant, healthy, present, and full of life you are. Many have said that their partners comment on how much sexier they are as they gain; if only we could have "partner goggles" instead of spending our time picking out flaws! Ask yourself, did you choose your friends and partner based solely on how beautiful they were, how much they weighed, whether they exercised a lot, or because they were clean eaters? Or did you find yourself attracted because of their personality, intelligence, humor, character etc.?

The five minute rant. Sometimes you just need to let all your emotions out. You are going through a tough process, so allow yourself five minutes to go on a rant when necessary. Be mad and upset; say or write the words you are telling yourself; have a pity party about how you are feeling; mourn the loss of what you thought should be—and then be done. Now take another five minutes to restate and reframe your thoughts. Reflect on what you have gained through the process of recovery. Think about the positives: more time for friends and family, new hobbies, less of a focus on yourself and your appearance, etc. You can also go to your affirmations.

> *Chassta*: I had my "five minutes," so to speak, and I am feeling fully recovered from it. Self-pity... one of the worst of all the human emotions. I just had to chalk it up to mourning the death of the person known as skinny Chassta and say hello to the fertile version 2.0. Cue the trumpets! Anyway, I know that the upped food density is helping a lot, and I am on the right path.

Letting go. Battling HA can be stressful. You no longer control or know what is going to happen or when. Even worse is not knowing the numbers that feel so important—how much extra weight is needed and how many months until recovery (or getting pregnant). It can feel pretty agonizing. All you can do is follow the HA Recovery Plan and let your body do the rest. We know it is not the answer you want, but it is the bottom line. To make this process less painful, try some activities like deep breathing exercises, meditation, walking, praying, or yoga. When you feel stressed or unhappy, give relaxation a try, just for a minute or two, and then let that turn into many more minutes (and ultimately peace and acceptance) as you become practiced at letting go. Not only will this help with feeling better in the moment, but training yourself in relaxation can also reduce the cortisol-induced suppression of the hypothalamus.

> *Paraskevi*: We spend our lives trying to make sense, understand, and learn who we are... but there is nothing to hold onto, except the experience of the present moment. We are born with health; our body knows what to do with all the nutrients, just trust the wisdom of nature and life. All this self-destructive crazy thinking is within our grasp to control and shift to something constructive; it has wasted energy that can be fueled into something that makes the world a better place. We need to be a new, better, happier generation of people so our children will reach higher than we did.

Dress for Success

So you are gaining weight. With this often comes the clothing conundrum—all of a sudden, or so it seems, your clothes don't fit. Growing out of your clothes may feel terrifying, but in truth it is a testament to your improving health and commitment to self-care. To make your recovery easier, it helps to get rid of the tops and jeans that don't fit anymore, shedding your unhealthy habits along with your wardrobe. Splurge a bit and purchase new clothing to flatter and even show off your new shape. If this is a difficult step to take, you can begin by thinking of your smaller outfits as "sick clothing," reflecting your inability to have a period at that size.

Replacing these too-small clothes is a step toward total freedom, your period, and your pregnancy (if/when desired). Say goodbye to mornings of trying to squeeze into uncomfortable outfits that then remind you of your larger size for the rest of the day. Donate or recycle the garments—do whatever it takes to get those sick clothes out of your closet, out of your head, and out of your life. If you cannot go that far just yet, box them up and put them away or ask a friend, family member, or partner to hide them.

Now, go shopping! Bring a friend because your judgment meter as to what looks good is probably broken right now. These new clothes need to be comfortable and make you feel attractive. Think elastic, flowy, stretchy—yoga pants or flattering skirts, with room to grow. Then you don't have to deal with a constant reminder of your changing size, or buy clothes again and again. And if you're hoping for a baby, these are perfect first trimester clothes too.

> *Justine*: I had a rude awakening when I put on a pair of pants that I haven't worn in a few months...ummm, yeah, those don't fit. I immediately threw them in the trash can, put on a different pair, and carried on with my day. While it was still a lingering thought, I went out and bought a new pair that same day. Side note: I learned a trick for buying new pants—in the dressing room, try them on with your back to the mirror. I know this goes against loving and embracing your body, but I think the dressing room is one of the hardest places for us to do that. I went by feel instead of look and that helped immensely!

Saying Goodbye to the Scale

Do you feel the need to weigh yourself once a day (or more)? Do you weigh yourself naked, after exercising, before eating? Does the number you see dictate how your day will go and potentially what you may or may not eat? If that number is low, are you happy? If the number is high, do you have a bad day and possibly shed some tears? If any of these apply, the scale has too much control over your life. Do not let a simple number define you, affect your mood, or alter your daily actions—whether that is with food, exercise, or socializing.

> *Steph*: When I was at my sickest, the scale was my lifeline. It was the measurement of my entire life. If the scale read the "right" number (meaning

> whatever weight my eating disorder voice told me to be at that day), it was a good day; a fantastic day. It gave me motivation to continue exercising and restrict the amount of food I was eating. On days that it read the wrong number, I was infuriated. I knew it meant a day where I had to eat less and exercise more. It was a day I would be hard on others and myself. It was a day where temper tantrums akin to those of a two-year-old occurred.
>
> I would like to tell you that the day I gave up the scale was the happiest day of my life. It wasn't. I was scared of losing my "trusty old friend" and terrified of not knowing, not being in control. However, not measuring made it easier to gain weight. My job was to eat and rest. There were no numbers on a box telling me I was doing something wrong. With time, as I recovered, I no longer cared about the scale. I looked healthy, I was still me, and I was not defined by a number. Instead, my life became full of happiness; one based on friends, family, and experiences.

In your journey to recover from HA, it is often helpful to get rid of your scale. If you are checking your weight frequently and watching the number rise each day, you will drive yourself crazy. You don't actually *need* to know your weight to beat HA; in many cases, it's better to let go of that number and just trust your body.

If you're not ready to stop weighing completely, try cutting down how often you step on the scale. If you are measuring daily, try skipping one weigh-in. Perhaps enlist your partner's help; have him hide the scale if you can't manage to avoid hopping on. Once you've accomplished not weighing yourself for one day, try for a few more. And then more, until you are no longer dependent on the scale at all.

There may still be times when your weight confronts you. At medical appointments you might be weighed so that your doctor can help you in your recovery or prescribe the right dosage of medicine (although this is rare, and the practice of weighing at doctor's visits perpetuates fatphobia in the medical system). It is okay to say that you do not want to be weighed! Another option is to step on the scale backward and request that you not be told the number. These simple acts take away the power of your weight to control your life or ruin your day.

Gaining the necessary weight for recovery is often easier when you are not fighting a rising, possibly scary number. In the end, we are confident that like many recovered HAers, you won't miss the scale and will experience a feeling of freedom from that little defining box.

> *Michelle H:* I really can't stress enough how life-changing getting rid of the scales has been for me. If anyone is wondering if they should, trust me, it's honestly been a huge, gigantic step toward recovery (both HA and my disordered eating). I realized earlier that I'm not letting a piece of plastic with digital numbers define who I am, and what a breath of fresh air that is. I know that my BMI isn't in what "they" say the healthy range is, but there is so much detrimentally wrong with the whole BMI theory. The more signals I see of my returning period, the more I'm convinced I'm doing the right thing. I still have rough days where it's harder to not be the size I was this past summer, but then the good things outweigh that a million times over. Looking back, I've come so far from the person who was waking up every morning drained and dizzy, not having any emotion but apathy. I was dying on the inside, but God has definitely turned my life back around and I finally feel like I'm in the land of the living again. So yes, it's worth it—it's all worth it.

Dealing With Comments

> *Steph:* I am not really sure what it is, but from the moment my husband and I started trying to have a baby until probably a year postpartum, every person under the sun thought it was their right to comment or ask about my body or weight. I think my favorite question was "How much weight did you gain during pregnancy?" Why was it my favorite? Because I never knew. I said goodbye to my scale years ago, let my doctor track my weight during pregnancy, and did not worry about it. When people asked and I told them I had no clue, they would stare at me in utter disbelief. What I always wanted to know was what gave them the right to question me about my weight all of a sudden? It seemed once we were trying to have a baby, everything about me and my body was fair game... uhhh, think again!

It is almost inevitable that once you start the process of recovery, people will make comments. They may range from "You look healthier" and "You look so much better now" to "Are you pregnant?", "How much weight have you gained?", or "Wow, someone's hitting the snack bar hard!" As if it isn't enough that you are trying to work through the mental and physical aspects of recovery, it now may seem that everyone from your partner to your coworker has an opinion on your body and feels the right to state it aloud.

These comments can be a double-edged sword. On the one hand, hearing that you look better and healthier may be encouraging and help you to continue down the path of recovery. Or they can be twisted by your HA mindset to suggest that people think you're "letting yourself go" and thus thwart your recovery. Do not fall into this trap—when people make these positive comments, they are genuine. You *do* look better and healthier! Do not take it as anything more than that. Remarks like "You used to be so skinny," or "You look so much better with extra weight" could make you angry, sad, or scared that your worst fears have come true and people have noticed that you are gaining. Or you can take them as a sign that you are another step closer to recovery. Regardless of how you feel about comments, you are most likely going to get them, so it is best to prepare yourself with a plan in advance. The first step is to do some self-examination and determine whether comments will help or hinder your progress. If hearing from your partner that you are sexier and glowing will encourage you to keep eating, then let him (and others who are aware of your recovery) know that positive verbal feedback will help you. However, if such comments cause you distress, ask people not to mention anything about your body or recovery at all.

While you may be able to influence what some say, you cannot control the words of everyone. Many people feel the need to make unsolicited comments about others' appearance. It is easy to be tripped up during recovery by an off-hand remark from a stranger, coworker, or even someone close to you, but keep in mind that the people making these comments are almost always thoughtless rather than malicious, and often stem from a place of being steeped in/trapped by the diet culture we live in. If a comment is encouraging and you are able to see it as such (as we hope you can), win-win! Thank them and keep the remark in your back pocket for a time when you are struggling. However, if the statement is unwanted or feels negative, it can be crushing. It can be helpful to think about a reply for the seemingly less than complimentary comments in advance. For example, if someone asks if you have gained weight you can use humor and say, "Maybe—I just can't stop eating Christmas cookies!", "Eh, who cares?", or joke, "I'm trying to gain weight to see what it feels like." You can turn the tables and inquire, "Why is this important to you?" or "What an interesting question, why do you ask?" You can perhaps get them to realize that their statement or question is rude by a simple "Excuse me?" Or if you feel like it, you can simply share that you're trying to get your period back or that you are trying to get pregnant and increasing your BMI increases your chances of pregnancy—they most likely won't make any more comments in the future! After the conversation, make sure to return to the positive thinking we talked about above. Don't let others' words get inside your head. Use your affirmations, remember why you are on this journey, and keep moving forward.

> *Casie*: I had a rough week where I was asked if I was pregnant by a male colleague at a conference yesterday and started to cry. So embarrassing. Granted, I have suddenly put on weight... and two other residents just announced that they were preggers. I just hope the crying means my hormones are finally coming along. On the other hand, my 85-year-old grandmother can't stop talking about how healthy and "sexy" I look. So I think we all need to focus on those types of comments, stand up straight, and continue doing what we're doing.

> *Clover*: Friends, family, and strangers commenting and questioning our weight and body parts seems to be common so I'd like to provide you with a few more tips and tricks (and a few down-right lies) to handle the topic. One tactic is to mention the situation yourself before anyone else gets a chance. Like, "Hey, everyone. Look at me, I gained weight!" LOL. Depending on the environment, I might randomly announce I had been trying to gain weight "just to see how it feels." Another approach is to reply with sarcasm; "Yes, I am gaining weight. I am trying to bulk up and get stronger as I prepare for winter." I would even say this if winter had just ended. On the other hand, sometimes it's not the comment that bothers you but the silence, which can be VERY loud, if you know what I mean. This is when I would just roll with it and remind myself of the ultimate goal and that my confidence doesn't (shouldn't) hinge on the opinions of others.

Summary

The task is fairly simple: increase food consumption and wait for the results. Unfortunately for most of us, this is easier said than done. We can't just wake up one day, change our habits, and go on our merry way. In order to recover, many of us need support. We need healthy coping mechanisms to guide us through the recovery process. When the going gets tough, turn to this chapter for assistance. Above all else, remember these key points:

- Transform your thinking through positive self-talk, affirmations, reality checks, and letting go. When necessary, give yourself the right to a five-minute rant, but then reframe those thoughts afterward.

- Get rid of your skinny jeans and other "sick" clothes in favor of outfits that are more comfortable, fit better, and have room for growth, such as yoga pants.
- Say goodbye to your scale. If you need, take baby steps to get there by slowly using the scale less and less. Lean on friends and family for support.
- If you need more help, find a counselor to guide and support you through this time.
- View positive comments about your body as the truth (they are) and use them as motivation. Be ready to fight back against unwanted comments and arm yourself with strategies to get through difficult conversations.

> *Lisa*: As I read through this chapter, so many things come to mind, but I will try to stay focused on the "weighty" issues. The big takeaway is that if you choose to take steps toward complete recovery you WILL expand… not only physically but mentally. This process can also be referred to as growth. According to Wikipedia, *"growth refers to a positive change in size, often over a period of time."* That would be our physical growth. Mentally, *"growth can occur as a stage of maturation or a process toward fullness or fulfillment."* I feel like these definitions are spot-on in regard to HA recovery. To take these thoughts on the mental aspect further, it seems that sometimes in order to experience growth we have to let go of the plans, the need for understanding, and the certainty of it all. Life is full of moments in which not everything will be understood. Not everything will have a plan (nor should it). Not everything will have an explanation. Growth comes from an ability to embrace these moments instead of drowning in the questions and unknowns.

To leave you with a few inspirational words, we asked the people on the Board what affirmations worked for them while trying to gain weight and recover.

> *Judith*: "This is my journey, and my journey is different."

> *Ami*: "What's the worst that can happen? You gain weight and get pregnant?"

> *Abby*: "I have learned to treat myself gently because with a few exceptions, I am doing my best. I will not feel guilty for caring for myself. I will not be hard on myself today. I love and approve of all of me—even those qualities I thought were not good enough."

Rachel: I used to counter my fear of gaining weight by simply thinking "that's the point."

Laurie: "There is NOTHING WRONG with the way you look"

Amanda M: "I am stronger than HA. I need to eat and rest now to make up for years of undereating and overexercising."

Natalie: I had more of a tough love approach with myself—I had to remind myself again and again how vain and superficial I was acting and that those who loved me didn't love me because of how I looked (nor did they notice if I was a little cushier)!

Sheeza: I used to say that our bellies are like hotels. If we nourished ourselves well, our babies would have five star suites and be super comfortable at their stay. Undernourished babies would be living in a nasty motel... Not fair.

12
The HA Recovery Plan: Exercise Changes

IF YOU REALLY WANT to get your menstrual cycles back (and have the best chance at pregnancy if desired), a multipronged approach is optimal. Part one of the HA Recovery Plan is to eat more, as we've discussed. Part two?

Exercise less. Or not at all.

Simple, right? Sure, except that it goes against everything we have been told for as long as we can remember. Why on earth are we suggesting you cut down your exercise or even completely stop it? For starters, the same reasons that you need to eat more. Right now your body is telling you that you are asking too much of it. The best way to cycle and become fertile again is to *do everything you can to rest and recover.* (If you were not an exerciser before but feel like perhaps you should add some workouts to make up for the extra food you're eating, we will say unequivocally that this is not the right time to do so.) "Doing everything you can" means eating more and exercising less (probably a lot less or not at all) while reducing stress. Working on all three variables at the same time means that eating and energy-related hormones will increase, and stress related hormones will decrease (from both reduced mental stress and reduced physical stress). You get a bigger bang for your buck—reversing multiple signals at the same time will help turn your reproductive system back on more quickly.

Particularly for those of us who are addicted to exercise, it is challenging to give up our workouts. We are used to the adrenaline, the "stress relief," the endorphins, and the thrill of beating a personal record. Often there is nothing else in our life that provides the same sense of accomplishment as our physical feats. It is generally tougher to give up exercise than it is to eat more, according to many who have followed the Recovery Plan.

You won't be working up the sweat you used to, and you'll probably miss that for a while, but at the same time, slower paced activities can be just as beneficial for your heart and overall health, if not better. Keep in mind that this is a choice for now; you will be able to go back to more strenuous activities in the future, with a better perspective on fitting them into your life. The really wonderful part about the decision to decrease or even stop exercising is that your *true* strength is revealed through the daily, willful act of letting go. Trust that your body will do what it was created to do and will heal completely, providing you with improved health, a period, and if you want, a baby/ies.

> *Carly*: I can't even begin to explain the importance of *cutting out all exercise*. Low-intensity exercise (e.g., walking or yoga) can be OK as long as you aren't going for hours or at max incline to compensate for cutting out your long runs, hour-long weight sessions, etc. I was at a very healthy weight when I started Clomid, but exercising 1.5 to 2 hours per day most days, and I didn't respond one bit until I eliminated exercise. If you are even questioning if you are doing too much... you are! I'm serious. Go all in! When I finally got my positive pregnancy test, I was only doing yoga once or twice a week. *That's it!*

> *Amy S*: You *can* do it—cut back on exercise, that is. Believe me, I never in a million years thought I could let myself gain weight and reduce exercise. *Never*!! These are the thoughts that got me through all this: (1) I want a baby more than I want to be thin; (2) I had very poor bone density results due to the lack of estrogen I'd had in my body over the years (my lowest E_2 level was 2 pg/mL!)—when I found out I thought, "Shoot, I want a baby, but I also want/need to be healthy. What good is it to be thin if I'm going to be breaking all my bones at a young-ish age, and who knows what will happen when I get older?" Even my mom, who is a dietitian who goes to conferences on osteoporosis, sat me down and said, "Amy, I know you want to have babies, and I want you to have them too, but what I want the most for you is to be healthy. Don't you want that for yourself?"; (3) I thought—if I have a daughter and *all* her doctors told her that not getting her period was really bad for her health and that the way to fix that was to gain weight and cut back on exercise—I'd be so sad if she put being thin above that; and lastly, (4) I thought if I would want that for my daughter, or even my friends, then why in the world can I not

> want that for myself? I owe it to myself. And on a lighter note, hey, I like being able to take breaks from exercise sometimes and eat what I want. And not be hungry.

How do you go from *needing* your exercise fix to letting it be just another part of your life? The journey is different for everyone. Some are so desperate to fix themselves (which usually stems from the burning desire for a baby) that they choose to go "all in" from the get-go and give up all high-intensity exercise cold turkey. On the other hand, for most of us, it is not that easy. So we slow down a tad, cut down exercise time a bit, and see what happens. But the longer we wait without results, the more we realize that even our three-mile runs (that used to be much more) are preventing us from recovering, and it becomes easier to stop running or exercising altogether.

> *Jennifer C*: Today was the first day in 17 years that I actually did not do any kind of workout and I was fine. NO crawling up the walls or out of my skin. NO bad moods. In fact, after work I spent a few hours with my parents just talking. My mom was in tears because she has her daughter back. I feel clear and strong. For those of you who feel like you have to work out every day or else you will hate yourself like I did most of my life, just let go. You deserve to feel good about yourself. No one can take that away from you. What I find works for me is I take every day as it comes. No tomorrow and no yesterday. JUST the present. Live in the moment. It took me a full year to really work on this, but I am so close to having my dreams come true. I realize if you want something badly enough, you're willing to work on the things that are in your way.

Exercise Plan

> *Amanda S*: My period came today!!! It has been over three years since I went off the birth control pill and learned that I had HA. I have gained weight over the last year, but the one thing that has changed recently was my exercise. I have not been to the gym in over a month due to being super busy with school and work. I am so happy and relieved that I feel like crying.

We almost don't need a whole section of the chapter for this; it's quite a simple plan. The quickest path to recovery is to cut out all intense exercise and either sit on the couch for a while, or choose less strenuous forms of exercise. In general, walking (not power walking), yoga (not hot), and similar activities are much easier on your body, and are ways to continue to feel active (if that is what you are seeking). But in some ways, the psychological need to exercise is perpetuating your problem. If you stop exercising entirely for a while, it may be easier to overcome the addiction as you learn what your life can look like without the compulsion to be active all the time. In our survey there were three factors associated with cycles returning:

- Reduction in exercise intensity.
- Reduction in exercise minutes.
- Immediate, "cold turkey" decrease in exercise rather than gradual.

As we described in chapter 3, we had asked our survey respondents about the intensity of their exercise at various points, on a scale of 0 to 10. The average score when someone had HA was a 7; in those who recovered natural cycles, that decreased to a 3.5. A score of 7 is equivalent to a fast run, with a heart rate between 160 and 169 beats per minute (bpm), very heavy breathing, and broken sentences if speaking. At 3.5, you would not be breaking a sweat, with light to moderate breathing. That's a big difference.

The second factor was a reduction in time spent exercising, with typically "high-intensity" exercise (running, cycling, aerobics, gym exercise machines, weight lifting) kept to less than three hours a week at the lowered intensity.

The last factor associated with cycles returning, and fastest path to that goal, was an immediate reduction in exercise. Our data show that the likelihood of recovering quickly is much higher if you go "all in" immediately—stopping high-intensity exercise completely during recovery—rather than gradually reducing exercise. These results are complicated by the fact that many of the survey respondents were trying to get pregnant and therefore started fertility treatments of some description. So the data describe the return of natural cycles prior to pregnancy or commencing fertility treatments. Of those who reduced exercise immediately, 61% had cycles resume prior to pregnancy. In contrast, only 46% had cycles return with a more gradual decrease in exercise ($p < 1 \times 10^{-3}$) despite waiting similar lengths of time. There are a couple of possible reasons for the discrepancy:

- It could be that a certain level of caloric excess is required that is not obtained while high-intensity exercise continues.
- Or perhaps even a small amount of cortisol from high-intensity exercise suppresses the hypothalamus.

Therefore, for many, it is not until high intensity exercise is cut completely that the healing process can begin. That is not to say that your cycles will not return with a gradual reduction in exercise, but it will probably take longer overall. Among survey respondents for whom cycles returned, on average it took two months longer for cycles to commence in those who reduced exercise gradually. This is yet another reason to go "all in" *now*.

> **Steph**: I don't know about you, but when someone tells me to do less strenuous exercise I want to know *exactly* what they mean. If left on my own, I might define less strenuous to mean not out of breath. So I want to be super clear. This may seem repetitive but if you are anything like me, you have to hear this again and again. When we say cut out all intense exercise, we mean no more aerobics classes (e.g., step, kickboxing, CrossFit, spin, you name it), no more running, no more sports (e.g., soccer, basketball, or swimming), and no more weight training sessions. Instead, less strenuous means *relaxing* yoga, Pilates, or walking. You should not get red, you should not be short of breath, and you should not sweat.

> **Deborah**: I'm hoping for a little perspective. I probably already know the answer, but I need confirmation. In reading about the "workouts" the rest of you are doing, I was reconsidering my "reduced" exercise routine. True, I am doing a LOT less, and not lifting at all. However, when I read "walking three to four times a week," my brain translates that into "frog-marching myself up a 12% incline at lightning speed"—which frankly, is far harder than jogging at an easy pace… but then I can tell myself I just "went for a walk."
>
> As for Pilates, here's the thing: the class I like to take is taught by this amazingly funny guy, but it is *hard*. I am dying in there. We move right into our "100s"… pumping our arms… and for 60 solid minutes every inch of my body is screaming "no more!" from exhaustion and pain (I thought I was in shape—but Pilates apparently exercises a whole new set of muscles I never knew I had). So while a nice relaxing and toning class is probably very beneficial, I found that mine were in fact making me stressed out and my butt and tummy hurt so much after I could barely laugh! Given that I'm not very good at relaxing, it didn't seem wise to keep going. So, I think I will switch to yoga. I'm sure Pilates is very toning, and good for people in general, but personally, perhaps not the best for me. Anyway, I am just trying to determine what a reduced workout week consists of since my assessment-radar seems to be rather skewed!

Of all the strenuous exercise we enjoy, running seems to have the biggest negative impact for those with HA; very few have been able to regain cycles while continuing to run. So if you are a runner, at the very least switch that out for some light elliptical (aiming for being able to talk while exercising;

Nico uses her elliptical time now as a way to catch up on phone calls), walking, or easy biking. Check out chapter 14 for some more tips on how to scale back and cut out your running.

> *Ellie*: The best advice I had (and the hardest to accept), was to completely cut exercise out of my lifestyle and eat a variety of foods. Sure, walking/biking is fine, if you're doing it for enjoyment and if that's too difficult, some light exercising sporadically (keeping heart rate down) is fine. But our society obviously has shifted to a high intensity interval training focus, which is exactly what our bodies do *not need* while attempting to get pregnant. Running long distances and exercises that keep the heart rate elevated are also detrimental for trying to conceive with HA. And eating low calorie foods just adds fuel to the fire. Your body is undernourished and overexercised, which equals *stressed*. The higher the stress placed on your body, the lower chance you have of conceiving.

> *Nico*: Once I was diagnosed with HA, I realized that I needed to cut down on what I was doing by *a lot*. So I made a pact with myself that I would only do one form of exercise each day instead of my usual two or even three, and that didn't mean ice hockey practice and then a game, it meant one or the other. *And* I had to take two rest days a week. I even tracked it on my blog so that I'd have some accountability and really stick to my plan. This reduction felt like a lot to me at the time, but it later became clear that even this more moderate exercise schedule was keeping me from ovulating and getting my period.

Supporting Evidence

There are no clinical studies that have specifically examined the question of how much exercise is reasonable with regard to HA recovery. However, there is plenty of evidence to support our suggestions. The most striking confirmation comes from a study we have mentioned before, where two groups of formerly sedentary women with normal cycles started a running program. The first group (12 women) increased calories to compensate for the exercise they performed (running an average of seven miles per day, five days a week); the second group (16 women) did not, and lost about a pound a week. The participants were observed for two months. Remarkably, even in the group theoretically consuming enough calories, only two experienced normal ovulatory cycles; the remainder were anovulatory or with luteal phase defects (LPD, chapter 19) (the luteal phase is the part of your cycle after ovulation). In the calorie-restricted running group (group

2), only one person had a normal cycle during the first month of training. In the second month, nobody had normal cycles. In fact, 75% of the cycles were anovulatory with delayed periods, which is suggestive of amenorrhea (the study was not long enough to confirm amenorrhea). At the end of the study, the patients were followed for an additional six months; all 28 resumed normal ovulation by six months later, but only upon reduction of training[1]. Unfortunately, no details were provided about the return of normal cycles other than they occurred after a reduction in running. The abnormal cycles, even in women who were adequately fueling in theory, strongly suggest that intense exercise like running is detrimental—and it makes sense that continuing to exercise intensely will hamper recovery.

Menstrual status in women starting a running program[2]

		Running + extra calories (Group 1, 12 women)	Running + caloric restriction (Group 2, 16 women)
		Number of women in each category (% in parentheses)	
Month 1	Normal cycles	2 (17%)	1 (6%)
	LPD	4 (33%)	10 (63%)
	Anovulatory	3 (25%)	5 (31%)
	Abnormal bleeding	5 (42%)	3 (19%)
	Delayed period	0 (0%)	1 (6%)
Month 2	Normal cycles	2 (22%)	0 (0%)
	LPD*	4 (44%)	2 (13%)
	Anovulatory	3 (33%)	12 (75%)
	Abnormal bleeding	4 (44%)	6 (38%)
	Delayed period	1 (11%)	12 (75%)

This table contrasts the menstrual cycles in runners consuming extra calories to make up for those burned during exercise compared with runners undereating to lose weight. The number and percentage of normal cycles versus those with various abnormalities are compared for the two groups on the right; the first month of training is shown at the top, with the second month at the bottom. Percentages do not add to 100 because women can fall into more than one category. *LPD = Luteal Phase Defect.

The high degree of abnormal cycles among exercisers, even with adequate fuel, has been substantiated in other studies. For example, one study found that among 24 runners averaging 20 miles per week 55% of cycles were either anovulatory or had LPD[3]. A decade later, a similar study including many different types of exercise showed 50% of cycles among exercising women to have abnormalities[4]. *These data strongly suggest that high-intensity exercise is detrimental to menstrual cycles, and will prevent their return no matter how much we are eating.*

> *Nico*: I have now tracked over 40 menstrual cycles in total, after each of my children was born. My luteal phase seems to be highly dependent on how much I'm exercising. I can't say for sure that my eating has been consistent, but that would certainly be my supposition as my weight has been stable after each pregnancy by the time I started cycling again. Here's the data:

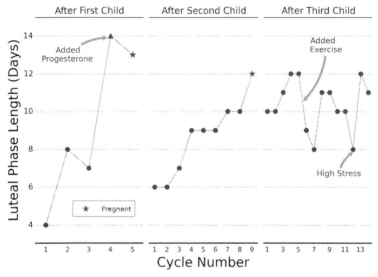

Luteal phase and exercise. The length of my luteal phase (LP) after my menstrual cycles restarted after each pregnancy is shown. After #1 (*left*) I got pregnant again on my fourth cycle. After #2 (*middle*) I got pregnant on cycle 9, and after #3 (*right*) I'm done! The arrow indicates when I increased my exercise after #3, and you can see the effect—my LP decreased from 12 days to 8. Added stress a few months later (a toddler with a broken leg) also did a number on my LP.

> Notice that after #3 was born, my LP was initially much longer than after my first two pregnancies, and improved even more, to my highest natural LP ever (12 days). I bet you can guess what the difference is—*very little exercise*! After #1 and #2 were born I was still playing ice hockey two to three times a week, biking to and from work a couple days a week, and lifting weights twice a week. After #3, all I could fit in was riding my bike maybe once a week and playing ice hockey once a week, plus chasing the kids around.

> After my 12-day LP post #3 (cycle 5), I started doing abdominal exercises every day to reduce my diastasis (separation between my stomach muscles, from pregnancy), and also added more high-intensity ice hockey two to three times a week. The length of my LPs immediately dropped (and that's with a few pounds of weight gain too, so I was not at an energy deficit). So for me, I'm pretty sure that exercise alone, even without an energy deficit, has an effect on my cycles.

In an observational study that followed two women for a year as they ate more in an attempt to resolve their amenorrhea (but continued to exercise), there were also ongoing menstrual cycle abnormalities. Both women increased their BMI and resumed cycling simply by eating more, but cycles were irregular, anovulatory, and/or had LPD[5]. These data support the idea that menstrual cycles can return with added calories alone; however, the cycles going forward are often not normal and are therefore associated with lower pregnancy rates.

A prospective study performed in Denmark further supports the idea that intense exercise can negatively impact cycles and increase the time needed to get pregnant for some. A group of 3,628 regularly cycling women wanting to conceive was followed for a year (12 cycles) or until conception. There was a strong correlation between increased amounts of intense exercise (e.g., running, fast cycling, aerobics, gymnastics, or swimming) and a longer time to achieve pregnancy, particularly with a BMI less than 25. On average, it took two cycles longer to conceive if more than five hours a week of intense exercise were performed, and any intense exercise *at all* was associated with a longer time to conceiving. On the other hand, moderate exercise (e.g., brisk walking, leisurely cycling, golfing, or gardening) up to five hours per week, was correlated with a shorter time to achieving pregnancy[6].

These studies reinforce our assertion that high-intensity exercise can be detrimental to the reproductive system. In other words, if exercise is messing up cycles in those who are eating a sufficient amount, imagine how difficult it is for a reproductive system that has been under-fueled and consequently shut down to restart under these conditions*.

We have found similar results among our survey respondents. Those who continued to perform "high-intensity" exercise (e.g., running, elliptical, Stairmaster, team sports, aerobics, cycling/spin), even at reduced intensity, were less likely to have natural cycles return. In those doing more than

---

* See chapter 28 for a discussion of exercise after recovery.

three hours per week of this type of exercise, only 30% regained cycles, compared to 54% of those performing less than three hours of these exercises at reduced intensity. That is almost a two-fold reduction in the likelihood of restoring natural cycles.

> *Lisa:* Oh boy. Back in the day, I definitely believed I was in the minority; I didn't need to gain weight and decrease my exercise. And if I had read about this small 30% I am certain I would have white knuckled that hope to my death. Heck, I almost did. As usual I had to find out the hard way. I continued with high-intensity exercise for two more years until I finally acknowledged that I was NOT in this special 30% and needed to temporarily cut my high intensity exercise. Committing to this earlier would have resulted in an earlier recovery…just like you are doing now! :)

Additionally, researchers examining changes in cortisol and other stress hormones found exercise at 60% or more of maximum intensity significantly increased cortisol levels[7], which then suppress the hypothalamus. No changes in cortisol were found at 40% of maximum intensity, so we therefore suggest keeping your heartrate (measure of intensity) to around 100 bpm or less, which is about 50% of max for the average person in their 20's or 30's.

> *Robyn Nohling, FNP, RD, MSN:* You don't need to wear a heart rate monitor every time you exercise. How cumbersome! The goal is to move towards a gentle, intuitive relationship with exercise that supports your body's mental and physical health both during the healing process and thereafter. A good rule of thumb for keeping your heart rate under 100 bpm is to make sure you can sing the lyrics to your favorite song out loud the whole time you're moving. If you get short of breath doing that, slow it down until you can sing without trouble.

If you want to continue with high-intensity exercise, take some time to seriously consider if the potential cost is worth it for you. We strongly suggest cutting out all those types of exercise for the time-being; in the longer term you can certainly add activities like running back into your repertoire.

All right, so let's say you bite the bullet and follow our recommendation (if elite runner Tina Muir can (page 185), you can too!). Without high-intensity exercise, the rates of recovering menstrual cycles are the same (around 54%), whether you do no exercise or perform light activities like walking and yoga. So if you feel like a leisurely walk (mind you, power walking up a 12% incline for an hour does not fit the bill), go right ahead.

Note that there certainly are people who exercise regularly and at high volumes while maintaining normal menstrual cycles[8]. However, there is *no evidence* to support exercising intensely and *regaining* normal menstrual cycles.

> **Stacey H**: It is different for everyone as to when you will cycle again. I started gaining in June 2012, slowly increasing calories and then slowly decreasing exercise. Five months later I decided to stop exercising altogether. A little over a month later I ovulated. That being said, when I wasn't exercising I did my best to just park my butt on the sofa, literally. I was nervous even walking the 10 minutes to town because I didn't want to freak my body out. Yes, your body needs that much rest! I think I would have ovulated earlier had I stopped exercising sooner.

Remind Me Why I'm Doing This

Believe it or not (and you probably won't until you go through it yourself), you will probably feel better physically with less exercise (mentally is a whole different story, which we'll get to in a minute), or at the very least, you won't feel worse. Your body will thank you for some time off to repair and rest. Those nagging injuries will heal, you'll feel less tired and more energized, and then as your hormones start increasing you'll feel all the positive effects of more estrogen as we described in chapter 10. Oh, yes, and you'll start cycling and/or respond to treatment better. (Although as we discussed, it is possible that you will have some time when you feel as if you have been hit by a truck, more achey and lethargic, as your body uses the newfound energy and rest to repair cells and organs that have been damaged over time.)

In the midst of this, however, there are probably going to be days where what we are asking feels *impossible*. Especially at the beginning, which is often when people slip up and go for a run or to the gym. Don't worry, one exercise session will not derail your recovery. Have an extra bowl of ice cream to make up for it, and take it extra easy the next day. Chapter 13 contains more tips to help ease the transition from the old "exercise-fanatic-you" to the new "working-toward-recovery-you."

When you acknowledge the benefits of exercise reduction, and put our recommendations into practice, you will experience a freedom you did not realize you were missing. As you pick up other activities, you might find that you enjoy not being tied to the gym or your running shoes anymore. You won't have to set your alarm clock super early to fit in your exercise;

you'll have more time to spend with people important to you, to accomplish neglected tasks, and to just relax and enjoy the amazing world around you. Your partner, family, and friends will enjoy the new, more relaxed you as well!

Finally, as we mentioned at the beginning of this chapter, remind yourself that the reduced exercise is for recovery. Once you begin cycling or get pregnant you can add back exercise (slowly!). All former HAers who wanted to continue to exercise after recovery or pregnancy have managed to do so, most while continuing to cycle. Post-recovery, however, the exercise comes second to the rest of our lives. There is less of a compulsion to exercise every day and more recognition that moderate exercise a few times a week is healthy (in fact, probably healthier than the daily exercise most of us did prior to recovery).

> *Helen*: Ladies, as the festive season approaches and I sit in a coffee shop with a praline cappuccino, I want to take a minute to thank this community from the bottom of my heart for giving me back the enjoyment of this special time of year! During my HA days I would panic about how to avoid eating and fit in training during the holiday. This morning as I listened to the rain bouncing off our windows whilst warm under a duvet with both my girls and not out pounding the pavements, I thought of you all and how blessed I am to have this second chance at life.

Summary

The second step in our HA Recovery Plan is to ask less of your body in the short term, by cutting down or cutting out your exercise. Let the extra food you are consuming go toward fueling and restoring the systems that have been put on the back burner for so long. The more you are able to rest, the faster the repairs can happen, and the faster your system will return to normal. Your body wants to reproduce—it is our species biological imperative—so give it a chance to rest and repair, replenish and restore before you ask more of it in the form of a pregnancy, or ongoing menstrual cycles PLUS exercise.

To reiterate, our short-term recommendations are to:

- Cut out high-intensity exercise like running, aerobics/spin classes, and other activities that get your heart rate above about 100 bpm.
- Engage in low-intensity exercise (e.g., walking, yoga) or no exercise instead.

- If you choose to continue exercising more than this despite everything we have shown you in this chapter, eat roughly an additional two calories for every one you expend during exercise while you are working to recover.

Temporary rest and repair, along with finding other ways to cope with and enjoy your life (chapter 13), will help you accomplish your ultimate goal: *the restoration of your health and fertility*. During this time, we hope that you too will find the freedom that comes from choosing your exercise rather than being controlled by it. Long term, our recovered HAers have found that they:

- Have a more carefree and relaxed attitude toward exercise—able to go for a day or two, or heck, a whole week, without an exercise fix and without crawling out of their skin.
- Understand the importance of taking a break when injured.
- Choose time with friends and/or family over getting a workout in.
- Fit exercise *into* their life, instead of working life *around* exercise.

> **Lisa:** WOW! I love this chapter (though deep in HA I would have hated it!). You know the old saying, "The truth hurts." I can only speak for myself, but reading the options to "decrease or even stop exercising" and "go for a day or two … without an exercise fix" in order to recover would have made me cringe when I was in the midst of HA. At that time, I was REALLY comfortable and enjoyed lengthy intense exercise. I had no concept of moderation and certainly had no need for "days off," even when injured. Did you also cringe or feel like you wanted to freak out when you read this chapter on the exercise solution? If so, you're in good company. Like most of us, you too will have to dig really deep to implement the exercise prescription suggested for recovery.
>
> Being a personal trainer didn't help ease my challenge either. Think about it. How many personal trainers do you know who gained weight and stopped exercising? As a result, I had to come up with a lot of mental tricks in order to keep a steady path towards recovery. More importantly, I was *very* purposeful in my decisions and actions every day. It was HARD instructing people, giving them killer workouts while I willfully sat on a bench (sitting and wearing flip flops was one way to decrease my activity while training). It felt like I was being tortured (LOL). The one thing I would continually remind myself (and still do) is that my physical appearance and inability to kick butt in the weight room or on the track did not diminish my ability to be an excellent spouse, best friend, or competent trainer. Just because my physique was changing didn't mean my brain

would suddenly fall out of my head or I would be less of a person, right? I think this thought process can be carried over into every area of our lives. We are way more than our appearance and physical abilities and yet we continue to cram ourselves into that rigid, narrow self-defining box.

13
There Is More to Life Than Exercise

WHEN YOUR LIFE REVOLVES around exercise, it is nearly impossible to envision your world without it. You live in a universe where the day doesn't begin, or is not complete until you have worked out. Exercise is your time, a way to stay fit, flush negative emotions, and relieve stress. You run, swim, bike, attend classes, play a sport, or engage in other exercise, because you love it, you have goals to meet, and there are races or competitions to be won. Exercise is not simply a part of your life; it is your life. When you define yourself, at least partly, by the exercise you participate in, being asked to give up these activities can feel unbearable. Maybe you could deal with eliminating a couple of sessions or reducing the time (a bit), but cutting it out altogether? No way! To add fuel to this fire, what if someone suggests walking, yoga, or Pilates instead?! Now that is just hysterical—how can one even equate these activities? No, no, this is all crazy talk. You cannot and will not do this; you are different, and you will find another option. This cannot be part of the prescription to regain fertility.

Have any of these thoughts crossed your mind? They certainly did for us. But as we pressed on toward the ultimate goal of HA recovery, a mental and physical transformation took place. We became individuals who could make time for a casual walk with a friend just to chat; we slept in instead of getting up early to ensure the daily workout was accomplished; we stayed out later because we had more energy (and didn't have to get up early); I guess you could say we slowed down enough to smell the roses. We acknowledged and embraced that life is not about how many calories you

> **Megan:** There are so many amazing things that have come out of this HA journey that it almost makes me grateful that it *did* happen to me. Hear me out: in addition to all of the health issues that have essentially reversed (dry nails, high heart rate, constipation, dry skin, night sweats, fatigue, AMENORRHEA, and so on), these four months have taught me patience, shown me that there's more to life than killing yourself at the gym, and improved my relationship with my husband *tremendously* (both emotionally and sexually)—we are closer than we've ever been. It's taught me to be more compassionate of others, to be more understanding, and I am calmer than I have ever been in my entire life.

> **Tania:** I think (and this is only my two cents' worth) that this "process" is meant to teach us how to relax and deal with stress without exercising it away... I believe that is why I am now dealing with this roller coaster ride of emotions (hormones!) that I didn't really deal with before. I think that it will make us all realize that it is OK to spend time at home with our babies and to realize that our bodies and exercise are not the end-all-be-all... that is what I am learning anyway.

So how do you get to a place where you are comfortable with reducing or eliminating exercise for the time being? Where you don't want to clothesline every person who runs past you, and no longer obsess over the fact that you "chose" not to work out for the day, the week, or even the month. Aaaaaaah! It is easier for some than others, which again is a reminder that we all have different journeys. Some of us quickly find that place where we are no longer bound by our training regime. Others take a little more time discovering that there is enjoyment in the new opportunities presented to them; they still miss their workouts, but manage to kick back for the moment recognizing that this is a willful and temporary *choice*. This is not a season of workouts; rather it is a season of preparation for your health, fertility, and potential future family. Regardless of the path you choose, this break from your regular workout routine will ultimately improve your health and well-being. It is not always easy, but it is absolutely 100% worth it.

> **Helen:** Honestly, honestly, the exercise thing gets better. It's a constant battle, but once you realize how much fun life is when it's not dominated by everything training-related you really won't feel as depressed! I began

this journey in 2008 and really only over the last three months has it become more normal not to train. I have cabinets of trophies and pages of pretty good times but it's meaningless. There is always someone out there training harder and performing better, and one day I promise you, you will realize that winning, training, and achieving are not real life achievements. Being a parent, a partner, and a "normal" person again are what make us whole. I am so fortunate I have a child whom I adore, but even during her first year I was so focused on competing again I lost sight of the real importance of life. In recent months I've realized that training, being skinny, and pushing myself to the limit should not define whether I'm a good person. True happiness is looking into your child's eyes and seeing that love back.

As you try to grasp the idea of a life beyond or without exercise and learn to be comfortable with the changes, we know that you may need more encouragement. Below we offer some strategies to help get you through this transition to your new normal.

Take it day by day. The simple idea of giving up exercise may seem daunting and worrisome. Even before you stop exercising and experience the world of relaxation, you may be feeling a host of emotions. However, until you have rested, you cannot truly predict how you are going to feel. So go ahead, try it out. Don't worry about a few days, weeks, or months from now; instead, make the commitment for one day. Today, make a choice to not exercise. Allow your body time to rest and repair. Plan to invest this free time in other meaningful activities: go to the mall with friends, read a good book, take up a new hobby, or maybe even think about sitting on the couch if you want (harder than it sounds but doable). Then when tomorrow comes, take another day off. On the other hand, if you are feeling overly anxious (like a pressure cooker), start out by taking "active rest days" with a walk, yoga, or Pilates.

> *Isla*: At the very least, you have nothing to lose by taking two weeks off, and even the most intense, highest level athletes do that in their off-seasons... Why can't we forgive ourselves for doing it for a few weeks/months to heal our bodies, or in preparation for pregnancy???

> *Lauren*: By fall 2013, I was going on two years without a period. I learned that HA also has negative effects on our heart, bone, and metabolic health. I knew what I had to do but *I just couldn't stop*. I prayed and I prayed for answers, and finally God gave me mine. You know what he did? He tripped me one day when I was walking down the stairs at work, and I

> sprained my ankle! I laugh because Nico always said, "If you injured your leg, you wouldn't try to work out on it; you'd give it time to heal." Well, the lunatic that I was, I attempted to work out on my sprained ankle, but I realized I was doing more damage than good. I finally recognized it for what it was: a sign that it was time to heal—my ankle, my reproductive system, my metabolism, etc. It was very hard but the community on the Board helped me through it. At first I told myself I would just give it a month off exercise, and if after a month I hadn't recovered, I could go back to my old ways. But you know what? After that first month, I didn't WANT to go back to my old ways. I was so inspired and truly, sincerely happier than I had ever been in my life, so I kept at it. Two months later, I recovered my cycles.

Focus on the positives. At the end of your rest day, make a list of all the things you were able to do instead of going to the gym. Even better, add more things that you would like to do with your extra time. When you find yourself antsy to work out again, use your list to reaffirm and remind yourself of the positives that have come from your rest time. To further encourage yourself, you could also add in what you disliked about your extreme exercise schedule: running in 10-degree weather with your lungs burning from the cold air and your nose getting frostbite, eating extremely late dinners because you were at the gym so long, having sore legs all day every day from your workouts, chronic injuries, and missing out on time with friends and family, for example. Or if you want to think about it another way, you can write down reasons that exercising is not good for you right now: my body is stressed and running when it's below freezing is more difficult; my body is tired, so exercising on five hours of sleep intensifies stress to my hypothalamus, etc.

> *Vanessa A:* Even if my body didn't want to do it, if I had set a goal in my head to get up at 5 a.m. and run, I would do it no matter what. A cold or flu wouldn't stop me. For about three years if it was Sunday afternoon and I hadn't run my 20 to 25 miles that morning I would feel so guilty! It is so nice to wake up and ask myself if I want to run, and if I don't want to, that's OK! I find that when I do run I actually enjoy it more because I am not just doing it because I feel I have to. I've also realized I am not going to become a contestant on The Biggest Loser if I don't exercise every day. I'm amazed at how my weight has stabilized, despite exercising far less and still eating more treats than I used to.

Enjoy mindful exercise. The concept of "mindful exercise" may escape you initially. For many of us, exercise when deep in HA is about how many calories we are burning or how far, how hard, and how fast we can go. There is an alternative, though, which is to alter the reasons you are exercising. Instead of focusing on calories and intensity, concentrate on the here and now, and the basic enjoyment of moving your body, even at a slower pace or for less time. Consciously working to change your attitude and approach toward exercise can make a world of difference to both your physical and mental well-being. For example, if you feel like taking a run, tone it down to a walk or jog and pay attention to what you are seeing and hearing. Make an effort to explore your surroundings rather than speeding past them. If you kick box or take aerobics classes, maybe introduce yoga or Pilates instead and really focus on how good these activities make your body and mind feel. If you play a sport, perhaps look for a coaching or volunteer opportunity where you can be of benefit to others instead of participating yourself. If you were longing for a high-intensity spin class, take your bike outside—enjoy the warmth of the sun on your skin and take in your surroundings; go for a leisurely ride with a friend and enjoy some conversation.

> *Anna*: Rather than trying to control my body with X amount of exercise and food per day, I'm going to try really hard to let my body make the decision when it's had enough to eat or whether I can really be bothered to exercise. I'm the first to admit it's easier said than done, especially because I have trained my thinking for so long to do whatever I'm doing until I have achieved my goal. I think I have pretty strong perseverance and stamina; now I need to redirect those qualities. I just came back from a swim. Rather than counting laps and watching time so that I could be reassured that I swam "enough," I used the opportunity to have a big think (mainly about how we can spread the HA message universally) and even had a chat between laps with a lovely old man who swam like a turtle. Previously, I would have gotten (silently) grumpy with him for breaking my rhythm. It's nice to slow down the pace of life and stop to smell the roses—dorky but true, I think!

Support. This has been said often, but it is worth repeating—have a strong support system, whether you find it in this book, in an online community, spiritually, or through friends, families, or professionals. You don't need to weather this alone. If you are starting to feel like you are about to fall back on the commitments you have made to yourself, it is in that moment that we encourage you to use your resources. Call a friend or your therapist, or jump online and read a blog article. Open this book and read some inspirational stories of others who have had similar struggles. Seek those around you to ground you and to remind you why you are working so hard. There is so much more out there waiting for you!

> *Jessica*: I started posting on the Board and the love, support, and solid information I received was more than I could have ever imagined. The amazing individuals who participate every day encouraged me, held my hand, were patient with me, and helped me to find the strength and courage to make and sustain changes. By late October 2013, I stopped all exercise except slow walking and gentle yoga. I also slowly added more to my diet, mostly in the way of healthy fats (and ice cream!).

> *Lisa*: I am big proponent of support systems during recovery. Not because we *need* assistance in order to recover but because "white-knuckling" the process alone is a waste of energy. My supports consisted of the following:
>
> - **God/prayer:** Having a personal belief system in God and regular prayer time refocused my thoughts on what is good, true, and lovely. I meditated on strength for recovery, hope, and the faith for restoration. Even when my faith was the size of a mustard seed, I was able to rest assured that there is purpose beyond what I feel I have messed up.
> - **HA Community:** I could not imagine my journey without these supporters. They listened, shared different perspectives, were relatable and resourceful, pivotal to my recovery, and became like siblings (or adopted kiddos … many are much younger!) to me.
> - **My husband:** He provided cheerleading, humor, encouragement, and jokingly reminded me when I'd gripe about how big I was getting, that I was "his little weight gain machine" (with a proud grin).
> - **Therapy:** It's interesting because when I suggest therapy to people, I often sense resistance to the idea of finding a "professional" (stigma-related, most likely). I remind my friends that we aren't seeking counsel because we are weak or broken. Instead, we want to better equip ourselves in dealing with this journey and possibly ease the challenges we confront and tackle. When I look back on it all, I realize that at a very young age when I started using unhealthy coping methods (e.g., controlling food) to deal with life's stressors, I stopped developing healthy ones. I never learned other ways to manage stress, anger, sadness, anxiety, and a host of other emotions. Gaining new coping skills beyond food restriction and overtraining is a process and the right therapist can help tremendously. Mine certainly did.

Support systems are healthy, will be used for the rest of our lives, and certainly make a positive impact on our journeys.

Learn new skills. Exercise has likely been a large part of your life. By giving it up, you may wonder, what now? Exercise may have served a purpose in allowing you to excel in an area, have time for yourself, or just have a hobby of your own. There is no reason why you cannot learn new skills in a different area to meet these same needs. It may seem difficult at first, but in time, you will find enjoyment and possibly a new passion. For example, taking a cake or cookie decorating class may be an excellent way to hone a new skill as well as add some calories into your day. Knitting or crocheting may come in handy for baby clothes or new fashion for yourself down the line. Reflect on your life and other activities you enjoyed in the past. How can you integrate those interests into your life today? Were you ever a Girl Scout? Perhaps you would be interested in becoming a troop leader. Did you like to write? Maybe start a blog. Take the energy and ambition used for exercise and divert it to another hobby or volunteer opportunity.

> *Brittney*: I know that exercise was a stress reliever for me, but I've learned other ways to deal with stress. Long, leisurely walks with my dog help. And I have a relaxing yoga DVD that melts away stress, too.
>
> *Nico*: In my HA heyday, just about all my free time was spent exercising—at least two hours a day. When I cut back to recover, I picked up a Beatrix Potter alphabet sampler cross-stitch I had started a few years earlier. I had only gotten to letter H before dropping it in favor of other pursuits. The stitching took me about 26 hours *per letter*—but having a goal of finishing gave me something much more relaxing and healthy for my body to do while still satisfying my competitive spirit. It is now finished and proudly hangs in my baby's room.

Experience the emotions. Exercise may have been your release or distraction from unpleasant emotions that now rise to the surface; or you might experience a variety of other feelings of inadequacy or self-loathing that can seem overwhelming as you work to recover from HA. But now it is time to recognize your emotions and work through them instead of avoiding them. Cognitive behavioral therapy (CBT), or its more practical cousin dialectical behavioral therapy (DBT), are a couple of therapy options (among many) that can offer some useful tools for changing your mindset. If you are struggling with your emotional health during this time, seeing a professional trained in one of these methods is highly recommended; individualized therapy can be a huge help in making mental changes that will release you from your eating and exercise compulsions. DBT[1] in particular offers a multitude of ways to address these emotions including:

- Understanding the emotions: identifying them and comprehending what they do to you.
- Reducing emotional vulnerability: decreasing negative emotions and increasing positive ones.
- Decreasing emotional suffering: letting go of painful emotions through mindfulness, and changing painful emotions through opposite actions.

It is important not to disregard your emotions. Face them and work them out so you can move forward.

> *Steph*: DBT has been a huge lifesaver for me. I was first introduced to it when recovering from anorexia and still use it in my everyday life. One of my favorite DBT skills is distraction. If I find myself fearful about weight gain, for example, I go to my freezer and grab a frozen orange (any citrus fruit works). It probably sounds bizarre, but don't knock it until you try it. I hold the orange and experience it in the moment—its smell, texture, and temperature. It is a grounding technique that helps bring some calm and serenity. Instead of focusing on potential for weight gain, concentrating on the sensations around that orange allow me to relax and come back to the present.
>
> I use my orange whenever I am distressed. Once I have calmed down, I can then use the other skills I have learned to identify, comprehend, and experience my emotions. I particularly remember a time when I was sitting at my desk a few weeks into recovery, trying to work. All of a sudden my heart started racing, I couldn't concentrate, and I felt the need to escape. Previously, I would have pushed this feeling away by refusing to eat or pounding the pavement. Instead, with the help of DBT, I took a step back. I observed the physical sensations occurring in my body (e.g., speeding heart, shortness of breath), considered the possible emotions I could be experiencing, and identified anxiety. I took a breath and asked myself why I was anxious—at which point I realized that the emotion was serving a purpose. It was telling me to pay attention because I was doing critical work. Having recognized this, I used my DBT skill of deep breathing to work out the physical symptoms, then told myself I would take a break and come back to the work in a bit. I actually went and got my nails done. I knew I had enough time to finish my task and that I would do it faster and better if I was kind to my body and took time to recuperate.

Summary

This chapter has offered some tips on implementing the HA Recovery Plan in terms of exercise, as well as adapting to the changes mentally and emotionally:

- Rather than imagining the rest of your life with no exercise, take it day by day; what can you do today to rest your body?
- Pay attention to the positives during this process; write down things you have time for now.
- When things get tough, try out new activities and don't be afraid to reach out for support.
- Do not hide from your emotions. Find appropriate methods, whether through CBT/DBT or other means, to explore and cope with them in a healthy manner.

> *Lisa:* Slowing down is an incredibly difficult concept to grasp. I did NOT want to slow down, gain weight, or decrease my exercise. What I was *actually* avoiding was the experience of discomfort. I initially thought gaining a few measly pounds and reducing exercise would get my periods back, skipping right over the discomfort part. Plenty of others have also tried this route unsuccessfully. What's the old saying, "Sometimes you win and sometimes you learn"? That was me. After this failed attempt, I let go of my "ideal" body, reached a BMI beyond what I had planned and significantly decreased my exercise—resulting in a lesson on getting comfy with the uncomfy. Five(ish) months of THAT attitude got me to where I am now—recovered.

14
Running Toward Recovery (with Steph)

During our time on the Board, we noticed there is something unique about the runners in the HA crowd. It seems to be more difficult to give up or significantly reduce the intensity of running than any other exercise. We thought that a chapter devoted to recovery for runners would be useful for those who classify themselves as such. Steph is a long-time runner and went through the process of reducing and eventually eliminating running in order to get pregnant. She shares her experiences below, including details on how she accomplished the not-so-small feat of cutting out running from her life for a while. Tina Muir is an elite runner for Great Britain who followed our Recovery Plan and cut out her running in order to regain cycles and conceive; we include some words of wisdom from her at the end of the chapter (page 185) to further help you if you are struggling with giving up your passion for the time being.

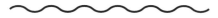

I am a runner. I love running. I love everything about running. It is my passion. I love running for fun. I love it for the opportunity to spend time with friends while hitting the open road and chatting for hours as we log mile after mile. I also love running for the competition. Whether it is a training run or goal race, I am in it to do better, push myself, and accomplish my personal goals. I care about the amount of time it takes me to complete a run and the pace at which I complete it. I train hard. I do what needs to be done. It is not a choice; it is a way of life. I go a little crazy without my runs and hate having to miss scheduled training sessions or races. I am addicted to running. I couldn't imagine my life without it. So when presented with the question of whether it was running season or baby season, I was bewildered. It is *always* running season, I thought. Now it just happens to *also* be baby season. *Right*?!

Unfortunately, if you have HA, you will likely find it cannot be both running and baby season. Or running and recovering your period season, for that matter. Running is going to have to wait. Rather, you need to sit on your bum and eat more. I cannot predict your reaction to being told to stop running in order to get your period back (or respond well to treatment), but for me it pretty much went something like this— "*Heck no*!!!!!"

When I was diagnosed with HA and told to stop running, I started a fight with the doctor right then and there in his office. I bargained, pleaded, and was downright mean and rude. Here was a professional giving me the answer to my problem and I all but stuck my tongue out at him. Turned out the doctor happened to be right; I could not both run and get pregnant. But at the time, given all I have just told you about my love and obsession with running, do you really think I just hung up my running shoes that quickly? No. Way.

So, I did what any other runner might do in the situation: I continued to run. My times got slower every day as if my body was telling me that it was no longer running season. But as frustrating as that was, I didn't care—I had a marathon to complete and I was not going to stop training. I had goals and aspirations. I had to stick with the plan. I started taking Clomid with a different doctor and told her I would reduce my running and keep it to 15 miles a week. To me this meant two miles during the week, thirteen on the weekend, and a few hardcore elliptical sessions in between. Well, neither my doctor nor my follicles thought this was such a good idea. My doctor simply stated that I was not going to get pregnant while running; my follicles showed it to me by not growing at a "normal" rate. My response was a few temper tantrums, followed by sitting on my butt and eating Oreo stuffed chocolate chip cookies (those were tasty) until I got pregnant. Actually, I was lucky and got pregnant fairly quickly after I quit running.

And today, now that I have a child of my own, I am running again. It is still my passion. I enjoy my training, I like pushing as hard as I can push, and I like beating my times. I still love running marathons. Since having my son, I have been lucky enough to run four marathons. My cycles were regular through each of them. **Because I now know how to fuel my body**

and my training appropriately. I know that I won't always beat my times, that I can't always stick to the plan, and that if I want to have another baby someday, I might have to let it be baby season over running season*. The process of eliminating running was not easy the first time, and I don't expect it to be a piece of cake if I have to do it again. Why is it still not easy?! I am recovered. I nourish my body. I take as many rest days as I might need, so why is it a big deal for me to just give up running for a while? To figure this out, let's take a look at why people are so in love (or obsessed) with running.

Love of the game. We love running for the power, strength, adrenaline, and excitement that it provides. Training for a race with friends, pushing the limits we never thought we could, and seeing times that were beyond our wildest dreams provide a high that is hard to find in other parts of life. Running offers a release. It helps with relaxation when we are angry or stressed and turns a sour mood into a good one. There are so many reasons to love running.

Identity. Do you identify yourself as a runner? Does it define who you are? Would giving it up be like losing a piece of yourself or your entire self? When I was in treatment for my eating disorder, I wrote in my notebook, "I am more than just a runner." This was a really BIG deal to me because, up until that moment, running and I were one and the same. I loved and still love the attention I get from running, whether it is someone congratulating me on a race, being impressed with my speed or distance, or asking me questions about running and how to get started. It is something I work hard at and it is something I am good at. It makes me feel special.

Running to control body size. It is often the case with HAers that running changes from something you get to do to something you have to do. When I was in the midst of my eating disorder, running was 100% something I had to do regardless of whether I was sick, tired, or hungry. Running came first because running was the answer to everything—emotional release, control, fulfillment, and most importantly, the ability to keep my weight at my self-imposed "magical number." When I was diagnosed with HA, I thought I was past all of that. I had recovered and gone months without running. But when I was told I had to gain weight and stop running, all of those same thoughts came rushing back to me and made me

---
* Upon editing this a few months after it was written, I can now tell you that I did not have to stop running the second time around and conceived two weeks before my fourth marathon.

wonder if I had ever really recovered. I thought, "Shouldn't I be able to stop running?" and "I don't run to eat; I eat to run." But it was just not that simple. I had to run or else… or else I would gain weight and the world would spiral out of control, according to the messed up society we live in.

If running (or other exercise, for that matter) is something you have to do, this is a red flag that you are mistreating your body and it is time for a wake-up call. Rather, running should be something you *want* or *get* to do. If you are running to work off what you ate and you have HA, it is very likely that you have an unhealthy relationship with food and running. Running has likely become a way to keep you "too thin for you" and is causing damage to your mind and body. When you are at this point, it is critical to stop running not only to have a baby, but to regain your health as well.

So what now? I have just laid out the reasons why it is so hard to stop running, but what good does that do? In fact, it probably makes you want to get up and go for a run, which means I am not really doing my job here. So let's move on. Now you have examined why it is hard for you to give up running, we can offer advice on how to stop for the time being. If you want, you can absolutely start running again at some point—perhaps after you regain regular cycles (although we suggest waiting for three cycles before increasing exercise)—as long as you make sure your running is fully fueled and pay attention to any effects on your cycle. Some Board members have resumed running slowly once pregnant; others have picked up running again a few weeks to months after the birth of their baby. But now? Now is recovery season.

If you love running. You can still love running even if you have to put it aside for the time being. It will still be there once you are at a healthier place to enjoy it. But it might not be enough to know that someday in the future you can return to running if you want. You are heartbroken and want comfort now! So ask yourself, why do you love running? Do you love it because you enjoy setting and accomplishing a goal? If so, what else can you do that will meet this desire? Can you throw yourself into your work? Can you find intellectually stimulating games to play instead? Can you take a class on baking, cake decorating, or playing an instrument? Can you complete a 2,000-piece jigsaw puzzle? No, these things are not the same as running. They may never give you the satisfaction you get from completing a running goal, but if they give you just enough to occupy your mind or make not running seem a little less difficult, that may be enough.

What if you love running for the release? You're in luck; there are a lot of ways to cope besides running. If you are angry, take a hot shower. If you are sad, cuddle up with your partner and watch a feel-good movie. If you are stressed, get a massage, see an acupuncturist, take a walk, or enjoy a night out with your partner or friends. There are many ways to cope. Running can seem like the *best* and *only* way, but the truth is there are other options. Maybe they aren't as good as running or maybe you'll find that you like them even more!

> **Ashley**: I actually feel less stressed and more relaxed than when I was running all the time. I think for me, it's because I don't have the stress/pressure to make sure I get my run or workout in every day. If I feel like going for a nice walk, I do, otherwise I don't worry about it!

If running is a part of your identity. There is nothing wrong with identifying yourself as a runner. If you ask a basketball player what they are, they will likely say a basketball player, but might also say man/woman/non-binary, teacher, entrepreneur, friend, you name it. The point is that you are not just a runner. There is more to you. Force yourself to remember this. Start with the basics. What is your profession? Do you have any siblings? Think of as many different possibilities as you can. It can help you realize that while being a runner is a part of you, it is only one part. This part has not gone away. Just because you cannot run at this exact moment does not mean you are not a runner. You are still a runner as well as a million other things. You have not lost any part of your identity; you are just taking a break. And maybe now is the time to change or add to the list and be a baker, reader, writer, or blogger. The sky is the limit.

> **Sophie**: You may surprise yourself and realize it is really nice to walk and notice things instead of running past them in a blur. Listen to your body! We all have different bodies, paths, and needs. Maybe look at this as a blessing in disguise—you can enjoy mornings in, time with friends and your partner, and not have to think about running at all hours and in all types of weather again. For me, I recall running in such cold I got an ice beard (what was I thinking?). Never, ever, ever again. And you have so many other qualities and virtues beyond running. You will find that part of the blessing of this process is discovering yourself again beyond ideas of being a runner, an athlete, etc. You will discover your spark again and find it worth all the runs in the world and more. Try to relax and enjoy. You will gain weight. Sorry, but that is what you need to do. But there's

> nothing to be afraid of. You will gain health, happiness, laughter, and fertility too.
>
> *Gypsy*: I wholeheartedly believe I will run again... but I believe right now my focus should be on recovering wholly, maintaining my body's trust, and finding other avenues. I need to realize that I am not in control and no matter how hard and how many times I try to take control (i.e., by going for a run), one of life's uncontrollable situations comes back to politely remind me that I'm not. When I started recovery, I went through a period of arrhythmia and heart racing—I think it was simply my heart balancing out between working its tail off to keep up with my running and learning what calming, exercise-free days needed from it. My words of advice are to love yourself and take time to truly listen to your body's needs and desires. It will take time, but slowly you'll come to realize what areas of your life need work. I've been learning that I need to focus on being completely present—not thinking about what's next or what just happened, but being completely here and now. I hope you are also able to allow yourself to love parts of your body today.

If you run to control your body size... how do you stop? Take those shoes off and don't look back. That's right, we recommend you go cold turkey. I am not going to say you are going to like it at first (in fact you are probably going to hate it), but it is worth it. You need to learn that you can eat, not exercise, and the important parts of you will not change.

Personally, even when people told me that I would be happier in the end, I still couldn't fathom being OK without my running. I loved running, I was passionate about running, but I also was still quite nervous about my body changing if I wasn't running. During these times it was important for me to remember the following. The same is true for you.

1) Gaining weight does not change my value in the world.
2) It is healthier right now to rest and eat than to do intense exercise, as that is preventing me from having my menstrual cycle.
3) I do not need to control my running or food to make me happy or help me cope.
4) I can be happy with a life that does not revolve around food and exercise.

I continued to repeat these mantras to myself. Some days it was easier than others but they helped me to make it through even the hardest days. Maybe just repeating mantras won't be enough for you. In that case, try going back to chapters 11 and 13 to choose other ideas that will provide you with skills to manage, whether it is support from a friend, talking to a therapist, or recalling your ultimate goal.

> *Tina Muir*: The rest of the world knows we as runners are crazy. We don't try to hide it, in fact, we embrace it . . . we love our sport, we are proud to call ourselves runners, and don't even get me started on the thrill of challenging yourself in a race. Except there is a minor (major) problem with running for some of us. If you are reading this book you are either missing your period entirely, or have very irregular cycles. I went nine years without a period, while I competed as a professional runner. All the while, I knew it wasn't healthy, that I needed to do something about it, but how was I supposed to stop running? Not. Happening. When doctor after doctor brushed me off with the comment of, "you just need to stop running," I would get more and more angry, "Yeah, just like that, would you like me to take off my arm and hand it to you when I do?"
>
> After I represented Great Britain and Northern Ireland in a world championship, my lifetime goal, something changed in me. I was determined to get my period back. I wasn't quite ready to stop running, but I did everything else I could. You know, all the things Google told you to do before you made the smart move of purchasing this book. Finally, about half a year later, I did stop running, after reading *No Period. Now What?* myself. Cold turkey.
>
> And it really wasn't as scary as I thought it would be. Sure, it was hard, and I did struggle with the idea of gaining weight after so many years of trying to look like the other elite runners I competed against, but I learned so much about myself and became a better person.
>
> The best part was less than a year after I stopped running, I gave birth to a beautiful baby girl, Bailey, who would be worth never running a step again for . . . but friends, I am running! I am back training, maybe not at full capacity (at this point I don't want to), and I still have my period. I won the Disney World Half Marathon in 2019, less than a year after Bailey was born, and I am up to running 70 miles a week, still breastfeeding, and I have a period! And a lot of it is thanks to the words in this book. Listen to them, they know their stuff. When I stopped running, my story went viral, even ending up in People Magazine! I became known as the Amenorrhea girl, but I was just happy to see this taboo topic getting the awareness it deserves. If you want to hear more about my story, I wrote a book about my journey to become a mother, and everything I did to get there. You can find *Overcoming Amenorrhea: Get Your Period Back. Get Your Life Back.* on Amazon (link at http://noperiod.info/resources). If this book is your manual, I can be your best friend cheering you on. Good luck, friends! I promise, it is worth it!

Summary

For many of us, running is a part of our identity. We need it whether it be for the competition, the elusive "runner's high," or to stay fit and trim. Asking a runner to give up their running is asking them to throw away a piece of their self. But, if you want to recover from HA, giving up running is a necessary piece of the puzzle for the time being.

To ease the transition, we suggest taking up different activities (e.g., knitting, walking, yoga, or volunteering) as well as recalling and coming back to your ultimate goal of recovery. We challenge you to take this step and discover a world where you can be your happiest without running. Once you have recovered your health, you *will* be able to get back to running (if you want to). But at that point, you will properly compensate for the energy you burn, take days off for your body to repair and recover, and your running will be in balance with the rest of your life rather than *being* your life.

> *Clover*: You want to know what I have? I have a big green plastic storage box full of medals and trophies, cool Clover race photos, awesome 5K T-shirts, recorded personal records, and … oh, you know what else I have? Osteoporosis and no kiddos.
>
> I've been "a runner" for over 30 years. Running is in my blood and I believe I was created to run, feeling the presence of God while doing so. I know that sounds a bit dramatic but I want to express just how big a part running played in my life because I am betting that you can empathize with my passion for it. With that said, please know that running wasn't the problem; running on empty and feeling like it was "the only outlet" was the problem. Would you believe me if I told you it was relatively easy to stop running when I finally made the decision to go all in? Being totally transparent here, it was in fact my second attempt at going all in that was easy. The first time, not so much. But when I did make the decision it was a breeze, for a few good reasons:
>
> 1) I realized I was literally killing myself—a slow self-destruction. Body systems were shutting down: my bone density was decreasing, I had chronic training injuries, random heart palpitations, etc. If running was a factor in my HA I would gladly give it up for my immediate and long-term well-being.
> 2) I knew the decision to stop running was temporary. In the grand scheme, six months to a year was a small sacrifice for the restoration of my health.
> 3) After 30 years of consistently running, not running was a mental test. And because I wanted to prove that I wouldn't be crushed mentally, I took and conquered the challenge.

Don't get me wrong, there were times I wanted to cry when my friends would talk to me about their fabulous runs and times. But really, what's the point of being consumed with those thoughts? Who gives two hoots if I am ripped and can run faster than anyone reading this book? Ha! You see, I was defined by being "a runner" and not only in my own mind but also by those who knew me (my husband, father, friends, and neighbors). While there is nothing wrong with having a reputation for being good at or committed to your sport, the problem arises when one continues to engage in spite of the adverse consequences. Running/training had become a need. It owned me and I simultaneously held onto it with a death grip (like something out of The Lord of the Rings ... "my precious"). Can you relate? If not, fantastic, but if you *can* relate and yet still don't want to make changes, I encourage you to re-read the quotes in this chapter.

P.S. Though I took over a year off from running and lifting, I can now run and train hard with my periods arriving like clockwork. Exercise doesn't own me anymore; I own it ... and hold onto it loosely!

15
Partners in Recovery

IF YOU ARE MARRIED, you and your spouse probably vowed something like "for better or for worse, in sickness and in health" during your wedding ceremony. Well, recovery from HA is one of the times in which you and your partner may rely heavily on those vows. Those of you who are not married can equally benefit from the information shared in this chapter, as it applies to all types of relationships. It is a widely held belief that successfully mediated conflict actually strengthen the bonds between people. Use the time during HA/REDS recovery and the challenges it brings as an opportunity to further cement the foundation of your relationships.

Over the years, there were many discussions on the Board about the role partners play in our journey to recovery. While writing this book, we thought about the times these well-intentioned people in our lives had a positive or less than positive impact. In an effort to get a better understanding of partners point of view, we compiled a series of 20 questions to ask the partners of our survey respondents, anonymously. Some insightful, touching responses are included throughout the remainder of this chapter.

The following information is intended for both you (although much of the first section is a recap of what you already read in chapter 5) and your significant other, or other supporters. They may want to read some or all of this book—but at a minimum, we encourage perusal of the next section, geared to equip your partner and others in your life to better support and understand you. The last section will help you to better appreciate your partners' perspective.

Our goal is to provide couples working toward HA recovery with ideas and actions that may be helpful, as well as those that may be less appreciated. Use the ideas as a starting point for understanding and conversation. For example, which suggestions would you like your partner to implement? Are there strategies either of you would *not* like put into practice?

While you each might not fully grasp the other's position, hopefully this chapter will foster more empathy, and your bond will strengthen as you continue to work on recovery.

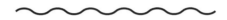

Partners, Start Here…

> *A perspective from a guy who has been there*: If you are reading this, obviously there is a problem. Perhaps your partner doesn't eat enough, works out for hours, gets angry if they miss a workout, hasn't had a period in years, and is rigid or inflexible with food, schedules, and/or activities. If you have ever made excuses for them as to why they won't eat out or go somewhere or is frequently claiming to be sick or not feeling well—keep reading. Chances are they have an issue with food (not enough) or exercise (too much) or a combination of both. I will tell you right now I won't even pretend to understand it; just like there are things about us our partners won't understand. Many of us prefer to deal with problems by finding a way to fix them, rather than talking about them. If we know "X" needs fixing, we will generally take care of it or find someone who knows how. The food and exercise issues in your partner's life need fixing: the toll they take on health and relationships is heavy and compounds with time. That being said, *they* will ultimately decide when or if they are ready to improve their health. If the choice is made to change, you can play a major role in the recovery process. If they refuse to acknowledge an issue right now—just wait. As health issues (osteoporosis, injuries, infertility, etc.) manifest themselves, hopefully the elephant in the room will be acknowledged, and a decision made to address the problem. If you are reading this book, more than likely your partner has admitted the existence of an issue and is taking steps to mitigate it. This is where you come in. The authors of this book have a tremendous amount of experiential knowledge and have spent countless hours researching HA and its recovery. In this chapter, they will give you a brief overview of HA and provide practical advice as to how best to help you help your loved one. You and

> your partner are in this together. The faster they recover, the faster you both will get on with living and moving forward. The physical damage is more than likely completely repairable, and once you are on the backside of this journey, your relationship will be stronger. Take a long game mindset and start now. – *Jim Roberts, husband of a recovered HAer*

As you are well aware, your partner is not getting a monthly period. They would like to restore menstrual cycles and are trying to find the best path to do so. What we've explained in previous chapters is that this lack of periods is probably due to a combination of stressors on the body; both physical and mental(chapters 1-3). The physical demands derive from undereating and restricting particular food groups, as well as exercise. The other side of the coin is high stress from life in general and from the "rules" associated with food restriction and overexercise. Based on Dr. Nico's experience guiding thousands through HA/REDS recovery, we've suggested an increase in both the amount and variety of food consumed, and a sharp decrease in high-intensity exercise for the time being, along with a decrease in other general life stressors (chapters 8–14). Tackling these tasks may prove difficult, particularly as many of us feel that we are most attractive and in control when we are "thin" and fit. We have to conquer a lot of fears in order to accomplish the tasks at hand. We tend to worry a lot about what you and others will think of us as our body changes and we lose some of our identity as "the fit one." We are anxious about managing stress without exercise. Most of all, we are afraid that we are going to go through this whole process and end up no better off than when we started, still with no period or no baby. We worry a lot. This brings us to your unenviable position. Your part in this process is to support your partner through the challenges being faced through the attempts to recover. You will likely find that extra TLC is needed, as well as reminders of how much you love and care for them, how attractive your partner is for reasons beyond physical appearance, and how important this endeavor is for your family and future health.

People provide advice to each other all the time: "What tires should I buy?", "Do you know a good accountant, mechanic, repairman, lawn service, lawyer?", you name it. So why not ask someone who has been a partner through the HA recovery process for suggestions? We polled the partners of those who are recovered and recovering from absent periods on a number of issues, and they shared their thoughts and advice on the recovery process. We include a number of quotes from this survey of recovery partners throughout the chapter, denoted by a "❖" symbol.

Understanding Missing Periods

Many of the partners who took our survey didn't know that being underweight (for an individual's particular body), undereating, stressed, and/or overexercising could result in the failure to menstruate and infertility. Therefore, we will take you briefly through the science behind these connections. For a more in depth understanding see chapter 5.

The body's ability to protect itself is remarkable. Much of our physiology is controlled by a small area of the brain called the hypothalamus. About the size of an almond, this region takes information from all over the body—how much body fat we have, how much we are eating (including the amount of fat, protein, and carbs), how much stress we are experiencing, and how much energy we are expending—and determines how much energy is available. If there is enough energy, and stress levels are minimal, the body can keep doing what it's doing. If there is not enough energy, or stress (including, perhaps, stress from exercise) is high, the hypothalamus shuts down various systems. Since fat storage and reproduction (i.e., menstrual cycles) are both unnecessary for survival, they are shut down first. Many take pride in decreasing body fat because that is what society has influenced us to believe is attractive. However, reduced body fat also decreases some classically female features: breasts, rear end, and thighs—along with our period. Our bodies don't want us to reproduce when energy is scarce, so periods grind to a halt.

There is more to this condition than the cessation of periods. The drop in hormones brings other side effects, including declines in sex drive and lubrication (yeah, sorry 'bout that), temperature regulation (ever notice that your partner is cold all the time?), hair and nail growth, bone strength (which won't always be evident until later in life), and more, including reduced athletic performance[1]. The side effects and health implications are vast.

Contrary to expectations, all of this can happen no matter what a person's absolute weight is. That bears repeating—it is very possible to lose one's period/experience REDS at **any** BMI. *An ongoing energy deficit, exercise, and/or stress can be the driver regardless of actual weight.* The technical term for all this is "hypothalamic amenorrhea" (HA): not getting a period because the hypothalamus (control center of the brain) has stopped communicating with the ovaries, which are therefore unable to grow eggs that produce estrogen, as they should.

So what to do about this? Depending on the particular combination of factors that caused your partner's HA (chapters 1–3), they will need to accomplish some or all of the following to regain cycles/health:

- A long-term increase in calories consumed to satisfy the hypothalamus that there is no longer an energy deficit; will most likely result in some degree of weight gain.
- A decrease in exercise amount and intensity.
- Elimination of major sources of stress.
- Reduction in restrictive thoughts and behaviors surrounding food choices and exercise to decrease overall stress.

Are you beginning to grasp why this is not a quick and easy journey?

Can You Fix This?

As a supporter, most of you will want to fix your mate's HA problem. Therein lies the dilemma. You cannot fix HA for your partner, but they certainly can. In many cases, when they complain to you about weight, fears, or the discomfort recovery entails, they are not looking for a solution, but rather for commiseration. Often, a simple "Yeah, it stinks," "It's *not* fair," or "I am proud of you" combined with a hug are all they are looking for. You can say a bit more if it feels right to you—such as you appreciate what they're doing, or notice how hard they are working at recovery. But unless they ask specifically for ideas for how to proceed, tread carefully on going further than just being supportive.

> ❖ I couldn't fix it, "but always made it clear that I was there to help her through it!"
> ❖ "This was the hardest part as I like to solve problems and help people, but only she could help herself."
> ❖ "Men are fixers. We are going to try and give our wives advice and make ignorant suggestions on what to do..."
> ❖ "Be patient. She needs you to listen to her and encourage her. Don't try to fix it, she is fixing it. Support her unconditionally, she will do the right thing."
> ❖ "I would not attempt to offer solutions when she continuously complained about how difficult things were and would just acknowledge that it's difficult."

"Skinny Jeans" Aren't Going to Fit Anymore

In order for your partner to address HA in a healthy and realistic way, they are probably going to gain some weight while eating more to refuel bodily systems. Depending on one's starting weight, the amount gained can be significant, which can be scary given our society's (unwarranted and unjust) abhorrence of those in larger bodies, and sometimes you might feel these emotions too. In general, the partners who took our survey expressed an appreciation for their mate's added weight, but in a few cases, concerns were expressed about "going too far." We would like to put those fears to rest. Our bodies are remarkably good at determining their own optimal size. We can achieve such freedom when we allow our body to lead rather than forcing it to be a size determined by modeling agencies, fashion designers, and Photoshop. It may or may not be a size that is lauded by society, but whatever it is, our experience has been that people experiencing HA/REDS and their supporters find the benefits far surpass any negatives. It is also important to recognize how much the focus our society has on appearance harms us all: financially (convincing us to buy products to "fix" our flaws), emotionally (constantly feeling negative about ourselves based on comparison to others or unrealistic standards), and clearly physically (hypothalamic amenorrhea for us, yo-yo dieting and its negative consequences for millions of others).

Regardless, your mate is likely going to have a difficult time with the idea of getting bigger. This can be more challenging if they are starting the journey in a body that is not visibly underweight. Not only because it can feel like throwing away all the work put in to get to their (/society's) desired weight, but also because of the continually reinforced messages that if we are not thin, we are not attractive/healthy/lovable. Your partner may be focused on increased belly and arm fat, going on a daily hunt for new cellulite, and generally looking for any possible flaws. However, you and others will notice positive changes instead, such as looking less drawn, healthier, and more vibrant. In our survey we asked respondents if their partners with HA appreciated hearing sentiments about weight gain. The common theme among the responses was those working on recovery had a hard time believing any positive feedback, but that it certainly helped them to stay the course. However, there were a few folks who mis-interpreted the well-intended comments negatively; others preferred not receiving any comments on their appearance at all. In such cases, more generalized support on lifestyle changes and non-physical benefits was helpful. The more you can reinforce that you see and appreciate your partner for way more than what they look like, the better!

Ideas to Help with Accepting Weight Gain

Verbal encouragement in the form of well-meaning compliments about physical attributes can be distorted, so we encourage focusing on intangible qualities (strong will, intelligent, reliable, flexible, motivated) and character traits (kind, selfless, trustworthy). Our survey asked if there was anything partners of those with HA found particularly helpful in providing support through the weight gain challenges. The following will give you a few ideas.

Positive feedback. Purposely gaining weight while reducing exercise can occupy our minds with critical thoughts more than ever. Encouraging comments from you, that are not appearance based or focused, can go a long way toward counteracting that negativity. Noting and appreciating the change in behaviors like added flexibility, new food choices, eating experiences, enjoying more time together without exercise, etc., can be motivating. The more you reinforce the benefits of recovery, the more likely the new habits are to stick around for the long term. In our poll, 80% of partners found expressing appreciation for positive changes in habits to be helpful. It might be worth trying a few approaches and using the response you receive to determine if you continue or not.

- ❖ "I remember commenting that she was laughing more often during recovery."
- ❖ "I kept saying I would love her no matter what weight or size she was, because she's so much more than her appearance."
- ❖ "Tell her about the good things she is doing for herself and the both of you as a couple. If she seems to relapse, ask why and try to talk through it."
- ❖ "Any mention of looking a lot better or buying new clothes to her meant she was 'too large.' So I tried more to comment on her new, healthier gym and eating habits."
- ❖ "If I was to go through the process of recovery with my wife again I would keep reassuring her that what she is doing is healthy!"
- ❖ "She likes when I recognize positive changes in habits."

Encouragement with eating. Sometimes it can be hard to purchase or order "forbidden" foods that are not on our daily menu, but if someone else goes to the store or makes the suggestion, we can begin to entertain the thought of getting out of our comfort zone and learn to enjoy the experience. There may be times where your mate decides or agrees to have a certain food, but mentally is still questioning the choice. Be aware of that mindset and keep reassuring them that they're making great decisions and it is the right thing to do. Other ideas include eating new foods together; going to nice restaurants; distractions before, during, and after eating; and perhaps even removing nutrition labels…

- ❖ "I suggested drinking milk shakes and eating more ice cream. Mmmm… ice cream. I gladly offered to suffer through her recovery by eating ice cream with her."
- ❖ "Just providing her with whatever I could do. If she wanted a Blizzard from DQ, I knew that was hard for her to ask… so I would jump to it as quickly as I could before she changed her mind."
- ❖ "This was not easy. I tried to remind her to find some things that were fun to eat or drink that would typically not be on her menu."

Support when buying new clothes. Having the waistband of too-tight pants cut into flesh all day long can be a constant reminder of the added weight. Buying better fitting clothes makes it easier to feel comfortable, push the weight gain to the back of our minds, and just live in our body. We recommend stretchy pants, skirts, and flowy tops that can double as first trimester clothes, if you are hoping for pregnancy. Making a suggestion to buy new clothes can be dicey, though; it might be better to wait and let your partner bring it up, then support the idea gently.

- ❖ "My wife hated the idea that her entire wardrobe would not fit and she would have nothing to wear. Every penny spent on new clothes was helpful."
- ❖ "Oftentimes, especially the clothing encouragement, she didn't want to hear any of it. She hates buying clothes for this season and when I tried to be supportive she preferred to not hear it at all."
- ❖ "Regularly telling her how good she looked as she gained weight back."
- ❖ "I encouraged her to go out and buy clothes that fit better right away. As she gained weight, her clothes didn't fit and she felt uncomfortable. When she went out and bought clothes that fit her again, she seemed to feel better about herself."
- ❖ "Shopping for new clothes in a bigger size was very, very hard for her. I went with her and helped find a lot of outfits that she looked great in and, more importantly, that felt comfortable."

Discussion of the ultimate goals. Getting pregnant and restoring long-term health are just about as worthwhile as goals come. Sometimes remembering the purpose behind the choices being made can help us to accept the temporary discomfort of both gaining weight and cutting exercise. Keep reminding your partner of these goals, regularly letting them know that they are doing an incredible job in working to achieve them.

- "I think that what finally sank in was that if she wanted to live the life she wanted, which included having amazing healthy babies, she would need to change her actions. I also let her know on a continual basis that she would be fine gaining weight to reinforce that even more. I think ultimately though it was that she knew she would not have healthy children if she did not gain and that wasn't fair to them or herself."
- "She stopped exercising first and this created more time for us. She then slowly began to be able to eat out and at friends' houses which opened up our social lives. She started to become joyful again as she started to eat more calories. She is so much more pleasant to be around."
- "Talk about the end result; focus on having a baby, something we both really wanted."
- "She had the rest of her life to work out and now it was time to rest her body."
- "Once my wife understood more of the science behind the issue, she bought into the concepts and things were much better. I periodically reminded her why she was decreasing exercise—for her long-term health—and how important it was to add kids to our family."

Challenges with Decreasing Exercise

Every HAer is different, but for the majority of us who exercise, cutting down on our workouts is harder than eating more (although not tougher than gaining weight). In many cases we use exercise as stress relief, and sometimes to "allow" ourselves to eat more in addition to controlling our weight. It can be difficult to decrease our workout time or intensity because many of us truly enjoy the way exercise energizes and strengthens our bodies. Or perhaps we are driven by a competitive spirit (even if just competing against our own personal records or goals) or appreciate the admiration we receive from others. So even when we know that cutting down on what we are doing will probably help us recover more quickly, it can take a while for us to come around to the idea that our exercise may be hindering our recovery. It is important for you to know that it is unusual for cycles to return while continuing to perform high-intensity exercise. Therefore, a drastic reduction or complete cessation of strenuous exercise is essential during the recovery process. As we have said, putting this into practice is hard. Support from you can really help ease the anxiety. Some suggestions on what others supporting their partners through HA recovery found helpful include:

Expressing empathy and support. We've already talked about the idea of positive feedback as far as weight gain—the same is true for cutting out exercise. Even if you don't completely relate, letting your mate know that you realize these are difficult changes being made, and continuing to express your appreciation for their commitment will go a long way toward helping them feel more comfortable with the reduced exercise.

> ❖ "Empathetically letting her know I realized how frustrating it must have been to not get to exercise as she wanted, but that I greatly appreciated and valued her sacrifice."
> ❖ "I tell her how proud I am of the sacrifice she's making for me and our family. For people who aren't active, they think of exercise as a sacrifice or a burden. For those that are really active—as she was—not working out is brutally hard."
> ❖ "I walked with her as an alternative form of exercise."
> ❖ "I took her on vacations away from the gym and made sure we did something "active" when I was able to get her to not go to the gym."
> ❖ "Letting her know that she was more than her exercise habits."

Finding other ways to reduce stress. Many use exercise as a pressure relief valve, a time to turn off the hamster wheel of thoughts in our head and focus on something else. Without exercise, that little hamster can be hard to tame; you can help by encouraging your partner to give lighter activities a try, as well as doing what you can to reduce other stressors—perhaps doing yoga or meditation together, for example.

> ❖ "Realizing that without running, her outlet for stress was limited, and looking for places to reduce stress in other areas (helping with dishes, cleaning, etc.)."

- ❖ "Expressing to her that I want her to feel good but take it easy while trying to recover. I encouraged the elliptical* instead of running. Running was too hard on her body."
- ❖ "Find alternative, less impactful ways to exercise."

Moderating your own activity. As challenging as reducing exercise is for those with HA, standing by while you go to the gym or out for a run is worse. That is not to say that you shouldn't go, but be mindful not to flaunt your exercise. For example, consider adjusting your routine to go at different times, so that your partner doesn't have to witness you exercising every day while they can't.

- ❖ "I just didn't push her to work out with me and tried to be supportive without being annoying about it. She didn't want to dwell on her decreased activity and I tried not to make a big deal about it."
- ❖ "Exercise was something we often did together. Not doing so has been tough, much more for her than for me. I miss our runs and my workout partner but believe what we are doing is for the best."

Experiencing Life

- ❖ "Go out to restaurants and have a good time. Order appetizers, dessert, and go for the full rack of ribs. Make her laugh. Conquer something together. *Taking emphasis off appearance* and having fun with the woman you fell in love with will make weight gain for HA recovery an insignificant concern for both of you."

Now here is something you can *do*. The more you can drag your partner out of the hole they want to hide in, the better. Spend more time with friends and enjoy activities together. They can learn a lot: first of all, that you are not ashamed to be seen with them (an illogical fear, but sometimes present nonetheless), which can be a big confidence booster; second, that despite thoughts that others will notice the weight gain, the reality is most people tend to be more preoccupied with the visit or themselves or the million other things on their mind than anyone else's appearance; third, there are many fun, enjoyable activities that can take the place of exercising; and finally, distracting with other pursuits that take the focus off weight and exercise makes the process easier.

Some ideas for activities might include getting to know the place where you live a bit better, going camping, learning an instrument, singing, taking

---

* Note: this is not necessarily the recommendation of the authors unless the elliptical workout is low intensity, equivalent to walking.

a cooking class together (with the added bonus of trying your dishes), exploring local museums, going on a vacation, and visiting with friends and family. If there has been something you wanted to try together, now is a great time to give it a shot. See this time as an opportunity you have been awarded to really have fun and enjoy yourselves together, making the most of what life has to offer you.

> ❖ "We took a vacation where she was able to see that seven days without the gym didn't 'kill' her like she thought! After that vacation she walked only."
> ❖ "We went out to restaurants more often. Had more date nights together."

Seeking and Encouraging Outside Help

Many of us pride ourselves on being strong and capable. We like to think that we can do anything we put our minds to; often we can, but this also leads to difficulties in asking for help, even when needed. If you don't feel like the support you are offering your partner is making a dent, another option is to seek additional help. This can include encouraging them to spend time with friends who can help guide through the emotions being experienced, to online support groups or blogging, to more formal support such as a therapist who specializes in disordered eating or infertility. It might be that you go to couples counseling if you are having a difficult time communicating and understanding each other, or it might mean that one or both of you go separately. Needing help doesn't make either of you less of a spouse or a person; rather, you've come up against a situation neither of you is trained to handle. Getting guidance from someone who does have training and experience is often a wise choice.

> ❖ "Get her parents or friends involved. She will have bad days. It will be hard on you. You will not always know what to say or do and sometimes there is nothing to do but listen. Know that she is under a lot of stress and that this is a HUGE deal and very scary for her. When my wife was having a hard/emotional day, I would let her mom or a close friend know so they could call her and be there for her too. I wouldn't tell her I instigated the call, but it did seem to help to have somebody, especially another female, to listen and empathize. Moms speak 'woman' a lot better than guys ever will."
> ❖ "Be patient, forgiving, and supportive. It's really hard to listen to this all the time, but 10 times harder for our partners to get through it. I would also encourage you to talk to others (not your partner). I

was surprised by how many other men I know who went through similar challenges. We need an outlet too; otherwise our partner will feel the frustration and that will not help them recover."

- ❖ "Encourage her to seek advice from and form relationships with others going through the same thing. The Board and other outlets are essential to crossing that final obstacle to realizing they're not alone and there is hope. As much as we as partners want to be there and help, there are some things we just can't relate to. The emotional, physiological, and hormonal obstacles involved in overcoming HA can simply not be fully understood by those not experiencing it. It's important for both sides to realize this."
- ❖ "It's OK for her to find support outside of your relationship. Doctors, therapists, and social workers are trained to treat these issues. Let her know that you're there for her every step of the way."

What Not to Say or Do...

Along with the support and help that you provide, there may be times when less is more. Unfortunately, there are approaches that can alienate your spouse/partner and drive wedges of misunderstanding between you. The principal way is by invalidating their feelings, which can result from rejecting, diminishing, making light of, or even ignoring sentiments. Whether they are rational or not, it is hard to control our emotions, and being told that we are silly for feeling a particular way does not make us feel the emotion any less; in fact, not being understood adds to the frustration. It is important you recognize that there may be times when your partner will be overwhelmed, sad, aggravated—you name it—about situations or perceived feelings that you just won't understand. For example, they might talk about being in a funk after a seemingly insignificant (to you) weight gain. Recognize that while you might not comprehend the "switch" of emotion being turned on, it is their way of working through this. One man said a mistake he made was "Telling her to just eat. I didn't realize it was more complicated than that"

In general, your partner might express more emotion than you are used to or are comfortable with. This can be a result of hormones. Or, more likely, it could be a reaction to no longer being able to use food restriction and exercise to manage negative feelings. Without these coping skills, we must search for new healthy ways to deal with varied moods, and surrendering to the emotions is part of the process.

The Long Haul...

The HA recovery process can be slow going (or seem like it). During this time, there are occasions in which people become impatient with their mate and/or the recovery journey. Make no mistake: health restoration is a marathon, not a sprint. Seriously, think double overtime and extra innings. Your mate did not get HA overnight and won't overcome it overnight. Patience is a virtue and the long game mindset is vital in overcoming the HA challenge. Remember this when frustration sets in (yours and theirs). Recognize that you may adjust more quickly than your partner does. It's always easier to acclimate to a new situation as an outsider, so you might quickly get used to the newer version of your partner who exercises less and eats more, and inhabits a somewhat different body. Just because these changes have started happening and are becoming normality for you, this may still be far from the case for them. It's quite possible that they are doing things differently, but feeling like an alien in their own body and still attached to old ways. Actions may change well before mindset catches up, and so the new habits may come into play whilst your partner still feels extreme angst and difficulty with it all. Be patient. Be tolerant. Be kind. And remember that this can be a long journey, and though they may be driving forward, the finish line may still be a while off.

- ❖ "I listened to the complaining, the fear, and the anxiety every day. A lot of tears. Each time I would patiently remind her why she was doing this, encourage her, and support her. I had to be the voice of reason because there was so much irrational fear during the recovery process. Don't lose your temper and just tell her to forget it and do what she wants."
- ❖ "Many times she became overwhelmed with anxiety about gaining weight, usually on a day where she didn't go to the gym. During times when we were supposed to be having fun, she would feel guilty and cry as we ate; I would just hold her and listen. I would listen about how scared she was of getting larger. And it would be the guilt from not working out that would trigger this, or if she saw she gained weight on the scale. I'd tell her—I would swear up and down—that she needed to. That she needed to rest. She needed balance."
- ❖ "The biggest challenge as a partner is to maintain a healthy relationship day to day yet at the same time not accept the controlled eating and over exercise. It is too easy to fall silent for the sake of harmony. Silence leads to resentment and misery long term. Stating

> the truth about my partners HA worked well when I could get alongside her and show that I understood the temptations and pull of HA. We could then slowly make changes to her daily eating patterns. (The everyday eating patterns are the most important to change and adjust in my view). I also needed patience. Change happens slowly. The wife I now have is more loving, thoughtful and caring for others than before she had HA. We have a beautiful child and having seen my wife blossom and become such an amazing mother is truly mind blowing. My wife is a better person for having gone through HA and recovered. I thank God for HA and the friends and support she has received to recover from it and the person she has now become."

Parting Thoughts for Partners

> That's probably way more information than you thought you needed or wanted. Let's face it, HA is not something many of us are even aware of to start with, but it has a profound impact on our lives. Hopefully the authors have provided some insight as to what is actually going on with your partner and your potential role in their recovery. Obviously there is not a one-size-fits-all approach here, but rather a buffet of suggestions as to how to support your mate as they seek to restore health. We cannot overemphasize the fact that this is a process, not an event. A process that, once complete, will strengthen and solidify your relationship for the rest of your lives. — *Jim Roberts, husband of a recovered HAer*

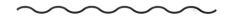

For Those With HA: Thoughts From Your Partner

All right, now back to those actually experiencing HA/REDS. We asked some questions of our partners in Lisa's survey that you might find interesting. The survey was completely anonymous, so we are confident that the answers are truthful. Hopefully they will help lessen some of your anxiety about your mate's reaction to what you need to do to recover from HA, and give you more confidence that when your partner compliments you, they really do mean it.

Do Ya Think I'm Sexy?

If Rod Stewart wondered about the physical attraction back in the day, why wouldn't we question it while we are letting go of the things we felt kept us attractive and sexy (weight control and exercise)? We asked in our survey, "Did you find your partner more or less attractive as she gained weight to recover from HA?" While this question may sound superficial (it is), nonetheless we asked it because it is a common concern. We know intellectually that our appeal is not contingent upon our appearance, but our culture has convinced us that size X is beautiful and anything bigger is not, messed up as that is. However, when we asked partners this question, the answers were exactly what we expected: all of the survey respondents selected either "found her more attractive" or that "the question [was] ridiculous." But our favorite response to this question was, "My actual answer is that I found her just as attractive as before. Seriously, why was this not an option?" The following remarks are from others describing their feelings about their partner's appearance during HA recovery:

- "The extra (lots of) pounds weren't overtly noticeable and just made for a healthier look. Also, this is a sexist question, as attractiveness should not be defined by appearance. Her personality did not change through her recovery from HA."
- "She is more attractive and I think has more of a sense of humor."
- "I am a butt guy and liked her larger rear end! Her recovery made her take a step back and realize how unhealthy she was and she got a better mindset because of it."
- "She looked sooooooo much better with more weight. The only problem was as soon as she was just starting to look better she would lose weight again. So frustrating!"
- "She lost a lot of weight when we got married. I was glad to see it back on."

We hope you're getting the picture here. Your partner is *not* as worried about weight gain and your appearance as you are, and really does think that you look at least as attractive, if not more so.

> *Melli*: I won't lie: it still feels hard some days to see my new self in the mirror (the bloaty PMS weekend I had did not help!); but I'm slowly realizing that I see something completely different than the rest of the world sees. My husband and I were shopping this weekend and I tried on a coat in a size that used to be "large" for me—and almost had a meltdown when it fit. I started grousing about how demoralizing it was, and my kind, sweet, patient, loving husband actually got mad and walked away. That stopped me in my tracks. I apologized for being so annoying, and he said he wasn't mad on his own behalf, but "I'm just trying to protect you from

yourself." He can't understand what I see in the mirror and like many of our partners, thinks I look better now than I did before. So ... trust those wise men and women, because they are so so smart (they chose us, didn't they?!), and they love us when we aren't very good at loving ourselves.

More Aspects of Recovery Appreciated by our Mates

Now that you have read the many quotes from other partners, you might begin to trust yours when you receive compliments. And, like most of those who took our survey, your mate will probably also appreciate your reduction in time at the gym and decrease in obsession with eating and exercising. The other changes in personality that often come along with the relaxation of our rules and habits are likewise noted and valued. For example, while our ability to maintain schedules, routine, and order, is often appreciated, some of us HAers took those attributes too far. We increased the intensity of it all—and order evolved into rigid behaviors. Here are some of our partners' words on what they welcomed about these aspects of recovery:

- ❖ "EVERYTHING. She is pretty much the person that I fell in love with so long ago (about 12 years). She even seems to be a better person today than she was when I met her; she seems more caring and loving to me and everyone else in her life now than the three or four years of the dark days."
- ❖ "She became happier and more fun to be around."
- ❖ "Her concept of what constitutes 'a big deal' changed dramatically. It helped put all the other things in life in perspective. She became more laid back which has increased the joy in our relationship."
- ❖ "Sexual response to me was better, like how it was when we first met before she lost weight. I think she became nicer, probably because she stopped being hungry all the time."
- ❖ "The relaxing of her 'rules' and return of her true personality."
- ❖ "She had more energy and didn't stress as much about not going to gym or what she ate."

Aspects That Partners Find Frustrating

Recovery isn't all sunshine and roses for us, and the same is true for those supporting us. Some of the aggravation stems from the same aspects that exasperate us; like not knowing how long the process will take. And yes, there is also some discontent when we are unable to let go of some of our HA habits and tendencies. What can you do about these issues? It helps to be mindful of those that can be problematic, and perhaps to make a conscious effort, now that you are aware of how these behaviors are perceived, to respond or act differently.

Unknowns and uncertainty. Our supporters would love to be able to tell us: "Well, if you gain X pounds this will all go away"; "Give it four (or five or eight) months and you'll be cycling again"; and most of all, if kids are a goal, they want to be able to say, "We'll have a baby this time next year"—because all of this is easier if you know that it will work out as you hope. Unfortunately, none of us knows what the future holds, which is just as annoying for our partners as for us. (Although we are confident that our statistics on recovery and what you will read about getting pregnant will help to ease your mind on these questions.) Some frustrations expressed included:

> ❖ "One tough thing about HA is that you don't know what the magic number is. If she knew, for example, that she needed to gain 10 pounds exactly, I think that would've been easier. But not knowing if it was 5 or 10 or 15 or whatever was really difficult. At first, she tried to inch up really slowly. It wasn't until she went "all in" that she started to recover. In reality, it wasn't a lot more weight, but she had to stop trying to manage it pound by pound for it to work. I think she'd often gain a couple of pounds, stop and say, 'This is probably enough; I'll see how this works out.' Then it wouldn't, she'd gain one or two more, and the cycle would repeat. Letting go of this way of thinking was hard, but ultimately it was necessary for her to recover."
>
> ❖ "I wanted the recovery to happen overnight. It took me a while to accept that it was a process."
>
> ❖ "It was an anxious time full of uncertainty as to whether the weight gain was going to work. The constant questions and worries were frustrating because we were having the same conversations over and over again."

Lingering HA tendencies. As we've mentioned, our partners love the new flexibility and relaxation of rules around eating and exercise that often accompany HA recovery. They tend to experience irritation when some of those old habits are hard to get rid of—just one more reason to go all in! Our partners were most vexed by:

- "… how hard it was for me to understand how she perceived her body, and why it was so hard to allow herself to gain weight. I am 100% sympathetic, but not understanding the mindset made it tough for me, and angry with our culture that 'teaches' the thin-is-great mindset she was dealing with."
- "… her seeing the recovery as a means to an end—to get pregnant. Recovery was short-lived and not permanent."
- "Her calorie counting. At first she wouldn't put the app down that counted calories. Once the app was gone, it was easy."
- "Rigidity with food choices and unwillingness to try something new."
- "The difficulty of changing her eating habits, which didn't really kick in until she got pregnant."

Negative self-image and low self-esteem. Our partners fell in love with us as whole people, not just what we look/ed like on the outside. They also focus a lot more on who we are as people than what we look like—why can't we do the same? No matter how much your body changes, or how little you exercise, you are still the person that your mate, family, and friends love. So do the best you can to love yourself as much as they do. It aggravates our supporters to no end when we fixate on how bad we think we look, rather than all the positives they see (inside and out). We have suggested to them that it is not helpful to invalidate your feelings by insinuating that you are being silly or irrational in your emotions. By the same token, brushing off and not believing their compliments makes them feel the same way. For example, HA recovery supporters were perturbed by:

- "Her not truly believing or perhaps perceiving her body how I see it with my eyes. Media reinforcement of celebrities that are clearly suffering from HA but apparently 'healthy' and 'fertile.' Photoshopping is the devil!"
- "How hard she was on herself. How she always thought she was "fat" (and that being larger was "bad") and so afraid of losing her abs and muscle tone."
- "The initial failure to believe or trust when I would say I didn't care if she put on some weight."
- "Her not accepting my compliments or putting herself down."
- "Her concern about what other people would think of her body. Never believing in herself."

Relationship concerns. Finally, despite what we may think to the contrary, our partners are invested in their relationships with us and care about maintaining them. Through all of this, connecting as a couple is more important than ever, particularly if you are hoping to conceive. Keep in mind that your mate is likely good at keeping a lid on feelings and may not know how to communicate emotions to you. One commented, "Understand that your partner feels just about every single emotion, heartache, and disappointment along the way that you do." Particularly regarding trying to have a baby, it was noted that, "Infertility can also be tough on the guys, although we have it easier than the women. I don't think you need to do anything, except to acknowledge that we hurt too." One great suggestion was:

> ❖ "Try to communicate to your partner more about how to be supportive, and maybe even gently explain when the attempt being made isn't working."

Parting Thoughts

Why are we so unable to love and accept ourselves? Why should society set the standard we need to follow in order to be acceptable? And why do we continue to compare ourselves instead of respecting and acknowledging the truths spoken by those who love us? These attitudes are thieves of our joy and ability to self-love. We not only steal from ourselves, but from our partners too. These wonderful people truly love us beyond the physical or abilities, beyond what is seen. Now it is time for us to do the same: to love and value ourselves.

16
Recovering Natural Cycles

Ashley: My period ended up coming *full* force yesterday morning! I didn't know what to do because I didn't have any tampons on hand! After rummaging through a bunch of purses and backpacks, I finally found an old one. Then I rushed to the store to buy some. My husband and I are going out to eat to celebrate and then to a basketball game afterward. Anyway, I'm still planning to eat as I have been and keep my exercise at low intensity until I get pregnant. I want to make sure my cycles continue!

Steph: Getting my period naturally for the first time in over 10 years was more exciting than when I first got it at the age of 12. At 12, I was a bit embarrassed and did not want to tell people. At 27, I couldn't wait to scream it from the rooftops and pretty much did! The day after getting my period, my husband and I were eating lunch with our friends at temple (probably about five couples at the table) when I beamed and announced to the group, "Today I am a woman. I got my period." I couldn't stop smiling as everyone congratulated me on my unexpected announcement.

Lacey: I had to come and update everyone—my period arrived today! I guess my conclusion that I ovulated was correct. Right now it's really light, more like spotting, but I have cramps and think it might amount to more. I'm so excited to see this day come! Now the real fun starts—baby making!

Stephanie J: Well HA I think I am beginning to kick your butt. I started to spot today, this is NATURAL period #2! I could not have done this without all of you lovely ladies and of course the extra 30 pounds LOL. So now every time I go to the restroom I do a little dance.

The Recovery Plan—Changing Your Habits and Your Life

> *Priscilla*: Getting my period last night stung, but today I am celebrating!!! To think where I was just six months ago, not to mention the last seven years of my life—it's astounding. I am very proud of myself for putting aside my desire to have what I once thought was the "perfect" body... I've come to the realization that this body that I have now is MY perfect body. It's the body that's finally going to allow me to have what I desire the most!!"

After you have implemented the Recovery Plan—been eating more for a while, cut out high-intensity exercise, worked at conquering negative thoughts and behavior patterns, and allowed your body some time to re-equilibrate—you will notice improvements. We've talked a lot about what these might be: changes like feeling warmer, noticing hair and nail growth, increased energy, etc. Other signs more directly herald the return of your menstrual cycle; specifically changes in cervical mucus that result from increased hormones as your body progresses toward ovulation (chapter 17). A week or two after one of these episodes of increased wetness, you may be very pleasantly surprised by the sight of blood!

> *Nico*: About eight months after I went off the Pill, I went on a three-week vacation to South Africa, where I had lived until I was 10. I spent lots of time with relatives, played a couple rounds of golf, and visited tourist attractions. My sister went too, and enjoyed telling all our family about her new pregnancy. Sitting through each announcement with a smile on my face when it was something I wanted so desperately for myself was not easy, but I managed. Finally, at my aunt and uncle's house, just after they had been told my sister's news, I noticed that my lower back was hurting, which usually happens the day before my period. I excused myself, went to the bathroom, and lo and freaking behold, BLOOD!! I walked downstairs with the biggest grin on my face. A grin that no one else can quite understand. So it really was true: I needed to eat more and sit on my rear end. No hockey, no weight lifting, no biking; all I was doing was playing golf and a bit of walking. I wrote on my blog the next day, "Don't know whether it's that I'm less stressed, barely exercising, or eating like a pig on vacation, but good old AF [Aunt Flo, my period] showed her face yesterday!"

It is like hitting the HA recovery jackpot the first time you ovulate all on your own, and getting your period is even more incredible. These results are a testament to all the changes you've made and the hard work you've put in, and it makes every second of feeling crappy worth it. The sight of blood when you go to the bathroom is confirmation of being healthy again!! Most of us revel in buying pads, tampons, or the more environmentally friendly cups or reusable pads for the first time in years, and even feeling cramps can provoke jubilation.

The initial euphoria of your hard work coming to fruition is often followed by a time of more questions: What can you expect from your cycles? Will they be "normal" right away? If not, how long will it take until they are regular? Can you start eating less and exercising more now that you're "working"? *When will you get pregnant?*? The experiences of others can allay some concerns and provide you with realistic expectations for what might happen over the next few weeks or months.

To begin, we will talk a bit about the signs that your first ovulation and period are imminent. After that, we will give you an idea of what to expect from your new natural cycles, and about potential modifications to your diet and exercise habits. We'll also discuss methods you can use to track your cycles, but part 3 will provide much more detail on what you should know when trying to conceive.

The Return of Your Cycles

It's been a while since we have discussed what goes on in our bodies during a menstrual cycle, so we will start with a quick refresher: As your hypothalamus wakes up, it will start to send out more frequent pulses of gonadotropin-releasing hormone (GnRH), which causes your pituitary gland to make more follicle-stimulating hormone (FSH) and luteinizing hormone (LH). This in turn begins the process of egg growth and maturation (chapter 5). One follicle will usually take the lead; as it grows, it starts to secrete estradiol (E_2), which causes changes in your body that aid in fertility.

It is useful to know that you will most likely ovulate before you get your first period. So if you pay attention to your fertile signs that we will describe here and in chapter 17, you may catch your first ovulation and get pregnant without ever having a period. It happens!

The most obvious sign that your E_2 is rising (i.e., a follicle is growing), is cervical mucus. The E_2 (and other hormones) cause an increase in amount and change in consistency of the fluid that is in your uterus and cervix. These alterations make the fluid more conducive to the meeting of sperm and egg. When there is no follicular growth happening, cervical mucus (CM) is sparse and either creamy or sticky in consistency. When E_2 initially rises, CM becomes more plentiful and runny. As the lead follicle matures, the amount of CM continues to increase, in addition to the consistency becoming almost like a raw egg white. There is often enough that you will notice it in your underwear; or if you dab at your vulva (area around your vaginal opening) after a bowel movement, it will be apparent on the toilet paper. If you pinch some CM between your thumb and forefinger and then separate your fingers, the fluid will stretch between them. This is referred to as egg white cervical mucus (EWCM), and it is often copious just before ovulation (although not for everyone).

Other ways to predict impending ovulation include checking cervical position and/or using ovulation predictor kits (OPKs—urine test strips that measure LH levels). Then ovulation can be confirmed by taking your temperature on a daily basis. Each of these approaches will be further explained in chapter 17.

In addition, be aware that as you work toward recovery it is common to experience multiple "patches" (a few days in a row) of EWCM before you actually ovulate. You might notice these patches about 14 days apart as your recovery solidifies. Why? Two weeks is the time frame in which follicles transition from the pre-ovulatory to ovulatory stage[1]. At the start of a normal cycle, there are quite a few small follicles in your ovary (approximately 10 to 20). As your FSH increases, these follicles begin to grow. Eventually one will push forward faster than the others and become "dominant"; this follicle then secretes additional hormones that stop the development of the others. Maturation completes, LH surges, and the egg ovulates.

What often happens as we are recovering, however, is that the wave gets started, but our hypothalamus is not yet able to follow through with the LH surge. When this occurs, the dominant follicle disappears and the whole process starts over again[2]. In some cases, it can take three to four waves of follicular recruitment and patches of EWCM—each about two weeks apart—before ovulation finally transpires. Some people also notice EWCM consistently for weeks at a time during recovery. If you are noticing EWCM, this is a *great* sign that you are on your way to recovery and a natural cycle! In addition, if you use OPKs regularly you might find that the line indicating your LH level fluctuates over time; this can be associated with the follicular waves. Some find that the test line on their OPKs gets darker as ovulation approaches—darkest a day or two before the actual event. Others see essentially no second line on the OPK until one day the test is blaringly positive.

> *Devon*: If you are getting a bunch of EWCM, you could just be gearing up to ovulate. Most here on the Board seem to have patches of it before

> getting their period ... it might just take longer for your body to get back in gear.
>
> *Lindsey W*: I regained my cycles, but it definitely takes time. Our bodies often have false starts, where you get patches of EWCM but don't ovulate. I knew I was on the way to ovulating when I started getting cervical mucus, but even then it took a month to ovulate and I had two false starts.

Length of Early Recovery Cycles

As we've discussed, your first ovulation (occurring prior to your first post-HA menstrual bleeding) and period after recovering from HA often feel like you got a hole-in-one. But as time passes and you get to cycle day (CD) 14 (the time for "normal" ovulation), you may start to become more anxious about when you will ovulate next. It is very common for the first few cycles to be longer than normal; in our survey respondents, the median time from the first period to the second natural ovulation was 25.5 days, with a range from 13 to 63 (http://noperiod.info/cycles and http://noperiod.info/second-cycle). Ovulation occurred by CD 45 in 87% of the respondents. In general, when ovulation occurred before CD 30, it was around the same time on the following cycle. When the second ovulation happened later than CD 30, the next (third) was 11 days sooner on average. The group exhibited a wide range, from the next ovulation occurring 30 days sooner to 15 days later (later ovulations were often due to added exercise). The wait to ovulate again can often feel interminable, and a long cycle means fewer chances to get pregnant. There are options to help speed up your cycles if you cannot stand waiting any longer, or if you have a couple of long natural cycles under your belt and want to shorten them to get more chances to conceive. These involve oral medications, such as over-the-counter soy isoflavones or prescription medications Clomid, Femara, or tamoxifen. We will discuss these in depth in chapter 21.

> *Nico*: When we returned from our trip, I walked into a second opinion appointment with another RE with quite a lot of hope. I was on CD 13 of my very own cycle! And it seemed that hope was not unfounded: when the doctor did an ultrasound I had ... wait for it ... a 14 millimeter follicle! I'd grown it all on my own. I was tickled; it looked like this might actually happen au naturel! Except that when I had another scan two days later with RE #1 there was no growth at all. Death of the eternal optimist.
>
> RE#1 then told me that injectable gonadotropins (FSH and LH to help mature the eggs that I could apparently not grow on my own) were

> my only option. We scheduled another appointment a week later. She did yet another ultrasound, and my follicle must have disappeared as it wasn't mentioned—but much later I found out that my estradiol had been 76, which strongly suggests to me that had I waited just a little longer I would have grown my own egg (my natural E_2 has been in the 20's or low 30's just about every time it's been checked.)
>
> *Charissa*: I'm on day 27 today and still waiting to ovulate. I've had patches of more fertile CM here and there, though still not really egg whitey. But my temperatures have been lower. I think this is the worst part of my cycles—waiting to ovulate when I think it's just around the corner. Any little thing can either give me great hope or get me really down. It's silly because I'm fairly certain I will ovulate in the next week. I just get my hopes up that it's going to happen sooner only to have them dashed... but I know I should just be really thankful that I'm cycling on my own and seem to be making progress.
>
> *Sarah Q*: I know how hard long cycles can be, especially waiting and hoping to ovulate earlier and then not getting pregnant. When I got my period back I maintained that weight for the first two cycles, but for the last one I actually cut my workouts to a bare minimum of yoga and gained a few pounds to see if it would make a difference. It did!

It is reassuring that whether you ovulate in a standard timeframe (before CD 21) or much later, like CD 45+, there is little difference in terms of pregnancy rate. There is also no difference in miscarriage rate (chapter 26). A late ovulation is not a problem after HA because there is a delay in initiation of follicle growth rather than ovulation. Once follicular growth starts, the process continues at a normal pace, so the egg development goes just as it should.

This was experienced by Dana[3], a regular poster on the Board, who had an ultrasound at CD 25, but her doctor stated that it looked as if she were around CD 5. She asked if there were any concerns about late ovulation with regard to egg quality and he said, "Absolutely not. With your lower hormones, you just coast in the early follicular phase for longer." She went on to ovulate eight days later on CD 33 and got pregnant.

> *Sarah Q*: I just wanted to chime in on the late ovulation discussion. In my first pregnancy I got my positive test after ovulating on CD 42, and this time I got pregnant ovulating on CD 64!! I am currently 11 weeks. So, as you can see, I have not had any problems with late ovulations and getting pregnant, but the waiting so long for ovulation to occur can be pretty frustrating!

Pregnancy rates by cycle day of ovulation

Cycle Day (CD) of ovulation	Number of cycles	Number of pregnancies	Percentage of cycles resulting in pregnancy*†
Normal (up to CD 21)	333	134	40%
Medium (CD 22–30)	129	37	29%
Late (CD 31–45)	55	18	33%
Very late (CD 45+)	51	15	29%
Total	568	204	36%

* The pregnancy rates are not significantly different between any categories; $p = 0.23$. The difference that you see between the rate at < CD 21 and > CD 21 is likely to be due to chance.
† Note that the pregnancy rates are potentially artificially high due to people being more likely to provide survey data for successful cycles. However, that bias would not affect the cycle day of ovulation information.

Resuming Exercise

You may be wondering about increasing your exercise after you've regained your natural cycles or made the decision to go down the path of medical assistance to get pregnant. Honestly, there is no one-size-fits-all answer. We can say that in general for those cycling naturally, we suggest not increasing high-intensity exercise until you have **three** cycles under your belt (http://noperiod.info/wait-three-cycles), and at that point, paying close attention to the effects that exercise might be having in terms of lengthening your follicular phase or shortening your luteal phase. We strongly recommend tracking your ovulation (chapter 18) for a good while into recovery so that you can monitor this. For example, if you had a 12-day LP (the time between ovulating and getting your period) prior to starting exercise, and notice that after introducing exercise, your LP decreased to 9 or 10 days, you might want to re-evaluate the intensity or frequency of your workouts, especially if you are trying to conceive.

For some, any high-intensity exercise can cause a short LP, which may need to be addressed if you want to get pregnant (chapter 19). For others, an LP that gets shorter over time can be a sign of cycles going missing again.

If you're trying to conceive and have decided to move forward with fertility treatments, you might not have the feedback that you can get from a natural cycle (e.g., longer follicular phase or short LP); however, if you are not responding to medication as you had hoped, that can be a good indicator that you are exercising too much (or not eating enough). We strongly suggest continuing to limit high-intensity exercise until you are pregnant (we will discuss exercising during pregnancy in chapter 25). Remember that the population studies in Denmark showed an increased time before getting pregnant with *any* high-intensity exercise[4]. Is it more important to you to get your exercise in, or to have a good response to your medications and the best chance at pregnancy?

> **Amy J**: I was diagnosed with HA in May. I struggled with the no exercise thing as my RE told me I could do 30 minutes of cardio three times per week and be fine. I found the Board and realized the truth. NO high-intensity exercise and eating more!!! I put on 15 pounds, stopped exercise, did five days of Femara, and my period came 33 days later. I responded to my second round as well! It was very difficult gaining that weight and not exercising. I had my moments of doubt, but reading the Board helped "talk me down." Foolishly I thought, "Hey, I'm cycling again ... it won't hurt to start exercising a little." I started doing 30 minutes of "light" cardio five days a week and, sure enough, it was CD 50 and no period. So I decided to relax and obviously got my answer. No exercise and two weeks later my period came. I did not do another round of Femara because I wanted to see where my body was. I did start taking my temperature and had a spike on CD 16!! I am now 4 days past ovulation and am in my two-week wait! I wanted to share my story for those of you who are doubting the process or considering exercising again, even "lightly." JUST DON'T DO IT!!! It's the best feeling knowing my body is working again. I don't love my size but love how much better I feel!

Changes in Eating Habits After Recovery

Once you start cycling you might be also be thinking about backing off on your recovery eating plan to some degree. Just as with high intensity exercise, we recommend continuing to eat at recovery levels until you've had at least three periods (http://noperiod.info/wait-three-cycles). Too often we get that first period, think "Yay, I'm recovered!," and then decide to restrict food to change body size . . . and the second period doesn't come. Waiting for three cycles allows your hormones to become more equilibrated and your body used to this new normal. It also allows you to discover more about your own cycle. Learn what your signs of ovulation are so you can loosely track when you ovulate (as well as when you get your period). This allows you to determine if you are having ovulatory cycles, as well as the length of your luteal phase, both of which are useful pieces of information.

After the third cycle, it is reasonable to start eating more intuitively. Intuitive Eating and the associated workbook by Evelyn Tribole and Elyse Resch are a fantastic guide to help you learn more about following hunger and fullness cues. At this point, instead of trying to eat all day every day, you can learn to follow cues and eat "normally." We continue to recommend eating regularly through the day, but start listening more to your fullness cues for deciding how much to eat.

You might switch out some (but hopefully not all) of the "fertility foods" for "healthier" options. Your weight might continue to increase some, remain the same, or perhaps decrease a bit (although if your BMI remains below 22 we do encourage you to continue to gain for optimal fertility and long term health), and you should still be aiming to eat around 2500 calories per day as that is the amount an active woman needs for full fueling. We do not recommend weight loss as a goal at any point after this process. Restricting to lose what you feel is "excess weight" or cutting out food groups again will put your body back into an energy deficit and/or reduce the hormonal signals generated by particular food groups, gives you a strong chance of losing what you have just worked so hard for. Dropping a few pounds is just not worth the potential of lengthening or vanishing cycles, especially if pregnancy is your goal.

If you are still feeling the need or desire to lose weight, please consider very carefully why you are feeling this way. If your finances allow, perhaps you could engage a body image coach to help you work through some of these issues; if not, spend a few weeks or months immersing yourself in the body positive, Health At Every Size world. Exposing yourself to others who have made the decision to reject diet culture and its toxic messaging can empower you to do the same, to embrace and appreciate your body for what it is and what it does for you rather than spending time and mental energy on trying to reshape it to meet society's damaging and unhealthy standards. It is also helpful to understand some of the mythology that has been created around body size and health or disease. We strongly recommend reading Health At Every Size by Linda (now Lindo) Bacon and Body Respect by Linda/o Bacon and Lucy Aphramor for excellent reviews of scientific studies around body size and health. Body Kindness by Rebecca Scritchfield is great for helpful suggestions and exercises for changing your own mindset, along with The Body is Not an Apology by Sonya Renee Taylor, You Have the Right to Remain Fat by Virgie Tovar, and More Than a Body by Lindsay and Lexie Kite. Links for all these books and more can be found at http://noperiod.info/resources.

One final comment on body size post-recovery: for the long term, it is likely healthier to be in a body that is in or above the "fertile zone." Studies of bone density as related to size generally find increased risk of fracture at lower BMI. One meta-analysis that examined prospective data from almost 60,000 people, with 250,000 person-years of follow up found strong correlations between fracture risk and BMI. Without knowing bone density, someone with a BMI of 20 has approximately a 20% increased risk of any type of fracture and 95% increased risk of hip fracture versus someone with a BMI of 25[5]. When bone density is accounted for (which is generally lower in those in smaller bodies based on decreased mechanical stress when carrying less weight), there is no independent risk of any fracture at a BMI of 20 versus 25, but still a 42% increased risk of hip fracture; this goes up to over a two-fold risk with BMI of 15. Is it really worth going back to your old ways? We would strongly argue that no thinness is worth that price.

Summary

It is an amazing reminder that you are healthy when you get your body to a point where you are having monthly natural cycles. Prior to the resumption of cycles, you may notice fertile signs occurring every two weeks or so; this happens as your body gears up to ovulate but isn't quite ready yet. This is a sign that you are on the right track. Once you do get your first period, it is possible that your first cycle or two may be longer than normal. The time to ovulation will decrease in just a couple of cycles if you continue with the Recovery Plan. If your cycles do not shorten naturally, some have chosen to use medications to encourage ovulation to happen sooner (part 3).

> *Lisa*: Surely you know Kool & The Gang's song, "Celebration"? OK, well, sing it with me now! "Celllllebrate good times, come on! . . ."
>
> This is seriously how it feels when you experience everything leading up to getting your period, and then actually start cycling naturally month after month after month (unless of course a pregnancy slips in stepping the joy up a notch). It's a huge celebration and should be. You've had an opportunity to REALLY get to know yourself and spent time with the uncomfortable and unknowns. You've waited, worked, and earned your healthy body back! The point of this is to help encourage you to think about sticking with the "natural way" a bit longer even when you believe nothing is happening. The reality is that changes *are* happening. The benefits emotionally, physically, and, for some, spiritually are BIG. And you will continue to benefit in every aspect of your life.

17
Tracking Ovulation and Family Planning

UNLIKE WHAT MANY THINK and what we often see in the media, the most important event in a menstrual cycle is not your period. The primo, number one most important part of your cycle is actually ovulation! The hormonal changes associated with ovulation are what provide the most benefit for bone density, heart health, and brain health. The event of ovulation is what allows for pregnancy. And tracking your ovulation regularly gives you a much deeper understanding of your menstrual cycles and their status. We cannot stress enough how important it is to track ovulation once you start cycling again. It is helpful for multiple purposes:

- Knowing when to expect your next period
- Knowing when to have intercourse for pregnancy if that is desired
- Knowing when to avoid unprotected intercourse if pregnancy is not desired
- Assessing the effects of added exercise and/or changes in eating (Chapter 28)

It's useful to have a clear understanding of what is happening around the time of ovulation to grasp why we are so strongly recommending tracking ovulation. In a normal, ovulatory menstrual cycle (go back to Chapter 5 for a lot more detail), the process is started by an increase in gonadotropin releasing hormone, GnRH, after the hypothalamus gets the signal to begin the cascade. The added GnRH leads to an increase in follicle stimulating hormone (FSH) secreted by the pituitary gland; FSH then is transported through the bloodstream to your ovaries and the process of follicular growth/egg maturation begins. As the egg and follicle mature, the secretion of estradiol increases by 5 to 10 times over your baseline level. *This increase in estradiol is the most supportive of bone density building.* Once the estradiol hits a threshold level sensed by your pituitary, that gland releases a large amount, or "surge," of luteinizing hormone (LH). This LH surge causes the follicle to burst and release the mature egg.

The egg then travels down the Fallopian tubes to your uterus, in case there are sperm present that might lead to pregnancy. But that's irrelevant for right now. What is relevant is what happens with the leftover follicle. The cells that were surrounding and supporting the growing egg don't disappear—rather, their function shifts, and they begin to secrete the hormones estradiol and progesterone to support the uterine lining in case of pregnancy. This new structure that remains behind after ovulation is called the "corpus luteum." The corpus luteum is the driver of the "luteal phase," time between ovulation and when your period arrives (Chapter 19).

Estradiol levels are maintained at a level that is approximately 3-5 times the baseline concentration; further supporting bone growth and maintenance. These levels are much higher than what is achieved with hormone replacement therapy or birth control pills[1], and one reason that natural cycles tend to lead to more bone growth than the outside hormones.

Progesterone levels increase by around 20-50-fold after ovulation. This rise starts almost immediately, with the highest level approximately 7 days past ovulation in a normal length luteal phase. This elevated progesterone has also been demonstrated to be associated with improved bone density[2].

If an egg is not fertilized, the corpus luteum typically degrades after about 12-14 days, and as it does both progesterone and estrogen levels decline back to baseline. These declining hormones lead to the menstrual bleed, and the decrease in estradiol is important because that is sensed by the hypothalamus and leads to the beginning of the next follicular growth process.

As far as knowing when to expect your next period, you can be certain that it is on it's way after you have confirmed ovulation; normally your period will occur 14 days later, but in about 30% of early recovery cycles, the period will come a bit sooner—this is called a "short luteal phase" and will be discussed more in Chapter 19.

Intercourse for pregnancy should occur in the days leading up to ovulation, with the day prior to ovulation being the most likely to result in pregnancy. And obviously, if you do not want to be pregnant, this is the key time to avoid unprotected intercourse.

Two large studies where participants recorded fertile signs and when they had intercourse found similar results. The highest chance of pregnancy was seen with intercourse one to two days before ovulation. The pregnancy rate ranged from 21% to 53%, depending on age[3]. There were no pregnancies attributed to sex six or more days prior to ovulation, or the day after ovulation and beyond. So, to give yourself the best chances of pregnancy, plan some sexy time in the days leading up to ovulation, using the figure below as a guide. Any time you notice the fertile signs we will describe, it is a good idea to have intercourse at least every other day, just in case. If you get a positive OPK, intercourse that day and the next is recommended.

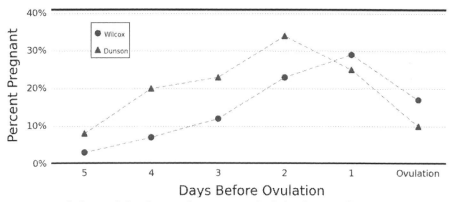

Intercourse timing and the chance of pregnancy. Analysis of two studies where participants recorded days when they had intercourse as well as temperatures and fertile signs, or provided urine for hormone measurement, found that there was a small chance of pregnancy with intercourse five days before ovulation, with the highest chance at one or two days before ovulation, depending on the study[4].

As you may already know, sperm can live for up to five days in fertile mucus[5] explaining why intercourse up to five days before ovulation can potentially lead to pregnancy. In addition, evidence suggests that if there are some sperm abnormalities, intercourse every day or second day (rather than less frequently) is optimal; with normal sperm characteristics, the frequency has little effect[6]. The volume of sperm decreases as the rate of ejaculation increases, but the total amount deposited remains about the same.

Finally, tracking your ovulation is extremely useful in assessing the effects of added exercise. We will discuss this more in Chapter 28—but the basic idea is that if you track your ovulation as you are adding back higher intensity exercise, you will know if the exercise is having the effect of either making your ovulation later, or shortening your luteal phase. Both occurrences would suggest that your body is struggling a little, and we would recommend keeping exercise where it is for another cycle, and probably adding some more food to compensate for the extra energy burned by added exercise

Signs of Ovulation

There are three major signs that ovulation is approaching that we will discuss in much more depth in the remainder of this chapter. Note that taking your temperature daily can confirm if or when you ovulate, but does not give notice of ovulation in advance.

- change in cervical mucus (CM)—specifically egg white-like CM (EWCM)
- change in cervical position (CP)—high, soft, and open
- rising LH, tracked through ovulation predictor kits (OPKs)

If you want to conceive, intercourse during the times when these signs all line up is imperative—not just right when you ovulate, but also in the days leading up to ovulation (pretty much any time you experience fertile signs). Your fertile signs will revert to normal after ovulation has occurred, closing the window for conception.

If you do not want to conceive, you probably do not need to be as diligent in tracking each of these symptoms, unless you want to use cycle tracking to avoid pregnancy. If you are using another form of contraception, a combination of cervical mucus with temperature tracking should do the trick for a general assessment of cycle health. You will likely get to a point over time where you can just note your cervical mucus changes and that will give you enough information about your ovulation and cycle. If you want to track to avoid pregnancy, *you must be diligent about tracking your ovulation and cervical mucus, to ensure that you avoid unprotected intercourse during your fertile window.*

Sign #1: Cervical Mucus

There are a number of physical signs one experiences as ovulation gets close. For many, there is an increase in vaginal discharge known as cervical mucus (CM) during natural cycles and sometimes when oral medication is used. The consistency of the CM changes throughout the cycle.

1) After bleeding ends, the CM is typically creamy, thick, and whitish; this is probably what you will experience as your hormones are increasing while you work toward recovery. You are unlikely to be fertile while experiencing this type of mucus.
2) The next stage, when your estrogen increases a bit more, is "watery" CM. This is clearer and thinner.
3) When estrogen increases further as your follicle grows, discharge can become more copious, clear, and stretchy. This is the famous egg white cervical mucus (EWCM), which looks and feels almost identical to an egg white. EWCM is the most sperm-friendly mucus; the little guys can live in it for up to five days[7]! You might experience just a day or two of this fertile mucus, or it can last for up to two weeks in some cases.
4) After ovulation, EWCM typically disappears; you may notice no more secretions, or you may notice sticky or creamy CM. Occasionally you might experience a small amount of EWCM, but not as much as prior to ovulation.

If you are using the oral medication Clomid to encourage ovulation (chapter 21), you might experience a thicker, less sperm friendly EWCM, or no fertile mucus at all. Taking cough syrup (containing guaifenesin only) to "loosen secretions" can be particularly useful when you are experiencing other fertile signs like a change in cervical position or positive OPK and are trying to conceive.

You may be wondering how the heck you are supposed to know if you're having EWCM, which lets you know you are gearing up to ovulate. First of all, you might notice EWCM in your underwear (i.e., notice that you feel wetter than you're used to). Another fairly simple way to check is after you go to the bathroom, particularly a bowel movement. You might see or feel EWCM dripping or stretching from your vagina. If not, use toilet paper to dab at your vaginal opening instead of just wiping and tossing (you might also find that as you dab/wipe you feel more slippery). Take a look at what's on the toilet paper. Notice the color and consistency of the mucus you find. While you're at it, pinch some between your thumb and forefinger and notice how it feels. EWCM will feel slippery. The last test is if you pull your fingers apart, does the mucus stretch between them? *That* is EWCM! This may all initially feel odd or gross you out, but it gets to be second nature over time (and you might as well get used to bodily fluids now; you'll be dealing with them a lot once you have a kid!).

> *Chrissy*: Ladies, I have to tell you—major, major EWCM—dripping! Methinks there is a chef up in my junk making a hollandaise and throwing out all the egg whites into my panties!! Ha ha!

If you want to get pregnant, and you've got the elusive EWCM, this is a good time to "get thee to the bedroom." You may not ovulate the first time(s) you experience EWCM, which can happen if you grow a follicle but it doesn't quite make it to ovulation as described in chapter 16. However, we still recommend some "storming of the castle." It can be fun to practice, and stranger things have happened than people getting pregnant without having a period first. We suggest intercourse about every other day when you have EWCM, or more often if you're in the mood (and perhaps more often when your other fertile signs line up as well). Be aware that some don't experience EWCM but rather just get more watery CM. It is feasible to ovulate without noticing classic EWCM; any time you notice a change in your CM consistency or amount, it's not a bad idea to do a little bedroom dancing.

Over time, you may be able to track your ovulation just by monitoring cervical mucus alone, but for your initial cycles we also recommend tracking your basal body temperature (see the "confirming ovulation" section later in this chapter) as that helps verify you have ovulated, as well as when that ovulation took place.

Again, if you want to avoid pregnancy, using contraception when you have any EWCM, or probably even watery mucus until you are confident about your cycle tracking is strongly recommended.

Sign #2: Cervical Position

Another physical manifestation of soon-to-be ovulation is that your cervix actually changes in both position and feel. During the early part of your cycle when you are not fertile, your cervix will feel hard, closed, and be easy to reach (low). In a textbook cycle this would be from whenever your period ends (because who wants to be checking for your cervix when you still have your period?) to about CD 11 to 12, or perhaps later when it's one of your initial cycles. As your more fertile time approaches, your cervix becomes softer, more open, and harder to reach (high). One method to check your cervical position (CP) is to lie in bed on your back with your knees up and feet on bed (as if you're going to do a sit-up), then use your clean index finger to reach inside your vaginal opening. A low cervix can often be felt fairly easily in this position; you might need to try feeling to the sides a little as it's not always right in the middle. Your cervix will feel hard, like the eraser on a pencil. To reach a high cervix you will probably need to bear down, in a manner similar to having a bowel movement. As you get closer to ovulation, your cervix will be much harder to reach and feel softer and squishier. You may also notice a difference when you're having intercourse, if you know to pay attention.

> *Clover, to the Board ladies*: "Cervix talk...OK...umm...well...I have 'a friend' who wanted me to ask this. She doesn't want me to mention her name, so don't ask. I am really, I mean 'my friend' is really perplexed as to what you should be feeling for downstairs. She has stuck multiple fingers sky high trying to find this 'cervix' thingy everyone is talking about. I even YouTubed, I mean 'my friend' YouTubed it, but can't figure it out. What exactly are you feeling for? Maybe she doesn't have a cervix. Surely I am not the only one who can't give her 'friend' this advice? LOL."
>
> Replies:
>
> *Priscilla*: Clover—Here's a link: http://infertility.about.com/od/trying-toconceive101/ht/cervixovulation.htm. It's not a video but I thought she explained it really well.
>
> *Chrissy*: To find my cervix, I have to go in, and then hang a left!!! I am crooked! At first I could never find it because I was going straight up, so you may be crooked too? (Ahem, ahem, *cough cough*, your friend that is.)
>
> *Judith*: Clover, please tell your friend I have never gotten the Cervix Talk either. I am very bad with stuff like that. Maybe that's why I don't have a baby, LOL! (*P.S. Judith had her first baby in March 2014, and her second December 2015.*)
>
> *Jaclyn*: Tips for Finding Your Cervix:
>
> 1) Wash your hands.
> 2) Squat down really low, with legs spread apart.
> 3) Reach your finger (I use my middle as it's the longest) into your vaginal opening.
> 4) Cough/push down/bear down.
> 5) You should feel something either soft (fertile) or hard (non-fertile).
> 6) You can also "scoop" some cervical mucus from the opening and examine it (especially helpful if you don't normally have lots of CM to analyze, as I never did).
> 7) It takes a couple of cycles to figure out the changes that occur during the cycle, but it should get higher and softer (like your lips) when you are fertile with stretchy mucus, and be lower and harder (like the tip of your nose) in the non-fertile or post-ovulation phase.
> 8) Don't forget to trim your fingernails!
>
> For goodness' sake...don't forget number eight, girls. Hehe!

Sign #3: Ovulation Predictor Kits

In addition to checking your CM and CP, ovulation predictor kits (OPKs) or fertility monitors can be extremely helpful in knowing when ovulation is approaching. These tests that you urinate on (or dip into urine in a cup) measure your LH and will be "positive" when you are surging, which means you will probably ovulate in the next 24 to 36 hours.

There are different brands available, at a range of prices—you can buy 100 "Internet cheapies" for about $20, get similar simple sticks at your local drugstore in packs of 20 for $20, buy much more expensive digital tests, or even fertility monitors that analyze actual hormone levels (http://noperiod. info/resources for some suggestions).

On the cheapies, there are two lines: a dark "control" line to indicate the test is working, and a "test" line that can range from blank to as dark as or darker than the control line depending on how much LH is detected. (The line will be darkest when you are surging.) The cheapies can be hard to interpret, though, so many like to start tracking earlier in their cycle with these sticks, and then later confirm a potential positive with a digital stick. The digital test will usually display a smiley face when your LH is above the threshold to start the process of ovulation. As returning cycles in HAers are often long, daily digital OPKs can become an expensive habit, which is why we recommend using cheapies until you suspect you are close to ovulation. The digital OPKS, particularly those that also detect estrogen and give a "high fertility" signal with a flashing smiley, can sometimes give false readings during HA recovery so we recommend cheapies as well.

As mentioned, a positive OPK usually (but not always) indicates you will ovulate in the next 24 to 36 hours, so intercourse every day for two to three days at this point is ideal for conception. Occasionally someone will get a positive OPK with a wave of follicular recruitment but not ovulate (one study found this occurred in about 10% of natural cycles[8]), similar to experiencing EWCM multiple times before a real ovulation (chapter 16). Getting a positive OPK and then not actually ovulating can be frustrating. When this happens, typically the next wave of recruitment is successful; your body just needs a little extra time to get sorted out. Keep treating your body with TLC and try not to get too down on yourself.

Occasionally, positive OPKs will continue for more than a couple of days. There can be a few different reasons for this: one is pregnancy; OPKs can detect hCG, the major hormone that embryos produce and what is measured by a home pregnancy test. Another is a consistent elevation in LH as often seen with PCOS. Finally, occasionally there are just random cycles where this happens. There have been two women from the Board with this experience—both did eventually ovulate based on tracking their morning temperatures. One had more than nine days of positive OPKs before ovulating; the other ovulated fairly soon after her first positive OPK, but continued to detect LH for a week afterward.

> **Steph**: The above are some great ways to tell if it is time to commence baby making, but it is not necessary to notice all three ovulation signs to get going. For example, you may find it hard to figure out your cervical position but that OPKs work well. Personally, I was never good at the cervical position approach and I didn't like OPKs or charting my temperature. Cervical mucus I could relate to and that was enough for me to know it was time to do the baby dance. Get to know your body and what works for you. This process can be stressful enough; if one way isn't your style, try another!

Confirming Ovulation

If you track your CM, CP, and use OPKs, you should have a very good idea of when ovulation is imminent. These signs all revert back to the non-fertile state after ovulation has occurred. You will notice much less CM and it will generally be back to the creamier variety, your CP will revert to low and hard, your OPKs (if you continue with them) will probably be negative again, and your temperature will go up.

There is some variation in these symptoms, so you will need to get to know your own body's signs. For example, you might experience EWCM for another day or two after ovulation or occasionally have a random small amount of fertile-seeming mucus sometime after ovulation, but if you do, the mucus is generally much less copious.

We mentioned that your temperature will go up after ovulation. Taking your temperature on a daily basis is the easiest way to confirm that ovulation has occurred. It does not help, however, with predicting when you will ovulate. "Temping" can be helpful, but it can also become another number to obsess over; it is important to decide whether it will be more useful for you to determine that you've ovulated or if temping will simply add stress to the process.

> *Nico*: I love data! Temping helped me feel a bit more in control and like I was doing something while I was waiting around to ovulate (and after I did). On the cycle when I conceived my first, I started temping a few days after my period ended and was using an OPK each day as well. I had absolutely no expectations that anything would come of it, but it was a way to pass the almost two months before we could get started on our IVF cycle. Imagine my surprise when I saw the two dark lines that meant I was going to ovulate! I freaked out a bit because my temperature was up that morning so I worried that we had already missed the window for getting pregnant, but my blog friends reassured me that the OPK was more reliable and we should get to the bedroom ASAP. I tested with the OPK again the next day and it was still positive, the day after it was negative, and the day after that my temperature went up. I had ovulated all on my very own!!!

The temperature you want to track is your "basal body temperature" (BBT), your lowest temperature in a 24-hour period, which occurs while you are sleeping. Both oral and vaginal temperatures are acceptable; see what works most consistently for you. Measurements can be in Fahrenheit or Celsius depending on your location; we will use Fahrenheit for the rest of our discussion.

The general consensus is that if you want to be able to accurately confirm ovulation, you should:

- Take your temperature first thing in the morning before getting out of bed because as you get up and move around your temperature immediately begins to increase.
- Take your temperature at the same time every day. You will note approximately a tenth of a degree elevation for each hour later you sleep. Use a special, more accurate BBT thermometer in order to detect the 0.3 to 0.4 degree shift that confirms ovulation. These can be purchased at any local drugstore. But if you already have a regular digital (not necessarily a BBT) thermometer, try it out before getting a new one. The major requirement is that it needs to read to the nearest 0.1 degree.
- Be aware that alcohol can artificially raise your BBT.
- **Don't worry if conditions aren't "perfect" when you temp each day; these "rules" are simply a guide. Feel free to experiment to find a method that works for you**.

> *Nico*: I know that some people do have to follow the "rules" for temping, but I found I didn't have to be quite so hard and fast about it. First, I just

> used a random thermometer I had that read to 0.1 degrees and it was consistent enough from day to day that I was able to pinpoint my ovulation with no problems. Second, I tried taking my temperature a few days in a row right when I woke up, then also after I had walked to the bathroom and sat on the toilet. They were the same, so the latter became my habit rather than waking my husband up with the beeping noise. (For some reason the people who made my thermometer decided that it should alert you every few seconds that it was collecting data, which is super annoying early in the morning!) Finally, my wake-up times varied from 5:30 during the week on the days I was playing ice hockey to 9:30 on the weekends, and I found that too didn't make a big difference. I'd subtract 0.1 from my weekend temps; earlier ones I'd just use as is. Alcohol, on the other hand, increased my temperature a lot, so I would just ignore my temperature the day after I'd had a couple of drinks.

In the days before you ovulate, your waking temperature will probably be between 97.0 and 97.5 degrees (it is often lower than that before recovery). It can be fairly consistent, varying by only one or two tenths from day to day, or you might experience much bigger changes, such as half a degree between different days. But after ovulation, your average temperature will be higher, by about three tenths of a degree or more. In the good old days, you had to graph your temperature on a piece of paper, but now you can use an online charting tool or get an app for your phone. Fertilityfriend.com (FF app) and Kindara are a couple of suggestions.

The first day of increased temperature is known as one day past ovulation (DPO). Three days of temperatures elevated above the "cover line" (the temperature range that divides pre-ovulation from post-ovulation; this will be shown in the charting app) confirm ovulation, particularly in combination with a positive OPK, EWCM, and/or a high, soft CP. Once your temperature has increased it is unlikely that further intercourse will lead to conception[9], so you can take a breather (if you feel like it).

It can be helpful to know that there are a few different patterns that can occur around the time of ovulation:

- A dip in temperature the day before or the day of ovulation is sometimes noticed.
- For some, temperatures show an immediate, sharp rise after ovulation has taken place.
- In other cases, temperature after ovulation increases slowly over the next few days.

The Recovery Plan—Changing Your Habits and Your Life

- Occasionally there will be a "fallback rise" in which the temperature will go up, then back down, then up again. Don't freak out if your temperature on what you think is 2 DPO is lower than you expect. Give it another day or two to confirm.

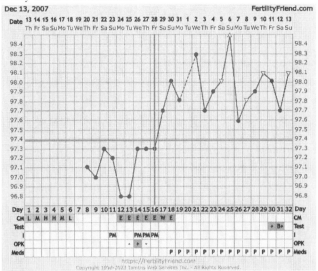

A Fertility Friend chart showing temperatures during a cycle in which conception occurred. The pre-ovulation temperatures ranged from 96.8 to 97.3, so the cover line was set at 97.4; post-ovulatory temps were between 97.6 and 98.5. The first line below the chart shows menstrual heaviness (L = light, M = medium, H = heavy) and cervical mucus (E = EWCM, W = watery CM), with two days of fertile CM after ovulation. The next line shows pregnancy tests with the first test (positive) taken at 14 days past ovulation, then a positive blood test the following day. The line below that shows intercourse timing (PM = evening), followed by OPK data, and the final line shows that progesterone (P) was used after ovulation. Image reprinted with permission from fertilityfriend.com.

After ovulation is confirmed, some continue to check their temperature every day; others find it too stressful to have that daily number to analyze and obsess over. If you continue to take your temperature, you may notice it getting even higher if you happen to be pregnant; this happens about 25% of the time. For the rest, there can be ups and downs, but staying above your cover line is encouraging. Most of the time, a dip back to the cover line or below suggests your period is on its way (less true if the dip happens in the middle of the luteal phase, though, where it can be associated with an embryo taking hold in your uterus, known as an "implantation dip"). It is possible to be pregnant but still have bleeding around the time your period is expected. If your temperature does not drop and/or your bleeding is different from normal, we encourage you to take a pregnancy test before proceeding with additional medications.

> *Gillian*: I am still hanging out waiting until I can take a pregnancy test. It's a real torture. I was thinking that house chores and three midterms would occupy me, but no... instead I am reading online about all the pregnancy signs and trying to listen to my body. I am so tired of waiting. I have no pregnancy signs whatsoever, nothing, zilch. My temps are between 98.2 and 98.6, but that does not really mean anything. My gut feeling is telling me that I'm not pregnant. All in all, sitting home all day studying and doing house chores is doing a number on me; I feel like I am sinking into a deep depression. (*Gillian was in fact pregnant when she wrote this, although the pregnancy ended in miscarriage.*)

In addition to (or instead of) tracking your temperature, a more reliable way to confirm ovulation is to get your blood drawn around seven days past ovulation and have your progesterone level checked. This can be done in natural or medicated cycles, although general practitioners are somewhat reluctant to order this test; a fertility specialist is more likely to do so. A progesterone level above 3 ng/mL confirms ovulation[10], although that is low; 9.4 ng/mL has been suggested as a lower limit for supporting a pregnancy[11]. If your progesterone level is lower than 9.4, or your luteal phase is less than 10 days long, chapter 19 offers some suggestions on ways to support your luteal phase. In general, progesterone levels do not correlate with LP length[12]; we have seen folks with progesterone well over 20 ng/mL with short LP.

There are now also urine tests you can purchase that allow you to check progesterone levels, and many of the electronic fertility monitors include testing for progesterone as an option. These tests measure a metabolite of progesterone called pregnanediol glucuronide (PdG), which correlates with blood progesterone levels. The levels that confirm ovulation are different from what is described above; information that comes with the strips you are using should provide additional guidance.

Pregnancy Testing

There are about two weeks between when you ovulate and when you can find out if the cycle led to pregnancy. By the time your period is late, pregnancy tests will almost certainly detect the human chorionic gonadotropin (hCG) hormone that is secreted by the implanted embryo, and you will get a positive result. If you do not want to wait until past when your period is expected, the most sensitive home pregnancy tests can detect hCG at about eight to nine DPO. The first few cycles you have a real chance at pregnancy are often quite exciting, so many like to test as early as possible. Keep in mind you could be disappointed by a negative result when in fact you are pregnant, if you choose to test early.

Having witnessed the results of the choice to test early or to wait until 12 DPO or later to test, we recommend the latter. Early testing is uncertain and can lead to avoidable stress and anxiety. If you do choose to test early, know that there are many who have gone on to have healthy pregnancies who do not get a positive pregnancy test until after 12 DPO. It's not over until the blood shows! Note that if you are taking progesterone supplements to extend your luteal phase (chapter 19), you may not get your period until after you stop the medication (although many do start bleeding while still taking progesterone, often at 15 to 16 DPO).

> *Emily, August 12, 2014*: Big Fat Negative… I tested early this morning around midnight just because that's when I got up to pee. Today is 13 DPO so plenty of time for implantation. I stopped the progesterone suppositories and took the estrogen patch off so I'm sure my period will show up soon. Anyway, I'll probably take a breather before we move on.
>
> *August 13, 2014*: I still hadn't gotten my period today about 40 hours after my negative test, so I tested again (14 DPO) and it was POSITIVE! Oh. My. Gosh. I'll start back on my suppositories and patch and call the clinic tomorrow. Can this be?!

When Things Aren't Working as Expected

When you are eager for pregnancy, getting to the point where you have a chance of pregnancy feels like such a relief, no matter if it's through natural cycles or starting treatment. You've made it to the starting line, finally! The first few cycles you're excited and hopeful, and if you get pregnant pretty quickly, thank your lucky stars. For many, it is simply a matter of ovulating and pregnancy happens pretty quickly, with minimal intervention. Others are not so fortunate. When it takes longer than you expect or plan for to get pregnant, it can lead to some pretty dark days, especially if you have a miscarriage (chapter 26). If you do happen to fall into one of these more challenging places, talk to someone. Sharing with a friend, family member who has been in a similar situation, or therapist can be helpful. Also consider infertility support groups, online support groups etc. There are a number of individual friendships that have stemmed from the Board, as well as a few smaller groups—one such group of five called themselves "the left-behinds," and commiserated at length about their shared trials in getting pregnant. (They all did get pregnant eventually, and a couple have now had additional natural pregnancies.)

> *Ann*: It's been forever since I posted, but wanted to jump on to share my good news. After three years of trying, I'm finally pregnant!! For those of you who don't remember me, I started posting in December 2008. I did two intrauterine inseminations, seven rounds of Clomid, a fresh cycle of IVF (ending in a miscarriage last fall), and two frozen embryo transfers after that. It was our last embryos that finally did it. I'm a little over eight weeks. I've seen the heartbeat twice now and all looks good. I had my exit interview with the fertility specialist last week and graduated to my OB (which has been my dream)! The best part is my due date is St. Patrick's Day (my husband is 100% Irish). I know it's still early, but this time around everything has been great. I'm lucky to say I haven't had any morning sickness ... just tired and hungry. Many of you have kept in touch or sent me sweet notes on occasion and it has meant the world! Being the last "Left Behind" was hard, especially since there were no tangible reasons why I wasn't getting pregnant. So ... I'm hopeful that this is it!! (*Ann's son was born in 2012 and her second son, also from IVF as she did not regain cycles postpartum, was born in 2014.*)

> *Jaclyn*: It's so hard when you are in the place of trying to get pregnant and wondering when or if it will ever happen. I have had (as many of us have) majorly depressed days, weeks, months ... and everyone at the time would say, "Go back to any old posts on the Board and you will see how down and out some of the women were before they got pregnant." Point being, you all will be in my shoes (pregnant) probably not too long from now, and it will feel just as crazy as it does to me right now. Yeah, it doesn't take away from the temporary major suckiness of wanting and not yet receiving—it is very painful and can wear you down—but it won't always be this way. I promise! One day you'll be doling out advice to someone else and thinking "This is nuts!" just as I am right now. Sure, I'm just six weeks and who knows, but I did make it to the "pregnant" part and I'm pretty pumped about that! It pains me to see the down, bummed out mood in some of you because I was just like that (we all were). You will get there! Don't give up hope. Never, never, never. And KEEP. GAINING. WEIGHT. It helps! I truly believe it was what made the difference for me. Not to mention that I couldn't care less now about weight gain ... really! Isn't it nice not to be constantly ravenous or tied to the scale or to your exercise routine or the "rules"? Ahhh ... it is so liberating and I'm

> thankful I had to learn all of that because it will make this pregnancy so much more enjoyable now that I won't be obsessing about weight gain and fitness. What a waste of time! *(Jaclyn's son was born 7.5 months later. Her second pregnancy was natural, on her first cycle of attempted conception.)*

Summary

This chapter has described many of the methods you can use to track and understand your cycle (true if you are using oral medications to encourage ovulation as well). These include:

- Paying attention to your cervical mucus; EWCM is common close to ovulation.
- Checking your cervical position; a high, soft cervix is receptive to sperm and suggests ovulation.
- Using ovulation predictor kits; a positive OPK usually precedes ovulation by 24 to 36 hours.
- Taking and tracking your daily temperature does not tell you when ovulation is coming, but it confirms when it has happened. This should not be the only method you use for tracking ovulation if you want to track for family planning (to either achieve or avoid pregnancy).

Remember that when HAers start menstruating again, cycles are often longer than described in textbooks; these will shorten over time, but if they don't, medical options to help will be discussed in chapters 20 through 22.

18
Still No Period?!

So here you are: you've followed the HA Recovery Plan; you're feeling "normal" (maybe even healthy and happy); and you're eating, relaxing, and participating in life. But despite all this, Aunt Flo has yet to make a grand appearance. You might begin to think, "This Recovery Plan is worthless! All I am is bigger, out of shape, and still infertile."

WAIT! Before you go run a marathon, give yourself a little more time. All is not lost. You *are* on the right track.

The HA Recovery Plan works. So why hasn't it for you? Where is your monthly visitor? Why are you not pregnant? There are a few possibilities as to why things aren't happening "down below" just yet and we will explore them. But before we do that, and before you use this book as your newfound footrest, let's examine the situation more closely. We are willing to bet that more things are happening than you may realize.

Signs of Recovery

Take a moment to think about your body. Have you been noticing more cervical mucus? Are your breasts getting bigger or possibly sore? Is your hair fuller? Are you much more willing to jump into bed with your partner? These are all signs that your body is gearing up for the big event. Before you know it, you will be ready to dig out and dust off that trusty box of tampons (or maybe think about a menstrual cup or reusable pads or panties to help the environment).

Beyond the physical signs, there are a couple of other ways to check how you are doing. The first is to see your doctor and get some bloodwork done. Doctors often like to check your estradiol (E_2) level, but we find that there is generally not a big difference in E_2 (or FSH) upon recovery, so do *not* be discouraged if your E_2 has barely budged. In agreement with this, the average E_2 in our survey respondents when they had HA was 19 pg/mL, and only increased to 22 after recovery. LH seems to be a better marker for how well your body is responding to the changes you have made, and often rises with HA recovery.

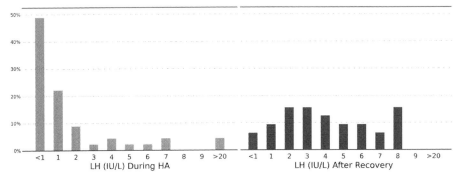

LH during and after HA. (*Left*) LH values when survey respondents were diagnosed with HA (40 participants). LH levels were less than 2 IU/L in 69% of our survey respondents (normal range is 2-12 IU/L). (*Right*) LH results after working toward recovery; here only 9% had an LH less than 2 IU/L.

The average LH of our survey respondents who provided information went from 1.0 IU/L during HA to 3.1 (more than triple!) after recovery. LH increases because your hypothalamus is starting to work again, sending out GnRH pulses. A higher LH level is an excellent sign your reproductive system is waking up.

Another way to get a sense of how your recovery is progressing is to do a Provera challenge. You may have already tried this during your initial diagnosis; you take Provera (or another progesterone equivalent) for five to ten days, and then wait to see if you get a bleed. Most do not respond when HA is in full force. However, if you try the Provera challenge again after making lifestyle changes and you *do* bleed, that means the lining in your uterus has been getting enough estrogen to grow to at least 4 mm. Bleeding in response to Provera is a big step in the right direction and bodes well for either recovering natural cycles soon or responding nicely to treatments.

Time and Patience

> *Leslie*: This is a very hard battle we are all fighting and when you feel like you are giving it your all and not seeing results it makes it even harder. Did you cut out all exercise? I swear that seems to get the best results for most with HA. Keep your head up and keep fighting because you will beat HA. It may take a few more pounds gained or more time but it will happen.

When you have followed the HA Recovery Plan for several months and are still anxiously awaiting that first spot of blood, it can be so tempting to give up. You might reason that if this plan hasn't worked by now, it is never going to work, so maybe you should just go back to your old habits. However, that is certainly not going to help matters. It is incredibly difficult to be patient during this process, but our bodies cannot heal overnight. Think about how long you were neglecting your body, how few calories you ate, how intense your exercise was, and/or how high your stress levels were. It certainly won't take that length of time to recover (our bodies are incredibly resilient), but by the same token, there is a lot that your body needs to repair. Patience is a key ingredient.

Think of HA recovery as recuperation from major surgery or an accident: you will notice small changes as your body heals, but full recovery can often take longer than you would expect or hope. Your body needs time, nourishment, and rest to heal mentally and physically. As we mentioned earlier, 60% of our survey respondents ovulated within six months of beginning the recovery process, and this was before the principles of "going all in" were laid out. Six months seems like an eternity when you want to be pregnant (yesterday) or want your period back. But in the grand scheme, six months is a small investment compared to what you will gain with total wellness, getting your period, and becoming pregnant if so desired. No loss there. On the other hand, if you are past the six-month mark and still have not gotten your period, the rest of this chapter will talk both about making sure that you are doing all you can to coax an egg down your tubes as well as what steps you can take next if you are done being patient. It might encourage you to know that of our survey respondents who restored natural cycles, 86% did so within a year of starting to work toward recovery, though many were not "all in" for this entire time. Overall time to recovery would likely be shorter if people were all in from the get-go.

> *Meg*: I'd been "working" on recovery for four years before I started cycling naturally. Before finding the Board, I had only gained up to a BMI

of 19.5 because that's what my doctors said was my optimal weight. Once I got that far without cycling, they said that it looked like weight was not my problem and that it must be grad school, stress, blah, blah, blah. But then I graduated and got married and was so much less stressed out. And still no period. Then I found the Board and you all convinced me that I should see what happened with a little more weight. That did the trick, although it took some time. I think that I gained the weight around when I started posting, so six(ish) months of *real* recovery before I ovulated.

Amanda M: I'm 35 and time isn't on my side so I started treatment while I was gaining and resting. Between November 2013 and May 2014 I did two cycles of Clomid and four of injections; then my RE wanted to do some exploratory surgery because they found fluid around my right ovary. I was SO bummed and frustrated!! But I had no choice so I sat back and waited.

Well, apparently being sidelined does a body good because about a month later I got my first natural period in 10 years!! I was shocked…still am. I honestly thought it would never happen. I trusted the process of gaining and resting, and I knew it could work. But sometimes I doubted that it would work for ME. But it did. I eventually got my body to a place where it trusts me again. It took three to four months of gaining and then sitting at the higher weight for another six months or so. I gained about 20 lb total.

Now that I have my periods back and can reflect on my journey to this point, I realize that my body is even smarter than I thought. I was in such a hurry to get pregnant, partly because I want a baby, but also partly because I wanted this whole uncomfortable process to be over as fast as possible. But my body knew that I had a lot to learn so it took its time healing so my mind could catch up. Don't get me wrong—I'm still a work in progress. But I have newfound respect and appreciation for my body and its ability to heal. I will never abuse it again like I did for so many years. I've learned to appreciate so many of life's pleasures: from little things like sleeping in on the weekends (instead of waking up at 5 a.m. to get my two-hour workout in) to bigger, more important things like having more time for friends and family, and making the most of that time instead of being constantly irritable and tired from lack of food and too much exercise.

The next question to ask yourself if you have not gotten your cycle back yet is: have you gone "all in" and committed fully to the HA Recovery Plan? If not, that is likely why you are not seeing results.

It is in no way easy to go all in. In fact, sometimes you believe you *are* all in, but still have limits and restrictions that might prevent recovery. Look back through chapters 8 and 12, read about what we are recommending, and ask yourself if you are truly doing as we suggest. Are you still exercising? If so, what are you doing? Are you running several times a week (this is not going to help) or are you taking a few slow walks (much more likely to move you toward recovery)? Think about your BMI and/or weight—have you drawn a line in the sand beyond which you will not allow yourself to go? Everyone's number or set point is different and if you aren't allowing your body to get there without interference, you are less likely to recover. And how about eating? Are you still controlling what enters your mouth? Are there foods you won't eat because they are "unhealthy," and is that limiting how many calories you're getting (even if unintentionally)? Are you still filling up with fruits and veggies? If your answer to any or all of these questions is yes, this is a great time to take a good look at where your priorities lie and how badly you want to meet your goals. Are you willing to endure some discomfort in order to reap the rewards? We encourage you to press on as you are now becoming more familiar with the work that needs to be done.

> **Tara R**: Hang in there! You can do this! It will all be worth it someday. This is the third time I've thought I ovulated and realized a week later (after getting my hopes up) that I certainly did not. I thought to myself, "I can't do this anymore. I can't stuff myself silly every day, give up all the exercise I love, feel like I look terrible in all my clothes, and STILL not ovulate. I can't, I can't, I can't!" But when I read that other people are struggling just as hard, it makes me realize that I'm not alone. We can do this!! We just need to stay focused and patient and remember how many things we have going for us outside of this realm. I'm going to keep making fun plans to keep my mind occupied (last week I took a jewelry-making class). (*Tara got pregnant naturally less than a month later.*)

Stress

> **Steph**: I started the process of trying to recover from HA in November 2011. When my period had yet to appear by February 2012, I had just about had it (yeah, I'm not the most patient person in the world). It wasn't even until February 2012 that I actually went all in. But between the discovery of having HA, needing to make unwanted changes in my life, and the baby that wasn't, I was sad, angry, upset, and stressed. Everyone says,

> "Just relax and you'll get pregnant," and they said the same thing to me. Why do people tell you that?! How can you relax when you are yearning for a baby and doing everything possible to have one but nothing is happening? Well, it is true that stress impacts your ability to recover and not only psychological stress as we typically think of, but physical (e.g., exercise) stress as well. So if you have truly implemented all the dietary and exercise recommendations and are yet to notice fertile changes, it may be that stress is the hurdle you need to overcome.

You may have heard of people losing their periods during a stressful few months and then cycling again when things calmed down, or about those who got pregnant on vacation after a long struggle. Why do we hear these stories? It's not to taunt you; these situations do occur and demonstrate how reduction in stress can have an impact on how quickly you recover.

This is all well and good, but then the next obvious question becomes: how can you de-stress while going through such a trying process? There are quite a few options that have worked for others that you may find helpful too. Granted, these suggestions may not resolve all your natural responses to stress, but they can impact your ability to cope in a healthy way. We already mentioned getting pregnant on vacation; getting away from all your typical responsibilities (and relaxing your restrictive eating habits and exercise routines) fits perfectly into the HA Recovery Plan. Think about other ways to reduce ongoing stressors in your life: if your job is pressure-filled, you might consider setting limits and boundaries on when/where you work, and find moments for yourself no matter whether you're at home or in an office. If your circumstances allow, possibly look into a position or career change. If family is causing ongoing angst, brainstorm with your partner or a friend how to make adjustments to decrease that anxiety or any other uninvited emotion.

Another option is to take a break from focusing on pregnancy and/or getting your period back. That does not mean you should stop following the recovery plan; it means that in addition you should find different activities to occupy your time and thoughts. Further ways of relieving stress among our survey respondents included prayer, meditation, spending time with family and friends, reading, cooking or baking, finding online support, and acupuncture.

In fact, acupuncture often comes up as a suggestion for stress relief and getting your period back. It can be a great way to relax and de-stress (but we have not seen acupuncture and herbs work as a replacement for the Recovery Plan.)

> *Steph*: I personally liked getting acupuncture. I spent the time envisioning and talking to my future child. I felt spiritual and connected. Do I think it is the reason I have a baby today? No. But it was helpful for my mental well-being.

If acupuncture is something you think you might benefit from, go for it. But understand that acupuncture alone, without any lifestyle changes, is unlikely to lead to cycle resumption. However, if you've put in the time and effort toward recovery, acupuncture just might help with the last step of reducing stress.

> *Lauren*: I do not think the acupuncture is what made me cycle this time around. I think it was eating more and exercising less. But I think acupuncture (every two weeks), in addition to acetyl-L-carnitine (nutritional supplement) and sleeping more, *supported* my lifestyle changes and perhaps helped me to cycle sooner than I would have otherwise. Plenty of people have recovered without acupuncture, so it's not required—I wouldn't spend your savings on it if it's a stretch to afford. Just keep doing what you're doing!

If you are interested in further support and expanding your recovery tools, both cognitive behavioral therapy (CBT) and hypnosis have proven to assist in recovery of cycles, especially in those who are at a size where their body is happy. In the classic study using CBT in women with HA we've discussed already, seven out of eight of those receiving CBT resumed ovulation compared with two of eight in the control arm[1]. Similarly, in the study using hypnosis to treat HA, a single session was followed by at least one ovulation in 9 of 12 women within 12 weeks after the treatment[2]. The paper describing the study offers a detailed description of the method used such that a competent practitioner of hypnosis should be able to replicate the treatment effectively. Finally, a few HAers have resumed cycles after starting prescription anti-anxiety medications. If your stress-sensing pathway is activated it can shut down your hypothalamus regardless of your energy balance and act as a barrier to resuming cycles[3]. A study in monkeys demonstrated increases in estrogen and progesterone to normal levels in "stress sensitive" animals after treatment with citalopram[4] (likely due to increases in LH[5]). There are some concerns about use of these medications while pregnant so make sure to let your doctor know if you are trying to conceive; another route may be a better choice in that case.

> **Leah**: I just got my period, like a heavy-flow-cramps *real* period. First one like this since HA!! Thinking about why after all this time of HA I would suddenly start cycling, I realized that a few weeks ago my doctor seriously upped my dose of Effexor because she said it needs to be higher to be effective for anxiety. (*Leah's cycles resumed a few weeks after increasing her antidepressant, 25 months after weaning. They have been regular ever since.*)

> **Anna F**: I have been on this board for a while off and on and I have had osteoporosis for a while and yet I did not get it! I have always been small and even now I didn't so much need to gain weight as I needed to stop eating lettuce and eat starchy carbs and fats instead to give my body real fuel. I also needed to seriously reduce the anxiety, which if you suffer from please know that can also impact getting your cycles back and not in a good way. Back then I kept thinking, "Well, my HA is different. I never exercise and I think running is only useful if being chased"—I cannot even explain how it felt to get my period for the first time possibly on my own. We worry so much about the little things we cannot control and in the end that's not at all what matters. Now if someone would remind me of this the next time I throw a tantrum that would be great. (*Anna worked on recovery for over five years, from May of 2008 until December of 2013. It was a slow process, and Anna ended up needing anti-anxiety meds and clomid to get her cycles back. She got her period in December of 2013 and got pregnant on the fourth cycle after that. Her cycles returned eight weeks after weaning.*)

Supplementing Recovery

For some, doubt may begin to set in when you've been all in for a good six months and still have no period. Depending on how much pressure you're feeling about getting pregnant or recovering your cycles for health reasons, you can wait for a bit longer (maybe look for support from others in a similar situation), or you can start exploring other ways to jumpstart ovulation. These include some ideas we've already mentioned: CBT, hypnosis, and anxiety medications. There are also nutritional supplements that have been shown to help with cycle recovery (acetyl-l-carnitine (ALC, http://noperiod.info/ALC), ground flax seed (http://noperiod.info/flax) and soy isoflavones, chapter 21). There are also a multitude of supplements that are suggested by other practitioners or online (http://noperiod.info/

supplements) that either do not help with recovery or may in fact be harmful, like vitex (http://noperiod.info/vitex).

Those supplements for which there is evidence for HA recovery are reviewed below. Other supplements do not have specific evidence for benefit in restoring missing periods, and are probably not worth taking. This is especially true for supplements that are supposed to "restore hormonal balance" with multiple ingredients. Often these are in doses that are unlikely to be effective, there haven't been studies on interactions between the ingredients, and the mechanisms are unrelated to HA.

It is also important to point out that many doctors will suggest birth control pills, hormone replacement therapy, or Provera/progesterone to "jump start" cycles. In our experience these do not work. All three provide levels of estradiol or progesterone that suppress FSH and LH production from the pituitary. After the medications are stopped, there is a small rebound in FSH and LH levels that could potentially be sufficient to start the follicular growth process[6]. However, as this rarely works, our supposition is that this rebound is very short-lived or doesn't reach a high enough level to actually cause the follicular growth process to begin and be sustained. There is no evidence we are aware of for menstrual cycles starting after BCP, HRT, or Provera in someone who has HA. The medical options described below work differently from this and have been shown to result in ongoing menstrual cycles.

After supplements, the next step would be treatments prescribed by your doctor. If pregnancy is not the goal at the moment, oral fertility medications, along with some other drugs that target various pathways, are a possibility for cycle restoration, as we will discuss below. Please be aware that these options should only be used *in addition to* the HA Recovery Plan. In other words, if your cycle has not restarted with adequate food intake, a decrease in exercise, and stress relief (plus time). These medications are not substitutes for fueling and resting. In addition, *before starting any medication or supplement*, please check with your doctor and read up on potential side effects and drug interactions. For example, ALC is not recommended in someone with a history of seizures, and interacts with Coumadin and Sintrom[7].

If pregnancy is your goal, the path would similarly start with oral medications to encourage ovulation. If you do not ovulate with those, typically the next step is injectable hormones (Chapter 22) or the GnRH pump if available, to cause ovulation and make pregnancy possible. If those options are not successful, in vitro fertilization (IVF) is a good option (Chapter 24).

If the oral medications do not cause ovulation, we would encourage you to give recovery a bit more time.

Nutritional Supplements

As far as nutritional supplements go, the first one to consider is ALC. Evidence from three small studies suggests that supplementing with ALC, available over the counter, can aid in recovery of cycles. In each study, participants were divided into two groups based on their LH levels; those with LH less than 3 IU/L and those with LH greater than 3 IU/L[8]. ALC had little effect on hormone levels in the women with the higher LH, but in those with the lower LH, both LH and E_2 levels increased significantly, indicating awakening of the hypothalamus. In the three studies, approximately 60% in the low LH group and 40% in the normal LH group ovulated at least once after three months of taking ALC per day[9]. The recommended dosage for ALC based on these studies is 1g per day, 500mg in the morning and 500mg at night. There was no increase in recovery with a higher dosage.

Another "nutritional/dietary supplement" that we suggest for HA recovery is ground flax seed. This recommendation is based on research into the "seed cycling" protocol that is often discussed online or possibly by naturopaths to "balance hormones." Seed cycling consists of taking flax and pumpkin seeds during the first half of the cycle (follicular phase, or from full moon to new moon if you don't have a cycle) and then sesame and sunflower seeds during the luteal phase, or between new moon to full moon. *There is no scientific evidence to support this protocol.* Looking into each of the individual seeds, however, one finds a number of potential benefits for flax seed in particular:

1) Fewer anovulatory cycles in normal cycling women[10].
2) Longer luteal phase with higher progesterone/estradiol ratio[11].
3) Reduced stress hormones and perception of stress[12].
4) A number of more general health benefits including improved lipid profile, reduction in risk of cardiovascular disease, decreased A1c in type II diabetics, and potentially cancer prevention[13].

We therefore suggest considering eating ground flax seed on a daily basis as an adjunct to recovery. The recommended amount is 10g (about 1.5 Tbsp) per day, based on what was used in the study looking at ovulation and luteal phase length[14].

Soy isoflavones (SIs) are another supplement with the potential to jump-start cycles AFTER your hypothalamus is normalized. Anecdotally there is about a 50% success rate in this case, which could simply be coincidence. There are no research studies that examine use of soy isoflavones for this application. Also, the SI do NOT work if you are early in recovery, and would not be recommended.

The isoflavones bind to and activate the estrogen receptors in your brain, making your hypothalamus sense a higher level of "estradiol[15]." You take them for five days so your brain senses this higher level, then stop, at which point your brain senses a drop in "estradiol." This mimics what happens in a natural menstrual cycle when the corpus luteum degrades (chapter 5), and if your hypothalamus is not suppressed anymore, then this can get the follicular growth process started. The rest of what happens in the cycle is your own body doing the hormonal work. If you are going to ovulate, you will likely do so around 7-14 days after taking the last pill. If you don't ovulate, we would suggest trying another round 28 days after the first. If that still doesn't work then either more recovery time is needed, or perhaps something a bit stronger, see below.

The recommended dosage is 200-250 mg of *active* SI per day (usually genistein and diadzein) for five days. Be mindful of the ingredients of what you are purchasing; some supplements will say, e.g., "100 mg isoflavones" but when you look at the small print it is only 13.8 mg active isoflavones. Please also note that a few people have recently disclosed feeling depressed while taking the soy isoflavones. If this happens to you, recognize that it is likely due to the SI and has been reported to resolve quickly. You should probably stop taking the isoflavones (and not take them again). If you have concerns or are experiencing depression interfering with daily functioning, discuss with a mental health professional to determine how to cope with the depressive symptoms.

Supplementation with actual estradiol could potentially work in the same way as the SI; unlike hormone replacement therapy where one takes estradiol consistently for 21+ days, possibly with progesterone added, a short five-day course of estradiol could potentially also make your hypothalamus sense a drop in the hormone (after stopping) and then jumpstart the follicular growth process, but this is pure speculation.

Medical Options

The next intervention to help get your period started is medicines that require a prescription from your doctor (although in some places they are available without prescription). These include the oral "ovulation induction" drugs clomiphene, letrozole, or possibly tamoxifen. Each of these medications, like the soy isoflavones, causes your brain to sense a drop in estradiol, resulting in your hypothalamus beginning the follicular growth process.

Clomiphene and tamoxifen bind to the estrogen receptors in your brain, blocking natural estradiol from binding, but do not activate the receptors themselves[16]. Your brain then senses a drop in estradiol and starts the follicular growth process. Letrozole blocks the conversion of testosterone to estradiol, thereby reducing the actual estradiol level and leading to the follicular growth process starting. We will only discuss clomiphene in this chapter as it has the most evidence for cycle restoration; further information about letrozole and tamoxifen can be found in Chapter 21.

The evidence for clomiphene being useful to get menstrual cycles started is found in a small study published in 2007. A new regimen, referred to as the "extended protocol (EP)" of Clomid was used to help people with HA recover their cycles[17]. There were only eight participants, but all eight recovered menstrual cycles and were still cycling six months later. The reason this works is that the menstrual cycle is like a perpetual motion machine; each step in the cycle is driven by the one before (chapter 5). Once your hypothalamus is no longer suppressed and the hormonal cycle starts, it tends to continue unless you resume underfueling and/or exercising on empty.

> **Molly S:** I haven't gotten my period yet, but I've noticed that I keep having "monthly" symptoms ... breakouts right around the same time of the month, lots of fertile signs ... but then nothing. I have come to terms with the fact that my body may need an extra push and I hope that I'm in a better place to start meds than I was this time last year. (*Molly got pregnant with twins on her next injection cycle. She tried three cycles at a BMI of around 20, which failed. At that point, she completely stopped all exercise, took a week's vacation from work, and fed her body! She started her fourth cycle up almost 10 lb, and sure enough, got pregnant with twin girls.*)

> **Laure:** At the end of June my period showed up after three months of Clomid. I cried I was so happy. Then at the end of July, I got another

> period, without Clomid. Then yesterday I started bleeding again. Still no treatment! I am *so, so, so, so* happy. My body is working again! These cycles were 35 and 36 days, so almost normal.

While there are no similar studies using Femara or tamoxifen with HA, it stands to reason that extended protocols of either drug would have the same end result, as the hypothalamus is stimulated just as with Clomid. Without the suppressive signals being sent by an energy restricted diet or exercise program, we believe that once the cycle of menstrual hormones is started by the medications, there is no reason for it to come to a halt again[18]*.

Another option is based on studies performed in the early 1990s that used a different oral drug called naltrexone to cause ovulation in women with HA. Naltrexone blocks the opioid receptor in the brain. Opioids like oxycodone, morphine, and other similar chronic pain medications such as codeine and Tramadol that activate the opioid receptor have been shown to reduce GnRH secretion[19], and thus shut down menstrual cycles. Therefore, opioid antagonists, which perform the opposite action, were initially demonstrated to increase GnRH signaling and cause ovulation in three women[20]. Results of two larger follow-up studies are shown on the next page. Approximately 75% of the women recruited to these studies ovulated with naltrexone treatment; Remorgida et al.[21] followed the patients afterward and found that menstrual cycles continued. As with the studies on ALC, Genazzani et al.[22] divided the subjects into those with low LH levels and those with normal LH levels (> 3 IU/L). Similar to ALC, an increase in LH levels was seen only in women with low starting LH, but ovulation occurred in both groups. We do not recommend naltrexone as the first treatment option, given that no studies have been performed in folks with HA since 1995. However, if you have tried the other methods we suggest without success, we think naltrexone is worth considering and discussing with your physician as it targets a different pathway. It is important to point out that the therapy was not effective in the three women in the Remorgida study who remained underweight (BMI < 18.5)[23], so naltrexone cannot be used as a shortcut to recovery.

---

* One potential (although unlikely) reason that cycles might not continue is mutations in the hormones or other proteins involved in the cycle.

Ovulation with naltrexone therapy

	Remorgida[24]	Genazzani[25]
Number of participants	15	Total of 30: 15 with LH < 3 IU/L; 15 with LH > 3 IU/L
Dose regimen	50 mg/day for 35 days; if ovulation occurred, continue for an additional 60 days	50 mg/day for six months
Number ovulating	8 out of 15 ovulated within 35 days	11 out of 15 in low LH group and 13 out of 15 in high LH group ovulated within 90 days
Number of cycles per ovulatory participant during study period	Between 1 and 3 in three months	Between 1 and 6 in six months

An additional treatment that sounds promising in restoring cycles is often found upon researching HA: leptin administration[26]. In one study, menstruation resumed in 75% of participants taking leptin[27], and many other hormone levels were normalized. Myalept (metreleptin) was approved by the FDA in 2014 to treat lipodystrophy, a chronic disease. Normally, once a drug is approved for use to treat a condition, doctors can prescribe it "off-label" to treat any other condition. However, in the case of Myalept, the FDA requires patients to go through an application process in order to acquire the drug. Therefore, off-label use to treat HA is unlikely. Another protein, kisspeptin, has been demonstrated to increase GnRH pulses in those with HA[28] but is not yet approved by authorities for patient use as of 2023.

Recommendations

The table below lays out our suggestions for the different options for supplementation, and cycle restoration AFTER your work on recovery is solidified. Probably the best way to assess this is by getting bloodwork done and checking your LH and estradiol levels. Another strong sign is if you are getting EWCM fairly regularly. Taking a course of Provera/progesterone can also be somewhat helpful at this point to assess whether you bleed or not.

Suggested supplement or oral medication protocols

Recovery State	LH Level	Supplement/Medication	Dosage Protocol	Duration
Just starting / early recovery	<3 IU/L	Acetyl-L-Carnitine	500 mg morning and night, daily (total of 1g / day)	Continuously until ~your third period, can be taken in conjunction with SI and Clomid**.
Solidly in recovery, no bleed in response to Provera*	3-5 IU/L	Clomid Extended Protocol (EP)**	50 mg for 5 days + 100 mg for 5 days[29]	One cycle during which ovulation occurs, then two additional cycles at 100mg/day for 5 days starting CD3. If no ovulation after two rounds of the EP, re-evaluate recovery work and/or try another method.
Solidly in recovery, bleed in response to Provera*	>5 IU/L	Soy Isoflavones (genistein and diazden)	200-250 mg / day for 5 days	Three ovulatory cycles, starting CD1 of following cycles. If no ovulation occurs on the first cycle, try a second round 28 days later. If still no ovulation, try a different option.
Solidly in recovery, bleed in response to Provera*	>5 IU/L	Clomid**	50 mg / day for 5 days	Three ovulatory cycles. Start on CD3 for subsequent cycles. If no ovulation, try a higher dose / longer timeframe.
Solidly in recovery, after trying SI and oral ovulation induction	>5 IU/L	Naltrexone	50 mg / day	Continue daily for 3-6 months

* It is not necessary to try another Provera challenge at this point, but if you do it can help guide as to which protocol to use.
** There is one study that found that response to Clomid in people with PCOS was improved when acetyl-l-carnitine was taken at the same time. If you are already taking ALC when trying Clomid, no need to stop. If Clomid does not work, you could consider adding ALC in addition to working further on recovery[30].

There are many factors that come into play when you consider medical treatments. Finances, insurance, whether your partner is on board, and how patient (or impatient) you are can all affect what the best plan is for you. How do you feel about waiting a few more months? Does the idea make you sick to your stomach, or are you able to enjoy this time of recovery? Is feeling stuck worse for your mental health than the stress that can come along with treatments? Make a plan that feels right for you. Something like, "Wait X more months for a natural cycle, then start a supplement or medical treatment." Often having a plan makes the waiting easier because you no longer feel like you're looking down an endless tunnel.

Why Me?

While you are waiting to get your period back, whether you're going "all natural" or trying various supplements or treatments, and particularly if you are longing for a baby, it can feel like all your work has been for nothing. What is the point? In particular, seeing others attaining your dream can be difficult. Facebook announcements from other runners, athletes, and those thinner-than-you seemingly pregnant at the drop of a hat can throw a damper on an otherwise pleasant mood. Or, a phone call from a skinny Fertile Myrtle (insert friend/relative here) announcing an "oops" pregnancy can likewise start a pity party. Sure, you "like" the sonogram on Facebook, and squeal about the pregnancy with the best of them; but that may be followed by a few tears or getting angry and taking it out on your partner, particularly if they don't understand your emotions. It is common to feel some sadness for yourself when you witness others easily experiencing the joy you are yearning for.

> *Judith*: My new mantra this year is "This is my journey—my journey is different," but, jeez, was that tested yesterday! My best friend has a beautiful two-year-old son, conceived on her first go despite being a super skinny runner whose husband smokes and drinks a lot. I thought it must have been a fluke, but apparently not—she just tried one more time, and yes, is knocked up with number two! Of course I am so happy for her, but it is incredible how some people literally can't help but fall pregnant, while it feels almost impossible for others!

But as they say, the grass is always greener on the other side of the fence. It is easy to look at these others with envy and wonder how they could possibly be pregnant or menstruating while you are not. Why couldn't you just be one of those lucky ones? In reality, though, if they share the same habits and fears as you used to, they are not lucky at all. HAers are the lucky ones. As much as the recovery process can feel awful, in the end it is liberating. Those who share our destructive habits but do not have HA may have been able to get pregnant, but will still have food, exercise, and stress issues after the baby arrives. People who have overcome HA have expressed appreciation for so many different aspects of recovery. Patience, ordering what sounds good at a restaurant, happier, no more "binges," time and energy to enjoy life, better athletic performance, mood, relationships, feeling warmer, improved relationship with your body, resurrection of libido, sleeping in, not scheduling life around workouts, desserts, healed digestive system, freedom around food, improved bones, deeper laughter, listening to what your body wants for food and when, not feeling out of control around food, less anxiety, discovering a more fun balanced person!

> *Carly*: When I finally got pregnant, I was seriously only doing yoga one to two times per week. That's it! I also want to say that *if you do this now, it will make your pregnancy so much easier*! When you crave empty carbs during your first trimester, you will be over the guilty feeling and just roll with it. You will be feeding a baby, and what you crave is what the baby needs. I especially say this about exercise. I didn't do a lick of exercise the past week; you know why? After a long day of work (on my feet—I'm a teacher), all I wanted was my couch and a nap at about 3:30 p.m. So, I did it! In a past life I would have felt guilty and, after I woke up, would have found some form of exercise to do. But if my body craves rest to nurture my little twins that are growing, then that's what I will give them.

Above all else, while you are working to recover, we encourage you to see the bigger picture. It is all too easy to get caught up in the endgame (pregnancy or the return of your menstrual cycle) that you do not realize how much recovery is doing for you and the people you love. If you take a step back, you will see the benefits of implementing our recommendations. You will notice you are overall happier (except maybe about how you think you look, but as we've said before, others generally don't agree with you), participating in day-to-day activities, supporting the people who love and/or rely on you, and improving your health. HA is a blessing inside a curse. The diagnosis of HA provides a necessary wake-up call: it tells you that you are hurting yourself and things need to change. Yes, you may have an ultimate goal that you are fixated on, and there is nothing wrong with that, but in the process you might notice you are doing a whole lot more than getting your period or getting pregnant; you are regaining your life.

> *Andrea R*: My grandparents visited us for the holiday and I bravely asked my grandmother how I looked/if she thought I was gaining too much weight. She started to cry. She said, "You have no idea how good you look now. I used to tell your mother that if you continued to lose weight you wouldn't live to see your children grow up. I am so happy to see you thriving and healthy again." There was a lot more that she said and the tears flowed. But it hit me hard because she is probably right. If I take *anything* in, and if for whatever reason I am not able to get pregnant again, at least this was a big eye-opener to get better for my children. I'm not saying this is any easier—I had another complete meltdown today over my body—but my children and hopefully future children are relying on me.

> *Jennifer C*: I have been feeling really strange the last month: nipples and breasts killing me, getting a really big, bloated belly, while my weight stays stable at my new number, and my exercise has come down to only walking for an hour five days a week. That is *huge* for me. I was on my walk this morning and I felt this surge of wetness. Then had really bad cramps. I went home to use the bathroom, and *I had my period*. After *20 years* without a cycle!! I hope this is for real and it stays monthly. You are all so right; all the discomfort and weight gain are so worth it. My bones are being protected. YES!! (*Jennifer was all in for nine months before starting fertility treatments; she used Clomid for her first pregnancy, but unfortunately had a miscarriage. She got pregnant again 13 months later, naturally.*)

Parting Thoughts

It is difficult to come to terms with the fact that you are struggling each and every day to regain your period or get pregnant and nothing has happened yet. You may need to just give it time (we know how frustrating that sounds but it is true), or you may need to examine whether you are truly going "all in." It is also possible that the underlying stress from this entire process is contributing to the problem. Things like going on vacation or taking a break from your regular/familiar routine, reading, learning something new, doing yoga or acupuncture may help reduce these effects, or it may be time to think about medical treatments. Regardless, do not think of this time as time wasted; it is time that is being well spent toward becoming healthy emotionally and physically for the rest of your life.

Elissa: When I think back to how I was with exercise and "healthy" eating, I can't believe I actually lived my life that way. I believe that HA was my wake-up call and, despite the emotional roller coaster that this has been, I am actually grateful for the experience because I found my way back to the person I truly am. You all can do it!!

Lisa: I remember back to the day that marked my fifth month all in and still without a period. I felt like a sausage about to burst out of its casing. I continued to excuse my physical transformation with unsolicited verbiage such as, "I'm, um...increasing my fat storage for pregnancy?" or, "Yes... I really stopped running and training after 30 years." Ironically, a week after the five-month mark *my period came*!!! I freaked out in a very happy, joyful way. Here is my Board post when my period arrived:

"For the first time in over 12 years I got my period today. I felt like crying...so very thankful. I am on month five(ish) of reduced exercise, a.k.a. walking (with a couple of random runs and heavy squats) and month two of increased calories and NEVER allowing myself to do any activity in a deficit. A month ago I started eating breakfast, which I had not done in about eight years.

I am still not comfortable in my skin but I am willing to be uncomfortable with my body for the sake of my health and the possibility of getting pregnant. I do not feel like I am out of the woods by any stretch of the imagination, but menstruating on my own is a very good sign.

Take note: I am 43 (old) and if my body can recover from the years of neglect I put it through, yours can too. In fact, I was pretty certain I was too old to recover from the damage done and age.

Lastly, by God's grace I stumbled onto this forum years ago, pestered Nico for specifics, slowly trusted the information provided from all the girls, and then later (much later) finally applied what has been PROVEN to work..."

Remember when I wrote I was "excusing" myself for the outward physical and lifestyle changes taking place? That stopped cold turkey after I got my period back (though I really dislike that I needed "the prize" before I was filled with the confidence I had not had up until that point). I share this experience with you in hopes that you might take away two things. 1) Although you might not see the healing taking place, have faith that something positive is indeed happening and when the time comes, you too will experience this joy. 2) I encourage you to look beyond what you deem imperfect and instead embrace the changes, apologizing to no one and owing no explanation for doing what it takes to reclaim your health. No longer being bound by exercise times and amounts, scheduled food, or food groups is true freedom. Freedom you deserve.

19
Luteal Phase

IN THE LAST CHAPTER we talked a lot about the first half of your menstrual cycle—what signs lead up to ovulation, and how to confirm ovulation. The second half of your menstrual cycle, between when you ovulate and when your period arrives (or not, if you're pregnant), is also important. During this luteal phase (LP), your uterine lining undergoes changes driven by a marked increase in progesterone and sustained higher levels of estrogen after ovulation to prepare for an embryo to implant and start a pregnancy. The higher levels of progesterone and sustained higher levels of estrogen also appear to be helpful for building bone density. For those with a history of HA, it is common for the LP to be short. This can potentially make it more difficult to get pregnant, whether you are trying to conceive naturally or with medications. There might also be less positive consequences for bones than with a longer LP; however, this topic requires more research. Surprisingly, there is a lot of controversy over what creates a luteal phase defect (LPD), and how, or even whether, to treat an LPD. We will share the evidence on both sides of this argument, as well as what you can do to lengthen a short LP.

A normal LP is between 10 and 14 days. During this time, the corpus luteum—the structure left behind when your follicle ruptures to release an egg—produces progesterone and estrogen that prepare your uterus for implantation. A normal LP allows plenty of time for an embryo to attach to your uterus and start producing the "pregnancy hormone," human chorionic gonadotropin (hCG). One of the effects of hCG is to support the corpus luteum and keep it from breaking down. This causes continued progesterone and estrogen production so the uterine lining can thicken further instead of shedding, as it does when there is no pregnancy and you get your period.

In an abnormal cycle with either a short LP (typically less than 10 days[1]) or where there is not enough progesterone to adequately prepare the lining (less than 8 ng/mL or ~25 nmol/L[2]), there is strong evidence that chances of pregnancy are diminished[3], and miscarriage rates are higher[4]. Unfortunately, abnormal LPs are quite common when recovering from HA (and even after recovery for some). Our LP is often the first sign that our system is in a borderline status. As we recover from HA, the LP is the last part of the reproductive cycle to return to normal. A short LP is obvious if you are tracking your cycles as we described in chapter 17. An LP with adequate length but low progesterone can only be discovered by getting your progesterone level tested, which is not common practice. Note that if you do have your progesterone tested during the LP, it is recommended to perform two tests three hours apart as progesterone is produced in pulses, although this is not standard practice at the moment. A single low reading (found in 15% of those with a normal LP) can merely indicate that a pulse is imminent[5].

> *Jamie*: I went in today and had two good-sized follicles, so I get to trigger tonight! I am having a progesterone test because I started spotting 10 DPO and had a borderline short luteal phase with the new Clomid protocol. I keep thinking that if I had used progesterone on those cycles I might have gotten pregnant. Oh well, I'm almost in a new two-week wait! I really hope this is it!

> *Allison*: My period is here with a vengeance. And at only 5 DPO. So now I am worried about short luteal phases. I know in many ways this is positive… it's the first time I've ovulated in at least nine months, so my period is a good thing. But it's hard not to still be bummed. My flow is heavy and my temperature is down today, so the bleeding is definitely not from implantation.

> *Lara*: Yup, my period is here. I just had a super short luteal phase. All of you who asked if I was doing progesterone supplements sure knew what you were talking about. I'm not too disappointed—this is the first time I have ovulated in so long. Now I know for next time to use the supplements.

In this chapter, we dive back into the research to get to the bottom of a common statement among doctors that "an inadequate luteal phase is because of a 'poor ovulation'," and that "you need to fix the ovulation problem; progesterone support won't help." This theory is based on questionable conclusions drawn in studies from the early 1970s. More recent research has shown that there are in fact fixable issues that occur specifically during the luteal phase, unrelated to the "strength of ovulation." Progesterone support certainly can help in many cases. However, if your doctor is unwilling to prescribe progesterone if your LP is short, we offer some alternatives that can potentially help.

Physiology of the Luteal Phase

> Lara: I asked my doctor about progesterone supplements and he said that they are pointless—that if a follicle doesn't produce enough progesterone then we have a bigger problem. I know most of you have done/are doing progesterone supplements. What do you think about his argument? I'm pretty nervous about having a short luteal phase.

> Lena: My RE doesn't want me to do progesterone either, even though I have had two short luteal phases on Clomid. She also feels that if the corpus luteum isn't producing enough progesterone, it is a "bad ovulation" and progesterone will not make a difference. She told me that the most common reason for a short luteal phase is not enough drive to the follicle in the follicular phase. She said it only helps for a very small number of people who do not make enough of their own progesterone. She thinks it just means you need a higher dose of Clomid—a bigger drive to the follicle early in the cycle.

Research studies in the early 1970s found lower levels of FSH and LH in women with LPD[6]. The low hormone levels were interpreted as inadequate follicular development, leading to today's "poor ovulation" theory. One could argue, however, that the LPD and lower hormones all had the same underlying cause (e.g., energy deficit), rather than the lower FSH and LH *leading* to LPD. Later research showed that in some women, LPDs were fixed by "strengthening" ovulation with Clomid[7], although other studies found that Clomid actually caused LPD[8]—this dichotomy neither supports nor disproves the poor ovulation theory. Injectable gonadotropins have also been suggested as a way to "strengthen ovulation" and cure LPD, as the amount of FSH and LH provided for the follicles to develop is greater than what is available naturally. However, progesterone support in gonadotropin cycles has been found to be even more important than with Clomid cycles[9]. None of this evidence particularly supports "poor ovulation" as the cause of LPD.

Data from our survey respondents show that there are similar rates of LPD (less than 10-day LP) in natural as well as treated cycles:

- Natural cycles: 30% of respondents had LPD in their first cycle
- Oral medications: 38% had LPD
- Injectable cycles: 18% had LPD (not significantly different).

The differences in percentages between natural cycles with theoretically inadequate ovulation and medicated cycles with "stronger ovulation" were not significant*, which also fails to support "poor ovulation" as a cause of LPD.

Further supporting the theory that LPD is not due to poor ovulation, a study in which women performed exercise during only the follicular phase or only the luteal phase found that both decreased luteal phase length. In fact, more women in the group performing exercise during the luteal phase, i.e., *after* ovulation, had short luteal phases than those who exercised before ovulation[10]. This latter finding demonstrates that the "strength" of ovulation has nothing to do with LPD in this case. If exercise was not started until after a normal ovulation, clearly the ovulation itself was not the problem.

Recent research has provided a clearer picture of what leads to LPD. Wuttke et al. found that luteal phase defects can be divided into three classes: hypothalamic LPD, small luteal cell LPD, and large luteal cell LPD[11]. Let's back up a little. As explained earlier, after the follicle ruptures to release the egg during ovulation, the structure that is left behind is called the corpus luteum. There are two different cell types in the corpus luteum that are involved in progesterone production during the LP: large and small luteal cells. The large luteal cells produce a baseline level of progesterone; the small luteal cells secrete additional progesterone in waves, with each wave started by a pulse of LH from the pituitary gland. The LH pulses do not stop when you ovulate, but continue throughout the rest of the cycle. It's been a while since we've discussed LH; recall from chapter 5 that pulses of gonadotropin-releasing hormone (GnRH) from the hypothalamus are the major signals that cause the pituitary to produce FSH and LH, also in pulses. During the LP, progesterone from the luteal cells prevents the hypothalamus from producing GnRH until the progesterone drops below

---

* The differences in percentage of survey respondents undergoing natural cycles or using oral or injectable medications with LPD were not significant ($p = 0.62$) partially due to only a few cycles in which injectables were used without progesterone support.

a certain level. When the GnRH pulse does occur, it leads to an LH pulse from the pituitary, which causes a progesterone pulse from the small luteal cells and an increase in progesterone. In case that all makes your brain a little fuzzy, here are the three key points to understand:

1) A constant baseline level of progesterone is produced by the large luteal cells.
2) Additional progesterone is produced by the small luteal cells in pulses.
3) The progesterone pulses are triggered by the hypothalamus when the progesterone level drops too low.

In hypothalamic LPD, the hypothalamus is overly sensitive to progesterone and is shut down by very low levels, so doesn't produce GnRH at appropriate times. This means the progesterone pulses don't happen often enough to keep the levels where they need to be. LH pulses were measured in women with hypothalamic LPD and found to be much slower than normal[12] (interestingly, exactly the issue when we have HA). When these women were given injections of hCG, which is chemically similar to LH, the small luteal cells were activated and produced more progesterone, and the LPD was eliminated[13]. This experiment proves that the LPD is due to insufficient LH, not a defect in the corpus luteum or "inadequate ovulation."

In the second form of LPD, LH pulses are normal, but the small cells do not produce progesterone. Progesterone support is therefore required to rescue the LP. With the final type, the large cells produce no progesterone, so the baseline progesterone level is too low. Injections of hCG cause the small cells to produce sufficient progesterone for a normal luteal phase[14]; supplemental progesterone also works.

It seems obvious that hypothalamic LPD is the culprit in those of us with HA. After HA recovery, even though the hypothalamus and pituitary work to trigger ovulation, it appears there is still a higher-than-normal sensitivity of the hypothalamus to suppression by progesterone, caloric deficit, and stress (exercise). Therefore, it is reasonable to consider treatment of an LPD in someone who has recovered or is recovering from HA.

What to Do About a Short LP

We said earlier that LPDs are treatable, and they are. But it is also true that in many cases, LPs will naturally lengthen over time as HA recovery solidifies, so you may not need to do anything. In our survey respondents with a short initial LP, 67% had their cycles lengthen naturally and went on to get pregnant with no progesterone support. In many cases there was an LP increase of four to five days between the first and second cycles. In those with a short initial LP, the average number of cycles to pregnancy was four, with a range from two to eight. There were a couple of people who had very short LPs (three and four days) who got pregnant the very next cycle. The remaining third used progesterone (typically prescription suppositories) to lengthen their LP and achieve pregnancy.

In those with borderline LPs of 10 days, 8 out of 10 got pregnant without using progesterone; the other two used progesterone during the cycle in which they conceived. One had her LP lengthen naturally prior to using the progesterone, but decided to take it when she was not getting pregnant just in case her level was too low, despite the normal LP length. The other went from an LP of 10 days down to 7, and used progesterone her next cycle, on which she conceived.

This evidence suggests that even with a short initial LP, pregnancy is achievable as the LP naturally lengthens over time. However, there are some for whom the LP remains short; in these cases, we suggest trying one of the methods below to provide the optimal chances of pregnancy.

Remedies to Lengthen Your LP

There are a number of options to potentially lengthen your LP, ranging from medications that can be prescribed by your doctor to over-the-counter supplements. The optimal way to lengthen your LP is with prescription progesterone or hCG booster shots.

- Prescription progesterone: Many forms of this medication are available: a vaginal suppository, cream, or gel; intramuscular injection; or an oral pill. There is no evidence suggesting any one type is more effective (although the oral pill is probably least effective[15]). The vaginal creams and gels are typically more expensive, so if you are paying out of pocket you may want to ask for Prometrium capsules that you can use as vaginal suppositories.
- Prometrium doses can range anywhere from 100 mg once a day to 200 mg three times a day. It doesn't seem to make a big difference unless your progesterone levels are extremely low, so we'd suggest 200 mg once a day. The pills are pink (100 mg) or light yellow (200 mg) gel capsules that can be taken either orally or vaginally. We recommend the latter due to improved absorption[16]. Insert the suppositories just

before bed so there is less leakage, and wear a panty liner—what leaks out is oily and hard to get out of clothes.
- If you use suppositories two or three times a day, it can help to lie down for 20 to 30 minutes afterward. It is not mandatory to do so, but you will get a lot of leakage if you have to stand straight away.
- Vaginal progesterone has been shown to increase blood progesterone levels by around 10-15 ng/mL[17].
- hCG booster shots: The final method that is occasionally prescribed by physicians to support the luteal phase (typically only after medicated ovulation induction) is human chorionic gonadotropin (hCG) booster shots. This is the most physiological way to improve an LP, especially hypothalamic LPD. These shots are often given a few times during the LP, e.g. 1500 IU at 3, 6, and 9 DPO.

> **Mandy:** How do you convince your RE to give you progesterone support? I can't get my nurse to prescribe me some. She says if I do blood work next week and my progesterone is low, then the doctor will prescribe it for me.

Some doctors are not willing to prescribe progesterone or booster shots, in which case it is worth trying other supplements that may positively affect your progesterone levels and luteal phase length. The options are:

- Ascorbic acid (a.k.a. vitamin C; 750 mg per day starting CD 1) was demonstrated to increase LP progesterone levels by almost 100%[18].
- Ground flax seed (http://noperiod.info/flax) has also been shown to increase luteal phase length by up to five days. The dose used in the study was 10g per day[19].
- There is a single, small clinical study that assessed the effect of the herbal mix FertilityBlend™ on the luteal phase, and showed a 50% increase in mid-LP progesterone as well as three additional days of higher basal temperatures[20].
- Over-the-counter progesterone creams have been shown to increase blood levels of progesterone by 1 to 2 ng/mL[21], and also to induce expected changes in the uterine lining[22] and HAers have used it to lengthen their LPs by one to two days. To apply, you rub a dime- to nickel-sized amount on your skin (arm or abdomen). This is not meant for vaginal use!
- Vitamin B Complex has a reputation for increasing one's LP, although there are no scientific studies documenting that assertion.

Studies in IVF patients have shown that progesterone supplementation can markedly increase pregnancy rates and decrease early pregnancy loss[23]. Studies in natural cycles are not as definitive but also support the claim that there is a minimum progesterone level required for a successful pregnancy[24].

In fact, in the study we mentioned where progesterone levels were improved by taking vitamin C, there was a higher pregnancy rate in the group taking vitamin C[25]. In the group taking no supplements, 22% of LPs improved, whereas 53% of LPs improved in the group taking vitamin C. All pregnancies occurred in those whose LP improved. Of course this is only one study, but taking extra vitamin C seems worth a try as it is simple, inexpensive, and has other health benefits as well.

If you choose to take progesterone in order to lengthen your luteal phase and become pregnant, it is currently common practice to continue the progesterone supplementation until late in the first trimester. This is well after the placenta has taken over progesterone production from the corpus luteum, which occurs at around seven to eight weeks gestation[26]. However, a couple of recent studies call that standard into question[27], with preliminary evidence suggesting that it may be prudent to continue progesterone only as long as needed. Once implantation has occurred the embryo starts producing human chorionic gonadotropin (hCG) that takes over the function of supporting the large cells in the corpus luteum from the hypothalamic-driven LH[28]. So if the pregnancy is proceeding routinely, progesterone from the corpus luteum is sufficient, driven by normally rising hCG from the embryo[29]. Recent meta-analyses find that taking progesterone likely does not impact miscarriage except when someone has a history of pregnancy loss and starts bleeding, in which case added progesterone can be helpful[30]. This is an evolving topic, so please discuss these questions with your physician.

Parting Thoughts

As we described, it is common to have a short luteal phase after recovering from HA. The LP does tend to lengthen naturally over time, but some do have naturally short LPs. In this case, especially if pregnancy has been attempted for a few cycles with no success, one of the following methods could be used to increase progesterone and lengthen the luteal phase:

- prescription progesterone
- hCG booster shots

- supplements (vitamin C, vitamin B, and FertilityBlend™)
- over-the-counter progesterone cream

Lisa: Losing your period is all fun and games until you get it back only to find you now have a short LP. Please know that this LP issue seems to be pretty random—it's hit or miss as to who develops a short LP among recovered HAers. Now before you start to put this on your worry list, take note that the encouraging part about a possible LP defect is that there is a good chance it will correct itself with no intervention; if not, as you have read, there are conservative solutions for the issue.

Part 3:
When it Takes More Than an "Oops" to Get Pregnant

> *Nico*: All in all, it took me 18 months from when I figured out I wasn't ovulating to finally getting those amazing two lines: pregnant. There were a lot of ups and downs. From the high of getting my first period to the low after my fourth failed injectable cycle when I was convinced that there was no way IVF would work either. I feared I was going to be barren forever and could kiss my dreams of a future with children and grandchildren goodbye. I'll cut the suspense and tell you that it was in fact a natural cycle that got me my first positive pregnancy test and baby.

Nico gained extensive knowledge as to what works to help HAers get pregnant through her own experiences, research, and years posting on the Board. She also garnered a better understanding of commonalities in treatment cycles that many doctors aren't aware of since they don't see many HA patients. In providing suggestions regarding medications in the upcoming chapters, we want to be clear that we are not medical doctors, and the information we offer is to help you be informed and understand the medical options. *Decisions on treatments should be made together with your healthcare provider.*

In this part, you'll learn about your fertile signs and when the best times are to have intercourse in order to conceive, whether you are trying naturally or with the help of oral medications. If you are choosing to use fertility treatments, we also include some general information that may be helpful for you to know. We will discuss the oral medications that encourage ovulation such as Clomid, Femara, tamoxifen, and soy isoflavones and what to expect during those cycles, as well as different options for dosing. We also talk about different experiences going through cycles using injectable gonadotropins to induce ovulation. Finally, sometimes even with working toward recovery or after recovering, the big guns of IVF are still needed; we will walk you through what a typical IVF cycle looks like and some points to consider. Ultimately, know that whichever method you end up using to get pregnant, the hard work you have put in to recover will absolutely boost your chances of success.

20
When You Need a Jump-start

THERE MAY BE a few different reasons that despite having followed the HA Recovery Plan, hopefully for a good six months, you decide to move forward with fertility treatments such as oral medications, injectable gonadotropins, or IVF. In some cases, natural cycles return but you still don't get pregnant. Sometimes cycles are super long (longer than 45 days), which means your opportunities to get pregnant are less frequent. Or perhaps, despite going all in with recovery, natural cycles are still MIA. Oral or injectable medications can help in each of these situations, but if your RE has concerns about egg or sperm quality (see the end of this chapter) or if other treatments have failed, he or she may counsel you to move on to IVF.

You can encounter mixed emotions when you start thinking about needing help to get pregnant. Initially, you will probably feel excited about the possibility of finally ovulating instead of just sitting around waiting. But there can also be some anxiety, self-doubt, and even depression. These emotions may intensify the further you get into fertility treatments. In particular, you might feel angry with yourself, or guilty, for getting into this predicament in the first place. But guilt and regret will do you no favors. Now is about your future and taking hold of the lessons you have learned and using them for good—being a healthy mom, and having a healthy baby in return.

Support during this time is essential; remember to keep lines of communication open with your spouse/partner. In addition, others in your life who have struggled with infertility (or those who haven't experienced infertility themselves but are empathetic and caring) can be a wonderful sounding board and shoulder to cry on. Online forums and blogs can provide a lifeline to those who understand, or, if you prefer face-to-face interaction, in the U.S. RESOLVE offers local infertility support groups, and similar groups can be found in other countries. Seeing a therapist can also help you work through the reality of the situation. With that being said, please know that you are not alone and you can and will get through this.

This chapter provides information useful for a variety of fertility treatments you might use. Sections include:

- Do you need to work on recovery first?
- Where do you go for help?
- What can you expect for pre-treatment testing?
- Should your partner be doing anything?
- What do you need to know about "diminished ovarian reserve" (DOR)?

Do You Need to Work on Recovery First?

> Sara: At the beginning I thought, yeah, my BMI is on the low side but it's still "normal." (It was 19.) Even though I couldn't get my periods back on my own I thought, no problem, treatment will work just fine. Well, I was wrong. After three Clomid cycles with no ovulation and five failed injection cycles (two canceled due to no response or overstimulation), I finally worked out that body fat has *everything* to do with conceiving as well as keeping the baby (when finally falling pregnant). I started gaining weight during my injection cycles and had the best response when I was at my heaviest. It was totally incomprehensible to me at the time, but I had to get to a BMI of 24 to finally ovulate naturally and fall pregnant. I shed many, many tears along the way and went through clothes not fitting and feeling horrible about myself for such a long time, but I finally realized that being at that very low BMI was not healthy—for my reproductive system or my body in general. Medical intervention is not an exact science; otherwise, everyone would fall pregnant on the first go. There are many on the Board who had to learn the hard way, including me. It's a harsh reality, but yes, gaining weight will help you get and stay pregnant. Once I got my positive pregnancy test, I never looked back regarding the weight gain and am a so much happier, balanced person for it.

Throughout this book, we have talked about the importance of gaining weight and reducing exercise. Now that you are about to embark on the path of medical treatment, we want to reinforce that message. Your doctor may suggest that your weight, exercise, and eating won't make a difference—that you will respond to drugs just fine, and they will get you pregnant. We respectfully disagree. While there is always a possibility of responding to meds and getting pregnant, in our experience, those who put in the time and effort toward recovery often respond far better to fertility treatment than those who have not yet begun the healing process. In addition, as you go through the journey of recovery, you gain firsthand knowledge of how to be truly healthy during and after pregnancy.

Along with the anecdotal data we have collected through our involvement with the Board, biological evidence suggests that recovery can assist in getting pregnant. Remember our old friend, leptin? It's the hormone produced by fat cells, and it is found, along with its receptors, in the uterus[1]. The receptor levels are highest at the time when an embryo would be implanting, between 5 and 10 DPO. In mice, leptin is required for implantation of an embryo—when mice are unable to produce leptin they cannot get pregnant[2]. The human system works similarly[3]. When you are in the throes of HA, especially if you are underweight, your leptin levels will likely be low. Gaining weight will increase leptin levels, and therefore, your chances of successful treatment.

> *Dana*: I conceived naturally on my third ovulation. I had done Clomid and injectables, but neither worked (no response to the one, over-response to the other) and I finally gave up. I stopped running completely, started eating a lot more, and, lo and behold, I ovulated all on my own.

> *Anna P*: After eight months without a cycle, I knew I had to start making changes. I cut back on workouts, started eating more, and gained over 10 lb in the next four months. I felt like I was doing all the right things and as nothing was happening, decided we were ready for treatment. We tried one round of letrozole and I didn't respond. Nothing. No ovulation, no period; nada. At that point, it had been a year without a period, so I decided to throw in the towel and go all in. My two times a week runs were going to be no more. I focused on Barre3 classes and walking when I felt like it, but did no high intensity exercise whatsoever. Within three months my period was back! After another 55 days with no signs of ovulation I saw my RE. He informed me that I had not yet ovulated and didn't seem close. My husband and I decided to try ONE round of treatment (which ended up being seven days of low dose injections). Well—somehow that one try worked and I am now almost 10 weeks pregnant. I can wholeheartedly say that it would not have worked if I hadn't gone all in, learned

> to relax, learned to trust the process, and learned to love myself. I know how hard this journey can be, but the lifestyle changes are so incredibly worth it. I am thankful I was able to learn so much about myself; I truly believe my journey with HA has made me a better, more thankful, person, and will most definitely make me a better mother.

Where Do You Go for Help?

If you are not already seeing a specialist to help you get pregnant, it can be difficult to know where to begin. First, if you are cycling naturally, the general guidelines are to try to conceive for a year if you're under 35 years old, or six months if you are over 35, before starting fertility treatments. This recommendation is based on evidence that in a vast majority of cases, it is just a matter of time before everything lines up and egg and sperm connect. The figure below shows how many cycles it took for our survey respondents to get pregnant. Yes, some people were successful in getting pregnant on their first try or two, but unfortunately that's not true for everyone. It can feel impossibly hard to be patient when you want to be pregnant, but remember, there are no guarantees with treatment cycles either. For that reason, we suggest that if you are cycling, you try naturally for at least six months before moving to treatment. Most insurance plans follow these time guidelines as well, so if you do make appointments prior to a year or six months, your insurance may not cover the costs.

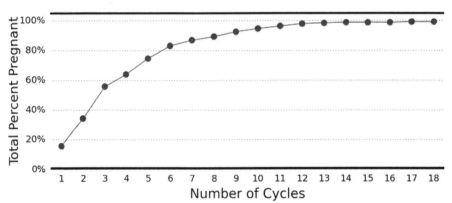

Number of cycles to achieve conception. This figure shows the percentage of HAers pregnant after one, two, three, etc., cycles, including both natural and medicated cycles.

There are two types of doctors that can help you once you decide that it is time to try something different and look at fertility treatments. Your obstetrician/gynecologist (ob-gyn) can do some of the initial testing and prescribe oral medications like Femara, Clomid, or tamoxifen (chapter 21). If those don't work, or if anything of concern is found in your testing, your ob-gyn will typically refer you to a reproductive endocrinologist (RE). These doctors tend to monitor cycles more closely, and can prescribe injectables or IVF if that is what you decide is right for you.

It is important to have an ob-gyn or RE with whom you feel comfortable—someone who will take the time to answer your questions and treat you as an individual rather than just another number. Given that there are specific issues encountered by folks with HA that differ from typical fertility treatment, you should look for a practitioner who will take your HA history into account. We'll discuss these variations in the upcoming chapters. If you find a practice you like but aren't feeling confident with the initial person you meet, do not be afraid to ask to see a different doctor.

> *Steph*: When I sought medical help for HA (before I even knew it was HA), I went to my ob-gyn. She did what she could, which was two rounds of Provera. Then she referred me to the RE in her office promising I would love him. Well, about two minutes into my appointment, I knew we just wouldn't click. I asked him not to share my weight and he repeatedly mentioned it. He was not sensitive to my feelings or reactions. Granted, his diagnosis and suggestions were spot on, but I couldn't work with someone who saw the process as so black and white, without emotion or struggle. He didn't get me and therefore I couldn't trust him or his recommendations. My dietitian Nancy Clark, recommended Dr. Janet Hall. At our first appointment, she listened to me as I told my story. She cared, she gave me a hug, she made me feel like we were a team and would get through this together. I loved her from the start. She offered similar advice to the first RE, but also support and empathy, which made it much easier to trust and listen to her.

> *Carol*: My appointment with the RE went really well. My husband liked him a lot too. He basically said, "Sounds like HA, you are doing all the right things, keep eating fat and not running," and he thought I would start cycling again very soon. He was just so confident I would get my cycles back on my own. It was amazing to feel so validated!

Pre-treatment Testing

If you are seeing an ob-gyn for fertility treatment, you probably won't undergo much of the testing laid out below. On the other hand, an RE may suggest some testing prior to going forward with oral medications. In most cases, however, these tests are performed prior to starting an injectable cycle. This is because injectable cycles are much more expensive so it is best to ensure that there are no other issues preventing pregnancy before moving forward with treatment. Typically, the tests include blood work, an ultrasound, and a hysterosalpingogram (HSG).

Ultrasound. A baseline vaginal ultrasound is performed, normally on CD 3. If you haven't had a period recently, your doctor may induce a bleed by having you take birth control pills or Provera, or will perform the baseline scan on a random day. The doctor or sonographer will look at your uterus and ovaries to make sure everything looks normal and that there are no leftover large cysts in your ovaries that can interfere with treatment. They will also count the number of small baseline (antral) follicles you have.

Your first CD 3 ultrasound can feel awkward if you still have your period. It's hard not to feel self-conscious, but keep in mind that those performing the ultrasound don't think twice about it so neither should you. We suggest wearing a pad instead of a tampon, or remember to take your tampon out just before the appointment, with a pad for backup.

Hysterosalpingogram (HSG). In this test, a dye containing a miniscule amount of radioactivity is injected into your uterus through a catheter, and the radiologist will follow the dye by x-ray. This will allow them to determine if your fallopian tubes are open, and also give a look at the shape of your uterine cavity. Both blocked tubes and an abnormally shaped uterus can affect chances of pregnancy.

The HSG can range anywhere from feeling just mildly uncomfortable, like period cramps, to very painful. You can take some ibuprofen beforehand to lessen the discomfort. Most experience mild soreness and are able to return to work immediately following the procedure, but for others it might be more painful, with residual cramps afterward. Make sure you wear or ask for a pad after this procedure, as you may experience some leakage of the leftover (fortunately colorless) dye.

> *Nico (2005)*: I had my HSG yesterday. It wasn't too bad. It took the radiologist about five minutes to find my cervix, which was interesting. Two things I found amusing: first, the tech who was helping draped my lower body entirely in towels. So all I was to the radiologist was a vagina. I thought it was a funny way of depersonalizing the procedure. Second, well, they got me all set up, catheter in the right place, balloon blown up, then the radiologist and the tech both left the room and came back

in wearing their lead aprons. I couldn't stop laughing for five minutes—the radiologist's apron was in a camouflage pattern! The test itself was fine—I felt a few minor cramps, but nothing unbearable. I thought it was neat watching on the screen. Yes, I'm a nerd like that.

Molly: I was really worried about my HSG, but it was fine. About one minute (maybe less) of acute discomfort and then an afternoon of moderate (but not horrid) period-style cramps. But it was good to know the tubes were in order...

Aya: The HSG made me sore! Ouch! But once it was over, no problems. I was thinking, if I can't take the pain of a shot of dye, how am I going to give birth? Everything looked great, so that was good. Next is chasing after my husband for a semen analysis—what a weird thing we have to do!

Jackie: My HSG was painful—the worst part was putting the catheter in and then filling with water... the cramps were bad, but I'm thinking they were worse because I was so tense. Also, my RE had me take an antibiotic starting the night before. It was super strong and about made me sick. Bleh!

Lisa (2009): I just had my HSG today. I was worried and thought it would really hurt because the RE recommended I take 800 mg aspirin beforehand. It was a breeze and I didn't take any meds for pain. A little pinching but that was about it.

Hysteroscopy. If any abnormalities are seen on the HSG or otherwise suspected, your doctor may order a hysteroscopy. In this procedure, your uterus is filled with a saline solution and a camera is inserted through your cervix. This part can be somewhat uncomfortable, so again, some ibuprofen before the procedure might be helpful. The camera can be used to visualize any potential polyps or fibroids, as well as to see the opening to the fallopian tubes. If polyps or fibroids are found, they can be removed at the same time. Removal is surgical and can require anesthesia.

Additional testing. Other testing can include urine and/or blood tests for sexually transmitted diseases, which can potentially make conception difficult, as well as genetic testing on you and your partner. If you move on to IVF, there is typically additional pre-treatment testing that will be required (chapter 24).

What Should My Partner Do?

If you end up going one of the medical routes, your doctor will likely suggest that your partner have a semen analysis done—there is no point in spending money for you to ovulate if his sperm aren't going to do the job. Generally, for this test, your partner will be directed into a small room with a selection of magazines and videos to help get him in the mood if necessary; he will then need to masturbate and fill a sterile cup with ejaculate. He will either leave the cup somewhere, or hand it to a designated person, so that the lab technicians can analyze the sample.

In a standard analysis, volume of ejaculate, how many sperm are present, what percentage are "motile" (swimming appropriately), and sperm shape (morphology) will be determined. If everything comes back normal, your partner will probably do a happy man dance and gush on about his super sperm for a few minutes. If results come back less than stellar, be kind to him; this can be a blow to his ego (even though his sperm quality is not totally in his control). In this case, in order to get pregnant, you may need to do IVF with ICSI (intracytoplasmic sperm injection), a procedure where a single sperm is injected directly into your egg.

Lifestyle changes can have an effect on sperm quality and quantity, just as our lifestyle changes can lead to ovulation. Some studies have found benefits to reducing or eliminating alcohol and tobacco usage, although others find no effect. Cutting out cigarette smoking would certainly have other advantages, so that might be worth considering. A number of studies and meta-analyses suggest antioxidant vitamin supplements (available over the counter) can help. Acetyl-L-carnitine or L-carnitine were found to increase pregnancy rates[4]. Other supplements that can enhance sperm parameters include vitamins C and E, zinc, selenium, folate, and carotenoids[5]. Wearing boxer shorts instead of briefs has also been suggested to improve sperm (due to lowering the temperature at which the sperm develop)[6].

> **Laura A. (February 2011)**: My husband's sperm analysis came back and it was not good. Count and motility were within the normal range (not great but not dire), but morphology came back at 1%!! I hadn't planned for this. Stupid as it sounds, I'd assumed all the problems were with me and once we'd sorted them out things would be OK. I have been crying all week and this is putting such a strain on our relationship. We have to wait a week to see the doctor, but from what I've read our only chances are IVF with sperm injection, or even donor sperm. I just feel like giving up. I can't see how this is ever going to work out for us. He

has now reduced alcohol to just two drinks per week, stopped sneaking cigarettes, and started taking lots of supplements (most important are vitamin C, vitamin E, zinc, selenium, and B vitamins). He's also drinking loads of green tea (antioxidants) and avoiding hot baths in the hope that this might make a difference. He was also ill with a flu-virus thing a few weeks before the test... God knows. Just feeling utterly helpless about it all.

Three months later: Some good news—hubby got his results back yesterday and they are great! His sperm count went from 16 million per milliliter to 102 million and morphology has gone from just 1% to 20%. Motility 60%. He has worked so hard and made so many sacrifices and I am very proud of him. I just want to say that lifestyle changes make a huge difference to men as well, so if anyone has male infertility factors, don't despair. We made all these changes ourselves. All doctor said was not to wear tight pants (boxer shorts instead)! Now it's just me to sort out... (*Laura got pregnant naturally 10 months later.*)

Diminished Ovarian Reserve?

On a completely different topic, quite a few HAers have been told that they might have diminished ovarian reserve (DOR) based on the levels of a hormone called anti-Müllerian hormone (AMH) in their blood. AMH is usually correlated to the number of small, resting follicles that one has; AMH < 1 ng/mL can mean few of these "antral follicles." To give you an idea of the normal number of antral follicles, one study performed ultrasounds on 652 healthy, fertile women[7]. The authors computed the 3rd, 10th, 25th, 50th, 75th, 90th and 97th percentiles of antral follicle count at each age.

Normal number of antral follicles[8]

Age	25th percentile	50th percentile	75th percentile
25	15	18	21
30	11.5	14.5	18
35	8	11.5	14.5
40	6	9	12

The concerns with low AMH are two-fold—1) a lowered pregnancy rate, even with IVF and 2) a decrease in the number of embryos available[9]. However, as we briefly discussed in chapter 5, levels of this one hormone are far from sufficient to diagnose DOR[10]. A correlation between LH levels and AMH has been demonstrated[11], therefore, caution should be used in interpreting AMH results particularly when someone has HA. For a DOR diagnosis, the follicles should be visualized and counted on an ultrasound; the expected number varies somewhat with age, but if you have more antral follicles than the 25th percentile shown above, that is promising. FSH is another hormone that is more classically associated with DOR; an increased level above 12 to 14 can be cause for concern.

Below you can see the information from our survey respondents diagnosed with DOR. "Low" AMH (<1 ng/mL) does not correlate in this population with extremely low antral follicle counts, and those who were trying to conceive were able to get pregnant, in many cases more than once. There were a few who had multiple miscarriages, but they persevered and were able to carry to term.

HAers with low AMH

Name	AMH (ng/mL)	Number of antral follicles	FSH (IU/mL)	Treatment / pregnancy history
Christa	0.61	8	12.5	First son conceived naturally with no problems; HA afterward. Regained cycles with weight gain and cutting exercise. Two miscarriages on natural cycles, then second son.
Kathryn	0.8	9	9.0	Gained weight and cut exercise; resumed natural cycles. Conceived first son on third natural cycle, conceived second on fifth natural cycle, with one miscarriage.
Kira	Lowest 0.72	6–10 per ovary	9.2 – 16.5	Not trying to conceive. Was told would need to freeze eggs immediately at age 24 due to potential low ovarian reserve. Responded perfectly to Clomid Challenge Test with natural ovulation, but moved forward with IVF to freeze eggs. Had a terrific response with 24 eggs retrieved and 11 embryos frozen.
Alaina	0.79	>50	Not measured	No natural cycles after weight gain and walking only for eight months. RE recommended IVF. Excellent response; pregnant, with seven frozen embryos for future use.

Name	AMH (ng/mL)	Number of antral follicles	FSH (IU/mL)	Treatment / pregnancy history
Candace	0.5, 0.8	10–12 per ovary	Normal	Pregnant on first cycle of Clomid + IUI.
Stephanie	0.76	20	5.9	Tried Clomid initially; two pregnancies in three tries, but ended in miscarriage. Two IVF cycles with no pregnancy. Back to Clomid; pregnant on first cycle.
Megan E.	0.32	Too many to count	3.8	Two failed rounds of Femara; pregnant on second round of Menopur injections. Her second was naturally conceived on her second attempt.
Stacey S.	~1.0	>15	~7.0	Four unsuccessful medicated cycles. Pregnant on third natural cycle (after a miscarriage). Second son conceived naturally following two additional miscarriages.
Jessica V.	1.2	Not measured	6.3	Two children, both conceived on first natural cycle attempting conception.
Tammy	0.5	9	7.2	No response to Clomid but pregnant on first IVF cycle.

Megan E: My AMH was 0.32 and FSH was 3.8. I did two rounds of Femara and two rounds of injections (Menopur). My RE said that he actually thought my AMH numbers were off because I had a lot of follicles so it didn't make sense. My first RE said that due to my AMH I should go right to IVF. The second one didn't blink an eye at the number and went forward with the other plan. (*Megan got pregnant with her first using Menopur. Her second child was conceived naturally, on her second cycle trying.*)

If you do have low AMH, you could consider taking a DHEA supplement, either 75 mg per day over the counter, or 25 mg per day of prescription micronized DHEA. DHEA has been shown to positively affect the number of eggs retrieved, the pregnancy rate, and the miscarriage rate in women with diminished ovarian reserve and low AMH in IVF cycles[12]. Many listed in the table above did take DHEA once DOR was suggested as a potential diagnosis for them. Optimal results are seen four to five months after starting supplements, so it is probably best to start taking DHEA now. If you do not have DOR or low AMH (below 1.05), no effect of DHEA supplementation has been proven[13], so it is not necessary for you to take it.

Parting Thoughts

This chapter has covered a smorgasbord of information that might be useful if or when you are going through treatment cycles. In the coming chapters, we will get more specific about the different types of treatments available to you. Finding out that you need medical help to get pregnant can be disheartening, especially after spending time and effort on recovery. It feels even worse when you must undergo treatment after treatment. Keep this in mind, though: over 99% of HAers who took the treatment path during or after recovery went on to become pregnant. Hopefully this will motivate you to press forward with patience (or develop it) while holding onto hope. By following the Recovery Plan, you are actively taking charge over what is controllable, and further treatment will bring you one step closer to meeting and holding your baby.

21
Popping Pills to Ovulate: Oral Medications

It's time to delve into the details of the different medications commonly prescribed to help you grow follicles and hopefully ovulate. One method of "ovulation induction" uses oral medications, including Clomid (clomiphene citrate), Femara (letrozole), and tamoxifen. In this chapter, we will cover the following aspects of these medications:

- An overview of how the medications work;
- Evidence that they can work for those who are recovering/recovered from HA, and how important efforts toward recovery are;
- Guidance on choosing which medication option to use;
- Information on various dosing protocols that have been studied;
- Whether it is necessary to induce a bleed prior to a medicated cycle;
- Timing of taking the pills;
- What to expect during a Clomid or Femara cycle;
- Information on soy isoflavones (over-the-counter supplements that work similarly to Clomid);
- What to do when oral meds don't work.

How Do Oral Ovulation Induction Medications Work?

This first section will describe how oral medications work to get your follicles growing so that you are on your way to ovulating, which is necessary to get pregnant. We'll start with a quick refresher on what happens in a normal menstrual cycle so that you can understand how the oral meds augment the natural process.

Just before menstrual flow starts and a new cycle begins, low levels of estradiol (E_2) and progesterone secreted by the corpus luteum keep GnRH pulses from your hypothalamus to a minimum[1]. The small amount of GnRH results in low FSH production by the pituitary and follicles in a resting state. Estradiol then declines further as the corpus luteum breaks down. This decrease removes the "negative feedback" control that E_2 has been exerting on the hypothalamus[2] and pituitary[3], and the FSH levels now rise. The increase in FSH starts the process of dominant follicle selection, and the journey to ovulation is underway.

The oral medications essentially mimic the decrease in E_2 that normally occurs with the corpus luteum breakdown. Your hypothalamus senses a reduction in E_2, which increases the GnRH pulses[4], leading to a rise in FSH and the start of follicular growth. It is important that you have changed your eating and exercise habits, and reduced stress, so that your hypothalamus is no longer suppressed by energy deficiency and cortisol and can make GnRH in response to the E_2 drop.

Clomid and soy isoflavones, two of the oral meds, both work in the same way: their molecular shape is similar to E_2 so they bind to the E_2 receptor in your hypothalamus, preventing E_2 binding. The hypothalamus no longer gets signals from the E_2 receptors, and therefore senses a decrease in E_2[5]. Tamoxifen works similarly, but exhibits an interesting property in the uterus, activating the E_2 receptors and causing thickening of the uterine lining[6]. If you find during treatment cycles that your lining is not increasing appropriately, tamoxifen may be worth considering. Femara, another oral medication, prevents the normally ongoing conversion of androgens to estradiol, lowering the *actual* estrogen level. The hypothalamus senses this decrease in E_2, with the same end result as the other oral meds. Just as in a normal, non-medicated cycle, this leads to increased GnRH pulses and FSH production so the egg maturation process starts.

Oral Medications and HA?

> *Kim*: Please don't be afraid to try Clomid or one of the other oral meds. I am obviously a little biased—Clomid worked for me and for so many other ladies with HA. As long as you have made the right lifestyle changes, then you certainly have a chance of responding. My changes before taking Clomid were dramatic; completely cutting all running (I replaced running with casual swimming three times a week) and gaining around 10 kg, making my BMI 23. I had minimal side effects and it was a very cheap option. In my opinion, it's definitely worth a shot before moving on to more invasive treatments not covered by insurance. Go for it! (*Kim got pregnant on her first clomid cycle.*)

Because the oral meds require a functioning hypothalamus, many doctors say, "Femara/Clomid (or tamoxifen) won't work since you have HA." This statement may very well be true if you have not made changes toward recovery, but once you have, you are removing or decreasing the signals shutting down your hypothalamus, and these medications have been proven to work, as our data indicate. Among our survey respondents, 110 tried oral medications; 80% ovulated on at least one cycle and 66% of those who ovulated achieved pregnancy. However, doctors unaware of the effectiveness of the Recovery Plan both in regaining cycles and increasing response to oral meds will often go straight to injectables. In our opinion, if you have put an effort into recovery, oral meds are worth trying, for a number of reasons. Compared to injectables, oral meds are:

- Less expensive—cost is not so much an issue if your insurance will cover the injectable medications, but if not, you're looking at a difference of $1,000+ per cycle.
    - Clomid, Femara, and tamoxifen cost around $1 to $5 per pill, with the number of pills depending on your dosage. Check your local wholesale store as they often have good pricing, especially if your insurance will not cover the meds. Soy isoflavones cost about $10 for a three-month supply. As a comparison, injectables are about $35 to $75 per vial if not covered by insurance and it is common to use 10 to 20 vials for one cycle.
- Less invasive—all you're doing is taking a small pill once a day for 5 to 10 days.
- Mentally easier—there is generally not much monitoring, if any, which means less time off work and less explaining to others.

- Lower chance of multiples—6% of Clomid/Femara pregnancies from the Board were multiples, with one set of triplets, versus 24% of pregnancies from injectables, including three sets of triplets, one set of quadruplets and one sextuplet pregnancy.

> *Kimberly*: I definitely have had issues with spending time away from work for RE appointments. I always make sure to get the earliest morning appointment, which varies depending on the office hours of the RE. My current RE will see me at 7:30 a.m., which means that I can get to work at a normal time, and no one suspects anything. However, this also interferes with my sleep, because I have to leave my house by 6:45. When I was seeing my first RE, I was ALWAYS late for work—I am talking walking in at 10 a.m., which is unacceptable. I made up some excuses about doctor's appointments, dental appointments, and various workers coming to my house. It was draining.

As mentioned, some doctors are unwilling to prescribe Clomid, Femara, or tamoxifen after a diagnosis of HA because they believe it will not work. However, our data and a few small clinical studies[7] suggest otherwise. Of the 329 pregnancies achieved by our survey respondents post-HA, 26% were with the help of oral meds, so clearly these drugs can work. We have data (next page) from our survey for 291 cycles in which oral medications were used: 80% Clomid, 20% Femara, and <1% soy isoflavones. The percentage of cycles resulting in ovulation, average time to ovulation, and pregnancy rate per cycle are shown below for Clomid and Femara. We have not included data for soy isoflavones as the numbers are too small, and we have no data for tamoxifen. Keep in mind when examining these data that a "normal" person has about a 32% chance of getting pregnant each month[8], similar to the pregnancy rate in our respondents who ovulated using either Clomid or Femara.

When you are seeing a doctor, it should be a partnership in which you are working together to try and solve your issues. It is totally acceptable to mention to your doctor that you understand the possibility these medications may not work, but you would like to try regardless. There are no downsides to trying other than time, and if you do ovulate and get pregnant you will save yourself a boatload of money and stress.

Ovulation and pregnancy with oral medications.

	Clomid	Femara
Number of respondents	97	25
Number of cycles	210	54
Percent of cycles with ovulation	**67%**	**61%**
Percent of respondents with at least one ovulation	75%	76%
Median day of ovulation	**18**	**17.5**
Range of day of ovulation	12 to 39	12 to 33
Pregnancy rate per ovulatory cycle*	32%	48%
Percent pregnant among those who ovulated*	**62%**	**84%**
Percent pregnant when using the medication*	46%	64%

* The difference in % pregnant is not statistically significant between Clomid and Femara due to small numbers using Femara; $p = 0.10$

We often think that because we ovulate and have intercourse or IUI at the appropriate time, we will certainly get pregnant. However, there is a huge element of chance. Do the sperm make it all the way to the egg? Can one of the sperm penetrate the egg's shell? Once inside, does the division and replication process go off without a hitch? There are so many steps at which this process can go awry. It can be disheartening when it seems like everything is perfect but you still don't get pregnant—all you can do is keep trying, and maybe consider a different method if what you're doing isn't working for you.

Out of those who ovulated with oral meds but did not get pregnant:

- 47% got pregnant naturally
- 37% used injectables
- 16% needed IVF.
- One person decided to adopt, but later did have a natural pregnancy.

Of those who did not ovulate with oral meds (21%):

- 20% got pregnant naturally
- 60% used injectables
- 20% needed IVF.

As stated, the chance of oral medications leading to follicular growth and ovulation (and pregnancy!) is much more substantial if you have put the Recovery Plan into practice and increased your BMI.

BMI, ovulation, and pregnancy when using oral meds

BMI	Total respondents at BMI	Number of respondents ovulating	Ovulation rate	Pregnancy rate in respondents who ovulated	Overall pregnancy rate†
<21*	67	45	67%	51%	34%
≥21	61	47	77%	70%	54%

* E.g., 67% of survey respondents with BMI < 21 ovulated. Of those 67%, 51% got pregnant (Pregnancy rate in respondents who ovulated column), giving an overall pregnancy rate of 34%, meaning of those who were at BMI<21, 34% got pregnant using oral meds.

† $p = 0.02$ (Fisher's exact test, two-tailed)

Interestingly, among folks who did not ovulate the first time they tried oral medications, those who continued to gain weight did ovulate on subsequent cycles.

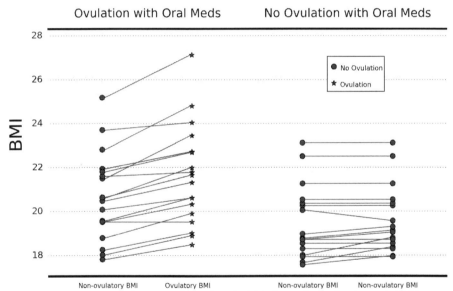

Ovulation after a non-ovulatory medicated cycle. This figure shows the change in BMI among people who did not ovulate on their first cycle of oral meds. (*Left*) Before and after BMI of those who ovulated on a subsequent cycle (19 people); (*right*) before and after BMI of those who did not ovulate (17 people). Almost everyone who went on to ovulate after the first failed cycle gained additional weight; those who did not ovulate either did not gain or did not get above a BMI of 19.5.

> *Belinda*: Here's a quick update from Friday's scan: it was day 15, and I had a 15.5 mm follicle and a few other 10-12 mm ones too, and a lining of about 9.5 mm, so as you can imagine, I'm very happy with that—in fact amazed! I have never had any response to Clomid before at BMI 20 to 21, so for me it was well worth getting to BMI 22, and I have to say I really

> feel great being here. As you've all been saying, it is so liberating being able to eat whatever, whenever, and not worry in advance about meals out, etc. I've got another scan Monday afternoon and am really praying things have moved on and I can trigger then. It's my birthday next Thursday and whenever my husband asks what I want I just say a baby!

So now that you see that oral meds can absolutely be successful once you've worked on recovery, we will discuss the different options.

Femara or Clomid or Something Else?

The most widely used oral medications to encourage growth of follicles are the prescription drugs Femara and Clomid. Tamoxifen is an additional prescribed option that is used occasionally. Soy isoflavones (SI) are an over-the-counter supplement not useful in regaining an absent period but potentially helpful in encouraging earlier ovulation when you are already cycling naturally. We will discuss SI toward the end of the chapter.

As far as the prescription options, we recommend Femara if your doctor will prescribe it. Recent studies find higher pregnancy rates in those taking Femara rather than Clomid[9] and there are fewer side effects, as will be discussed below. If your doctor will not prescribe Femara, Clomid is certainly a reasonable choice. Tamoxifen is another possibility that works similarly to Clomid, with comparable ovulation and pregnancy rates[10]. We will not discuss tamoxifen further as it is not a common treatment for HA and we believe Femara is a better option; however, if your doctor prefers it, tamoxifen is a rational choice with fewer effects on the uterine lining than Clomid. It is likely that much of what we describe in the remainder of the chapter would apply to tamoxifen.

Unfortunately, none of these drugs have undergone extensive testing in people with HA, so we have to infer from other populations what the benefits and drawbacks might be. The clinical literature suggests that Femara is the better choice for those with unexplained infertility or PCOS[11], common study populations for ovulation induction drugs. Pregnancy rates using Femara were anywhere from 30% to 70% higher in multiple studies and meta-analyses[12], depending on the study. Among our survey respondents, recall from the earlier table there was a non-significant but similar trend of higher pregnancy rates with Femara.

A different avenue of exploration suggests that Femara may be the better choice for biological reasons:

- Femara does not affect the estrogen receptors in the uterus, whereas Clomid can lead to a suboptimal uterine lining (in 41% of cases[13]).
- Clomid can affect cervical mucus (CM), potentially making it less hospitable to sperm.
- Femara has a shorter half-life than Clomid, so it is out of your system by the time ovulation occurs, whereas Clomid can remain in your blood for weeks after taking it.
- There is potential for an accumulation of the negative effects of Clomid on your lining and CM over time.

The final consideration is that there is a potential to conceive multiples when taking any fertility medications. Among the pregnancies Nico has tracked from the Board, 6% of those using Clomid conceived multiples; six sets of twins and one set of triplets. So far, there have been no multiple pregnancies among Femara users, which is another good reason to choose it (and to use the lowest dose at which ovulation occurs).

Based on these lines of evidence, our recommendation is to start with Femara if your doctor is willing to prescribe it. Reasons that some doctors hesitate to prescribe Femara include:

- Femara is FDA approved to prevent breast cancer (because it decreases estrogen levels), but not to treat infertility. The lack of approval is not because Femara doesn't work or is dangerous, but because the company that makes it has decided not to perform the large clinical trials that would be required. However, there have been dozens of clinical studies performed using Femara to encourage ovulation, and thousands who have used it effectively, so many doctors will prescribe it.
- Another issue is that a small study in 2005[14] (never fully published) found a slight increase in mild birth defects when Femara was used. However, many larger studies since then have found no increase[15] so the consensus is that the results of the first study were incorrect and that Femara is safe to use to achieve pregnancy[16].

Potential Dosing Protocols for Clomid or Femara

The typical dosage protocol for Clomid or Femara is to start with a baseline dose for five days, beginning three to five days after a Provera-induced bleed begins. If the first round of these oral medications doesn't lead to ovulation, Provera is used to shed any lining that may have developed, and another five-day round is given at a higher dosage. This continues until a standard maximum level for each drug is reached. However, researchers have gotten creative and come up with other protocols to try if the standard five-day regimen isn't working. Many of these studies have been performed in people with PCOS because it is much more common than HA—but folks from the Board have tried many of these protocols (listed below) with success. There isn't strong evidence for a particular protocol given that most have been tried in only 5 to 100 study participants; however, these are options that can be discussed with your doctor to determine a good plan for you.

Clomid or Femara dosing protocols:

- Standard (typical starting protocol, referring to the standard five days of taking these medications): 50 mg Clomid or 2.5 mg Femara for five days (or 20 mg tamoxifen[17]).
    - Conventionally, one starts these medications between CD 3 and CD 5. We will discuss the options below in the section "Medication Timing."
- Medium standard: 100 mg Clomid or 5 mg Femara for five days (or 40 mg tamoxifen[18]).
- High standard: 150 to 250 mg Clomid or 7.5 to 12.5 mg Femara for five days (or 80 mg tamoxifen[19]).
- Extended protocols (EP; oral meds taken continuously for longer than five days):
    - Clomid: 50 mg for five days directly followed by 100 mg for an additional five days[20], or:
    - Continuing a standard protocol of Femara or Clomid for 7 to 10 days[21].
- Stair-stepping (a.k.a. "piggybacking"): Taking additional Clomid or Femara after no response to the initial five-day dose, with no bleed during the break[22].
    - Additional medication can be taken around CD 12 to CD 14 if an ultrasound shows no response, or later in the cycle (e.g., CD 28) if no ovulation has occurred.
- Short protocol: 50 mg of Clomid for three days[23]. This would likely work with Femara as well*.
- Combination protocol: 5 mg Femara and 100 mg Clomid for five days*[24].

---

* Protocol has not been used by any HAers on the Board to date.

The dosing we suggest depends on whether you're already cycling naturally, and whether you respond to Provera. With Clomid, the less you use the better because of its effects on your lining and CM. There aren't the same lining concerns with Femara; however, for this drug, higher doses lead to ovulation of more follicles and therefore a higher chance of multiples[25], but interestingly, a possibly lower pregnancy rate[26]. So in both cases, it seems that the optimal dose is the lowest one to which you respond. The table below shows varied situations and the dosing we recommend in each case. If no ovulation is seen, increase either the dose or the length of time taking the medication; both have shown success in clinical studies. However, no study has been performed to determine which type of dose increase (amount or time) is more effective, so we cannot offer specific guidance.

Suggested oral medication protocols

HA degree and Suggested Protocol	Femara	Clomid	Soy isoflavones
Cycling naturally: low standard protocol	2.5 mg for 3 to 5 days	50 mg for 3 to 5 days	150 to 200 mg for 5 days
No natural cycles but Provera response: standard protocol	Medium protocol†: 5 mg for 5 days	Standard protocol: 50 mg for 5 days	Not recommended
No natural cycles, no Provera response: Extended protocol	2.5 mg for 10 days[27] OR 5 mg for 5 days + 7.5 mg for 5 days	2 mg/kg/day‡ for 10 days[28] OR 50 mg for 5 days + 100 mg for 5 days[29]	Do not use

† Doses increase more quickly with Femara than Clomid due to fewer concerns with lining thickness.
‡ Rounded to the nearest 25 mg.

In 2007, a study was published in which a new regimen, an "extended protocol (EP)" of Clomid was used to help women with HA recover their cycles[30]. The study was small, with only eight participants, but all eight recovered menstrual cycles and were still cycling six months later. The women were not trying to conceive, but ovulation is ovulation; the same protocol can be used with the intent of getting pregnant. In fact, many on the Board and in support groups have used the Clomid EP over the years since the paper was published, and either gotten pregnant or restored natural cycles. Recently, more have been using a Femara EP instead of Clomid given the overall benefits of Femara.

The medication protocol from the study was:

- Cycle 1: 50 mg for five days followed by 100 mg for five days (10 total days of medication).
- If ovulation occurred, then cycle 2: 100 mg / five days, and cycle 3: 100 mg / five days.
- If no ovulation, then cycle 2 was a repeat of cycle 1; cycle 3: 100 mg / five days; cycle 4: 100 mg / five days.

All eight commenced natural menstrual cycles after completing the three (or four) rounds of medication. If you do not bleed in response to Provera, we recommend 1) continuing to work on recovery! and 2) using an EP of either Femara, Clomid, or tamoxifen. With the increased time on one of these medications, estradiol is sensed as low for a longer period, providing more of a push to the hypothalamus than the standard oral protocol. In one study, the Femara EP resulted in a higher pregnancy rate than the standard protocol likely due to more mature follicles, with no difference in rate of multiples[31]. After a few rounds with successful ovulation, you could consider a cycle without medication to see if natural cycles have resumed, as in the Clomid EP study[32].

> *Amy H*: Basically, you do 50 mg Clomid for five days, then immediately follow with 100 for five days. In the study, it jumpstarted periods for many ladies with HA. I'm giving it a shot because I've gained almost 10 lb, reduced exercise, and have signs and symptoms of my hypothalamus getting going, but may just need a little boost to ovulate.

If you try a standard protocol and do not show any signs of follicular growth at a monitoring ultrasound after CD 12 or have not ovulated by CD 28 in an unmonitored cycle (no fertile signs like changes in cervical mucus or increases in temperature), it is possible to take a second or third round of medication without inducing a bleed first. On the Board we call this protocol "piggybacking," while researchers have termed the idea "stair-stepping"[33]. The additional medication gives the follicles another push of FSH to start growing, almost like what happens in some natural cycles where there are multiple waves of follicular growth before an egg finally matures[34]. What we generally recommend is to begin another round of medication if you have not ovulated by CD 30, aren't currently having fertile signs, and have a negative pregnancy test. Another possibility is to use Provera to hopefully get a bleed and then start a new cycle fresh (if you don't bleed by eight days past the last pill, you can go ahead and start the meds too).

> *Juliet*: Let me look back through my ridiculous notes... OK, I finished 100 mg Clomid on August 31. I had ultrasounds on September 5, 8, and 10: all showed nothing bigger than one 14 mm follicle. I started 150 mg Clomid September 10, and I had three large follicles on September 14 (last day of 150 mg). They seriously came out of nowhere! (*Juliet got a positive pregnancy test at 12 DPO.*)
>
> *Kristin*: So, I had my ultrasound today after piggybacking five days of Clomid with four more. I had two nice, big follicles at 18 and 19 mm but my lining was only 6.2 mm. My doctor said I should trigger in two days but my chances for pregnancy are low because of the lining. I am bummed. I am still doing the hCG shot though! (*This cycle ended with her period, and Kristin's third and fourth children were ultimately conceived naturally.*)

Unfortunately, there are no hard and fast rules with regard to what dosage protocol to choose. There have been a few studies comparing lower doses to higher doses for each medication, but none comparing the various alternative protocols, and in particular, no studies that examine whether the dosage or length of time the drug is taken is more important. It really is up to you and your doctor to determine what you are comfortable with—just remember that if you try one protocol and it doesn't work, increasing dosage or the length of time you take the drug are both options that have been successful for others.

Inducing a Bleed Before Starting Medications

It is not absolutely required that you have a bleed prior to taking one of these oral medications. If you try Provera and don't bleed, you can go ahead with an extended protocol of either Femara or Clomid; your hormone levels and uterine lining are in essentially the same baseline state as post-bleed anyway. If your doctor does an ultrasound and your uterine lining is thin (i.e., less than 4 mm), the same applies. There are also people who have not done either of these but gone ahead with Femara or Clomid regardless (one had a lining of 5.4 mm and successfully ovulated with no bleed first), usually with reasonable success. There were 52 cycles in which our survey respondents used Clomid or Femara without a bleed first. Both the rate of ovulation and pregnancy were similar to cycles in which a bleed was obtained. In addition, there was a similar trend as above with ovulation more likely at a BMI over 21. Be aware that if you take Femara without a bleed first you may experience some spotting, as the drop in estrogen can cause shedding of a small amount of lining.

A recent study found a much improved pregnancy rate (27.7%) when women with PCOS started Clomid with no bleed after an anovulatory cycle as opposed to either a natural bleed (4.5%) or progesterone-induced bleed (6.6%)[35]. This startling difference in pregnancy rate was found across three treatment groups but could very well be PCOS-related as the authors suggested[36]. Despite this, the study does support the claim that a bleed prior to beginning oral medications is not required. Another well-known RE proposed that the PCOS-specific mechanisms were perhaps not what was driving the increased pregnancy rate and that starting ovulation induction without an initial bleed should be more commonly instituted[37]. There is not enough data to make this a strong recommendation, but it is perhaps warranted depending on the specifics of your situation. These findings provide further support for piggybacking, as we described above.

Medication Timing

It is common to start taking your oral meds on CD 3 (CD 1 being considered the first day of red blood), although it can vary from CD 1 to 5. There are some small studies that suggest that if you're taking Clomid, starting earlier in the cycle may be preferable[38] (see next page). Beginning sooner gives more time for the follicle to mature and also more time between the last pill and ovulation, allowing for better growth of the uterine lining. Femara is typically started on CD 3. There have not been any clinical studies comparing different start days for Femara treatment; however, there is no reason to think that it would be detrimental to start a few days earlier or later. If you are starting meds without a bleed, just assign your starting day as CD 3.

Effect of Clomid timing on lining thickness and pregnancy rate

Study and protocol	Test dosing protocol and results			Comparison dosing protocol (normal protocol) and results		
	Clomid dosing days	Endometrial thickness	Pregnancy rate	Clomid dosing days	Endometrial thickness	Pregnancy rate
Biljan[39]: 100 mg	CD 1–5	NA	26.7%	CD 5–9	NA	0%
Badawy[40]: 100 mg, 5 days	CD -3–1‡	9.1 ± 0.23 mm	20.9%*	CD 3–7	8.2 ± 0.6 mm	15.7%*
Takasaki[41]: 50 mg †	CD 1–5	9.7 ± 1.5 mm, > 8 mm in 19/20 subjects	NR	CD 5–9	6.7 ± 1.8 mm, > 8 mm in 3/21 subjects	NR
Gol[42]: 50 mg	CD 3–5	10.3 ± 1.39 mm	14.1%	CD 3–7	9.52 ± 1.96 mm	10.0%

* Differences in pregnancy rates were not statistically significant.
† Study performed in women with thin lining (< 8 mm) (41% of all subjects) after one round of 50mg Clomid taken CD 5–9.
‡ Dosing commenced three days before the start of the subject's periods.
NR = Not Reported, NA = Not Applicable, i.e., not assessed.

Going Through a Clomid/Femara Cycle

Once you and your doctor have decided whether or not to get a bleed before starting your cycle, what dosage to use, and what cycle day to start on, it's time to get cracking! Many will take the pill(s) at night just before bed in hopes of sleeping through some possible side effects; others will take with a meal. Determine what works best for your lifestyle, and then take your medication at approximately the same time each day. In a way it might feel anticlimactic—you just take a pill or two each day and that's it. Then, of course, there's more waiting. You may read about some doctors prescribing estrogen supplements after finishing Clomid (less so with Femara as it is not known for having a potentially negative effect on your lining), with studies overall suggesting a positive effect[43].

> **Steph (2012):** The past week I have been enjoying the fun-filled experience of taking Clomid, a medication that is supposed to help you ovulate. When I asked my doctor about side effects, she said they vary from feeling nothing to an extreme form of PMS, with hot flashes, bloating, mood swings, and cramps. I figured, given my experience on Provera, I would

> at least get "lucky" on the bloating. Sure enough, just hours after taking my first dose, I began to feel as if I were a beached whale. Wednesday and Thursday I was so bloated after I ate and drank that I could hardly move. On Friday I had an emotional breakdown over whether we should have chicken for dinner. And on Sunday and Monday I had intense lower back pain, which I have decided means that something must be working. But these "symptoms" could all just be in my head—I have been known to be indecisive about dinner and I was tired from work, bloating could have been in my mind or from overeating, and back pain could be from a strain of sorts. I don't really know. Some of my friends tell me it is absolutely the Clomid; others say it might also be a little bit psychological. I will never know, but it is just how I feel and that is OK.

Many start on oral medications with little to no monitoring other than tracking ovulation signs and symptoms on their own (chapter 17). It is perfectly reasonable to start with no monitoring, as in many cases follicles will grow and ovulate with just the extra help from the oral meds. If you have a couple of cycles with no apparent ovulation, or with signs of ovulation but no confirmation by temperature change or getting a period, you will probably want to adjust your dosage as well as potentially get to the next level of monitoring, which is a mid-cycle ultrasound or two. After an ultrasound, your doctor might recommend taking a trigger shot (chapter 23), which results in ovulation of adequately sized follicles 90% of the time[44]. With Clomid or Femara, a recent study found that the optimal follicle size at which to take the trigger shot was between 23 and 27 mm[45]. Earlier triggers can work, but there is no downside to waiting a couple of days, so we recommend that you wait.

Other Options: Soy Isoflavones

Soy isoflavones (SIs) are a supplement with the potential to jump-start cycles AFTER your hypothalamus is normalized. Anecdotally there is about a 50% success rate in this case, which could simply be coincidence. There are no research studies that examine use of soy isoflavones for this application. Also, the SI do NOT work if you are early in recovery, and would not be recommended.

The isoflavones bind to and activate the estrogen receptors in your brain, making your hypothalamus sense a higher level of estrogen. You take them for five days so your brain senses this higher level, then stop, at which point your brain senses a drop in "estradiol." This mimics what happens in a natural menstrual cycle when the corpus luteum degrades (chapter 5), and if your hypothalamus is not suppressed anymore, then this can get the follicular growth process started. The rest of what happens in the cycle is your own body doing the hormonal work. If you are going to ovulate, you will likely do so around 7-14 days after taking the last pill. If you don't ovulate, we would suggest trying another round 28 days after the first. If that still doesn't work then either more recovery time is needed, or perhaps something a bit stronger, see above.

The recommended dosage is 200-250 mg of *active* SI per day (usually genistein and diadzein) for five days. Be mindful of the ingredients of what you are purchasing; some supplements will say, e.g., "100 mg isoflavones" but when you look at the small print it is only 13.8 mg active isoflavones. Please also note that a few people have recently disclosed feeling depressed while taking the soy isoflavones. If this happens to you, recognize that it is likely due to the SI and has been reported to resolve quickly. You should probably stop taking the isoflavones (and not take them again). If you have concerns or are experiencing depression interfering with daily functioning, discuss with a mental health professional to determine how to cope with the depressive symptoms.

Supplementation with actual estradiol could potentially work in the same way as the SI; unlike hormone replacement therapy where one takes estrogen consistently for 21+ days, possibly with progesterone added, a short five-day course of estrogen could potentially also make your hypothalamus sense a drop in estrogen and then jumpstart the follicular growth process, but this is pure speculation.

Ovulating and Getting Pregnant!

When you want to conceive, it is important to time intercourse appropriately, so we're going to summarize our suggestions for how to do so (go back to chapter 17 for more details):

- Use OPKs starting from about three days after your last pill so that you know when you are about to ovulate.
    - Do not start earlier or you could get a false positive as the drugs cause your pituitary to produce LH. FSH and LH drop after you stop taking the pills, then rise again as the egg matures inside the follicle, which is when you get a true positive OPK that heralds ovulation.

- Pay attention to your cervical mucus; often an increase in amount and change in consistency is noticed prior to ovulation.
    - Clomid is known to affect cervical mucus, making it thicker and harder for sperm to swim through. To counteract this effect, some take expectorants (cough syrup with guaifenesin only) to help thin the mucus. You can also use sperm-friendly lubricants such as Pre-Seed or ToConceive, which you can find online.
- You can also check your cervical position; this can help corroborate the OPK and CM.
- Taking your temperature each morning when waking is useful for confirming ovulation (along with a progesterone blood test approximately seven days after ovulation).
- Remember that it is not uncommon for HAers to ovulate "late."

Cycle day of ovulation

Ovulation day	Percent ovulating	Cumulative percent
CD 12 to CD 14	21%	21%
CD 15 to CD 18	37%	58%
CD 19 to CD 27	35%	93%
CD 28+*	7%	100%

* Ovulation by CD 36 with the exception of one person who ovulated on CD 39.

Renee: I've been away from the Board as I mourned my canceled cycle and decided I needed to start focusing on living my life for now and not focus so much on tomorrow—easier said than done. Well, I'm here today because if I update you with sad news then I also have to update you with the good: out of nowhere, I got a smiley OPK this morning on CD 33! What?! What caused me to test, you may ask? Well, I grossly decided to check my CM at work yesterday because I felt like something was up. The first time I checked, it was lotiony. Then, right as I was leaving, I went to the bathroom and... egg white slip-and-slide! It was the most I've ever had on the tissue!

On the ride home, I wondered, "Are those ovary pangs I feel? Nah. It's in my head. Couldn't be." But something was going on. So I took a cheapie OPK when I got home and it seemed like maybe it could be positive. Either way, I was determined to be baby making last night and my husband knew it!

This morning, I got up, took the ClearBlue Easy OPK and got a smiley! My first ever! So, ladies, I'm being cautiously optimistic that I could

> have a shot this cycle after all! (*Renee's daughter was in fact conceived in this originally canceled cycle.*)

When Oral Medications Don't Work

It can be incredibly disheartening when your fertility treatments don't result in ovulation, especially after you've put in time and effort toward recovery and are dealing with the emotional repercussions of your changing body. It all seems worth it if it means you get your natural cycles back, or at least respond to the meds. But when you're not receiving any positive feedback in the form of getting even a chance at pregnancy, you can understandably feel like all your changes were for nothing. You may want to just say "forget it" and go for a long run or cut out some of your extra calories and lose a few pounds. It's normal to feel this way. And it's OK to be angry too. If you go for a short easy run or hit the gym to get some of that anger out for a day or two, it's not going to derail your recovery. But once you have a chance to regroup and think about it, you realize that if you're not responding now there is no way you would have responded X pounds ago, or by pushing your body however hard you were. Maybe all that's needed is a little tweaking of your protocol. In addition, perhaps you need to gain a little more, or further cut the intensity of your exercise. You may feel like your body has naturally leveled off at whatever BMI you're at, but especially if you're under a BMI of 20, or even 22, you should consider adding extra calories to see if you can increase your weight a bit more (review the BMI, ovulation, and pregnancy table earlier in this chapter).

As far as when to give up on oral meds and try something else, that will depend on your circumstances. Most doctors will recommend no more than six months on one particular protocol (in one study, 75% conceived within the first five cycles of Clomid[46]). If you do not have success with oral meds, it might be worth taking a month or two off to see what your body can do on its own, and then move forward with an oral med/injectables combination cycle, injectables alone, or IVF.

> *Natalie C*: So after a weekend of really thinking things over about what route to take after the failed Clomid round, I have come to a place of peace and surrender. I was really sad that Clomid didn't work, but I know that this was just not my time yet. I talked with my nurse who talked with my RE, talked at length with my husband, and also saw my acupuncturist for her opinion. My RE really wants me to move on to Menopur

> injectools with IUI. I was very hesitant at first but then my acupuncturist actually encouraged me to try them along with the acupuncture. My husband is fully on board and even though we are paying out of pocket, we think this is the next step for us. So next cycle I will start Menopur! (*Natalie conceived using a combination of Femara and Menopur, unfortunately with two miscarriages along the way. She is currently pregnant with her second, conceived naturally.*)

Summary

If you are at a point where you want to attempt to speed up the process of getting pregnant, oral drugs can be a good first choice. We recommend Femara as the first oral medication to try if your doctor is willing to prescribe it. Studies in women with PCOS or unexplained infertility generally show a higher pregnancy rate with Femara, as well as fewer negative side effects as compared with Clomid. In addition, there was a somewhat higher pregnancy rate among our survey respondents using Femara vs. Clomid, supported by similar findings in studies comparing the two drugs[47].

Suggested medication protocols to discuss with your physician:

- If you are cycling naturally but want to shorten your cycles, we recommend a standard protocol of 2.5 mg Femara or 50 mg Clomid for three to five days (or soy isoflavones).
- If you bleed from Provera or the equivalent (or have done so in the past), we also suggest a standard five-day protocol of 5 mg Femara or 50 mg Clomid to start.
- If you do not bleed from Provera, we would advocate trying an extended protocol, perhaps 1) 5 mg Femara or 50 mg Clomid for 10 days, or 2) 5 mg Femara for five days followed by 7.5 mg for an additional five days, or 50 mg Clomid for five days followed by 100 mg for another five days.
- If you don't ovulate on your first round, you can piggyback a second or even third round of meds without getting a bleed, to encourage ovulation. Typically, the dosage is stepped up a level for the subsequent round.

Once you have determined your protocol and taken your meds, you will want to watch for signs of ovulation, as reviewed above. Hopefully this will do the trick and get you pregnant (or cycling again, if pregnancy is not in the cards right now).

Lisa: So you're thinking about popping some pills now? If you have put in the work, increasing your BMI and body fat (a.k.a. estrogen-pumping machines), while decreasing stress (both mental and physical), and have sat with this for the recommended time, then you have two great options: 1) press on, waiting for your body to do its thing naturally; or 2) give the pills a go.

And while you contemplate the best choice for you, ponder this expression: "You reap what you sow." Ever heard it? It's pretty reflective of the HA journey. When we sow seeds in soil, we don't immediately reap the goods, right? We have to wait patiently, work hard, provide nutrients to the soil and persevere in order for the seeds to take root, grow and produce. Before you make the next decision, ask yourself: are you doing what it takes to reap a harvest?

22
Shooting up: Injectables

THE NEXT STEP up the assisted reproduction ladder is daily injections of the hormones your brain is unable or unwilling to make. These medicines cause follicular growth, egg maturation, and ovulation. Some doctors suggest "injectables" as an immediate treatment plan for a person with HA, regardless of BMI and exercise habits. In other cases, time and effort have been put toward recovery but restoration of natural cycles or response to oral ovulation induction medications isn't sufficient, so injectable hormones are the next step.

> *Jaclyn*: I just want to encourage you to do everything you can BEFORE even considering injectables or IVF. I did both of those before reverting to more weight gain and then Clomid and Femara (which is what got me pregnant). I really wish I hadn't jumped into either. I thought injectables would give me a better chance—I think they ever so slightly increase your chance but not enough to make the extra expense and time spent monitoring worth it if you can respond to either Clomid or Femara. I would recommend trying six ovulatory cycles on the oral meds before thinking about injectables or IVF. I bet you'll get pregnant long before you need either of those! I'll remind you that I didn't get my positive pregnancy test until I gained to a BMI over 22. I had ovulated from both Clomid and Menopur (injectable) prior to this at a lower BMI—I just didn't get pregnant.
>
> *Julie*: I always though infertility was my biggest battle to face. I never stopped to think that beating it with an RE and ovulation medications

> rather than weight gain possibly led me into a much bigger battle with prematurity and the fight for my sons' lives and health.

For those who have yet to take the leap toward recovery, injectables can seem like a panacea—getting pregnant without having to change a thing. But those of us who have gone through the work to recover express a thankfulness for the journey, no matter the outcome. There is a deep appreciation echoed for the emotional and physical healing that takes place, which no amount of injectables could do. From the outside, it might appear that the person who gets pregnant without making any changes with weight or exercise is lucky. But are they? What they don't get to experience (when opting to jump straight to injectables without making significant lifestyle changes) is the freedom from being bound by exercise and food. That monkey on our back lingers; we have seen it steal joy and occupy time that could be focused on the gift within once a pregnancy occurs. Additionally, these "lucky ones" miss out on long-term restorative health benefits. So yes, it is possible to use injectables to get pregnant without working toward recovery, but they are not a magic bullet and often do not lead to pregnancy in those who are still too thin, underfueling, and/or overexercising (four failed cycles for Nico!).

> *Chrissy*: Just offering up another perspective on the weight gain. I WAS that girl who conceived at a BMI of less than 20 for my daughter, using Menopur. Yes, I had gained a few pounds before conceiving, through eating better and more calories, fats, etc., but never went "all in." I tried to convince myself I was doing so well and I was on the right track, but never truly freed myself of the food restrictions. Throughout the pregnancy I continued to control my calories, trying to have the perfect weight gain, week by week, trimester by trimester. Well, it didn't happen. I under-gained. But I would go for my prenatal assessments and the baby was thriving—growing at more than the 75th percentile every time! Even when I brought up my lack of weight gain, the doctors brushed it off saying, "Your baby is great, everything is fine." I gave birth to a healthy, robust 7 lb 14 oz baby at just over 39 weeks, having gained only NINE pounds!
>
> What happened? Within two weeks my BMI had dropped below 17. I was trying to breastfeed my daughter but it only lasted four weeks before she had lost weight and I had lost weight, as I was scared to eat as much as I was hungry for. My poor body wanted calories and, while I was eating over 2000, I was not eating enough to sustain myself or a baby. My point? Eating and control issues do not go away just because you get pregnant.

They do not! In fact, I think there are studies that show that relapse of an eating disorder is quite common in pregnancy. Beat the control demons before you get pregnant! It is SO important! I was sicker after delivery than before I got pregnant.

Jessica: A few other ladies have already said this, but gaining weight before injects is not a waste. In fact, what would be a true waste is to use injectables before your body is truly ready. There are many examples of women who went to injects at BMIs of less than 22 and did not respond well (long cycles, lots of small follicles, not pregnant). Even if your insurance does cover the injectables, they will not work optimally if your body isn't ready. Regardless of monetary costs, injects have a pretty large physical and emotional cost (at least in my experience with them). So even if they are "free" in terms of money, they are not free in terms of time, side effects, emotional rollercoasters, stress levels, etc. That is not to say that they are a horrible experience or anything, but I would tell anyone who is considering them to try to get their body (and mind) in a truly healthy place first. I did three cycles of injectables at a BMI of 19 to 20. Each cycle was long (20+ days of injections) and resulted in follicles that were still considered pretty small. All three attempts ended with emotionally crushing negative pregnancy tests. While my weight was OK from a medical standpoint, I was still stressing my body by pushing too hard with exercise and being very "careful" with my food choices. I also ran through each and every cycle, not knowing any better, which I don't think helped my cause.

Anyway, all of this is to say that even if you do go down the injectable route, please, ladies, please give your bodies the rest and energy they need to be able to respond to the meds, grow follicles, and support implantation and a healthy pregnancy. And even if injectables do work without recovery, our children deserve mothers who have truly healthy minds, bodies, and spirits!

After my third negative cycle, I decided that it didn't make sense to just keep repeating the process and expect a different result. I decided to take the advice on the Board and rest and nourish my body in a new way. I haven't run since August and have stuck to only walking and yoga since October.

I am now at a BMI of 22 and am currently waiting for a bleed to start my fourth cycle. Is it still difficult some days to accept that this is truly healthy for me? Absolutely! Do I fear that I won't get the response I am hoping for? Definitely. However, I can say for sure that I feel so much stronger and calmer mentally than I have in a really long time. I am able to laugh and enjoy other people and have long stretches of time where

> I don't even think about food (which for someone who literally thought about food every waking second of every day during the worst of my eating disorder, that's a huge deal). My husband says that this is the most beautiful I have looked in years and that he is having more fun with me now than he has ever had (and we've been together over 10 years). *(Jessica got pregnant on her fifth injectable cycle, second after going all in.)*

If you've truly put in your all toward recovery, but have not resumed natural cycles or responded to oral meds, injectables are a good option. The extra push from the injected hormones will hopefully lead to ovulation and the pregnancy you're longing for. Please know that even if you aren't cycling naturally yet, the work you have put in means you are extremely likely to menstruate after pregnancy (chapter 27).

There can be even more trepidation associated with starting a cycle of injectables than you felt with oral meds—the idea of giving yourself a shot can be very intimidating! Additionally, if you have put in the time and effort to recover, but have not gotten natural cycles back or responded to the oral drugs, it can lead to feeling even more hopeless and "broken." In many cases there is also added stress and pressure if you are paying out of pocket for your medicines and monitoring (these cycles are not cheap!). All of these feelings are normal; you may be able to process and deal with them with the help of friends, family, or an online or real-life support group (like the Board), or you may find that talking to a therapist who specializes in infertility issues is what you need.

> **Steph**: With me, what you see is what you get. For better or worse, I am an open book. So when my husband and I were dealing with infertility, I was extremely open about it. I blogged constantly about our journey, but I also talked about it with the people I knew in real life, which in some cases can be even harder to do. But I found that many of my friends had experienced some level of infertility and were happy to talk to and support me. My husband and I would joke that I somehow attracted people coping with infertility. I would go out, meet someone new, and end up in a conversation that somehow led to a discussion of how we were managing infertility. These people ended up becoming true friends. You can't go through this alone, from infertility to newborns. You need others, so go ahead and open up. I am not saying you have to let the world in (although I did), but don't be afraid to talk about it; you may be surprised by the response and to learn that infertility is way more common than you realize.

Before You Get Started

Before moving forward with an injectable cycle, it is advisable to ensure that you and your partner have no other issues preventing pregnancy. This often means undergoing a few more tests before treatment begins. You may have had some of this testing done during your oral ovulation induction cycles, or your doctor may not have suggested the testing until you decided to try injectables. We described the tests in detail in chapter 20, but as a reminder, they are:

- A baseline ultrasound to ensure that your uterus and ovaries are ready for a treatment cycle.
- An HSG to confirm that your tubes are open and your uterus is normally shaped.
- A semen analysis for your partner.
- Possibly, urine and/or blood tests for sexually transmitted diseases, as well as genetic testing on you and your partner.

Injectable Gonadotropins and HA

> *Nico*: As you read through this chapter, you will notice a lot of very specific advice about injectable cycles, and you might wonder what our qualifications are to offer these suggestions. This is a very reasonable question to ask. The advice and suggestions are based on the study of many research papers, as well as the observation of hundreds of injectable cycles through my interactions on the HA Board. The experience I have garnered from my years posting on the Board is generally not documented in the medical literature. In addition, most healthcare providers only treat a few patients with HA and therefore are not aware of much of what we tell you. My hope is that the information will help you and your doctor devise the best possible plan for your specific situation.

If all looks good after the testing, you're ready to get started with the injections! When doing a cycle of injectables, you are essentially taking your own hormones out of the picture. You inject a combination of FSH and LH (or FSH alone), starting around CD 3, and those hormones cause eggs to grow and mature. When the follicles containing the eggs are large enough (typically 17 mm or bigger[1*]), you will be instructed to take your trigger shot (chapter 23) to cause the final maturation of the egg(s); ovulation will follow about 36 hours later.

That makes it all sound really simple. Unfortunately, there are many parts of an injectable cycle, and many cycles, that are not so straightforward. First, there are decisions about what medication and dose to take. Of course, your doctor will have his or her plan, but as we've said before, most doctors don't see many with HA so are not necessarily aware of some unique aspects to our hormonal pictures. One of these aspects is the low LH. This means that one of the injectable medications like Menopur or Repronex that include both FSH and LH seem to work better than those containing only FSH (e.g., Gonal-F, Follistim, Bravelle, or Puregon).

- In HAers with an LH level below 5 IU/L, cycles using FSH alone have led to a much higher rate of cancellation. Among our survey respondents, when we compared cycles (113 in total) from those using FSH-only medications (even in combination with low-dose LH) with those using Menopur or Repronex, the cycle cancellation rate was much higher (29% versus 11%, p <0.01). The cancellations were a result of too little response, over-response, or follicles stalling.
- If your LH levels are well into the normal range, say 5 IU or above, it probably doesn't make much of a difference whether you use a combo med or FSH alone (we don't have sufficient data in those with LH > 5 IU to examine this question).

These medications come in different forms: some are powder in a vial, to which you add water to reconstitute the drug; and others come in a pre-filled syringe or "pen" that lets you adjust dosing. For the vials, doctors will typically prescribe full or half vials (vials of Menopur or Repronex normally contain 75 IU of FSH, plus 37.5 IU LH), where dosing is given based on the FSH amount. The pens allow a bit more flexibility, often with the ability to adjust dosing by 12.5 IU at a time.

Injectable Dosing Protocol Options

Now that we've covered the medications to consider, the next step is to talk about the different ways these meds can be administered.

---

* Note: For reasons that are not clear, optimal follicle sizes are different based on the method used to grow the follicle. Natural follicles tend to rupture at between 20 and 30 mm. As we mentioned in chapter 21, sizes from 23 to 27 mm have been shown to be best for follicles on oral medication cycles. For injectables, follicles 17 mm or greater will ovulate with high probability.

- The most common is called the "low and slow" protocol; the idea is that starting at a low dose and increasing slowly will lead to development of just one or two dominant follicles, which is ideal.
- Another method to consider is an oral med/injectable combination; here, the oral drug primes your system, and the injected FSH and LH give your pituitary the boost it needs. This is our recommendation for reasons outlined below.
- The least common method is the step-down protocol. Here, you start with a high dose to get things moving, then drop to a lower dose to avoid overstimulation.

The combination of oral meds with injectables is currently infrequently used with HA, although research shows that this protocol can reduce the amount of gonadotropins needed, as well as decrease the chances of overstimulation and a multiple pregnancy[2]. Therefore, a combination of oral meds and injectables is our recommendation for your initial cycle. We will, however, discuss the low and slow protocol first, as the same dosing scheme is followed during the injectable portion of the cycle when you pursue a combination protocol.

Low and slow protocol. When you're following a low and slow protocol, think of your first cycle as a test run to find the dosages that work best for you. There is a good chance that you'll get pregnant, but you also might not, so in some ways it's easier to think of this cycle as a trial. You and your doctor will learn from what happens, and can then adjust dosing for subsequent cycles if needed. You start with a dose to which you probably won't respond (although a small number do respond at these low doses)—but what it does is prime the follicles and start changes that are undetectable via blood work and ultrasounds commonly used for monitoring. Some doctors will start as low as half a vial (37.5 IU), but it is more common to start with a full vial (75 IU). This is what we recommend as a starting dose unless you have a large number of antral (baseline) follicles (more than 15), or you have had at least one natural period, in which case a starting dose of 37.5 IU might be more appropriate.

> *Katie*: I was slow to start. I do not remember the exact numbers but my E_2 barely rose after the first four days at 75 IU (one vial) of Menopur. Then my doc increased my dose to two vials and my E_2 went up to 103, then 300-something, and just kept rising. The key is to find the dose that you will respond to. All in all, I was only on Menopur for 10 days my first try and 9 days the second try when I got pregnant with my twins.

> **Stacie:** I did my first Menopur cycle last month. I was a slow responder and we finally upped my dose to 150 IU, but I ended up with eight follicles and we had to stop the cycle. I was a little heartbroken. This cycle we held the dose at 112.5 IU the whole time and it did the trick. As of yesterday I had one big, beautiful 18.5 mm follicle. I'm going in for my IUI tomorrow morning!

It is important to start at a low dose, to which you probably will not respond, because of the large number of follicles typical with HA. These small follicles are just waiting for a push from hormones to develop (hence the common confusion with PCOS), making it easy to overstimulate. When this happens, three or more follicles grow big enough to contain mature eggs, which often means your cycle may be canceled (for fear of triplets or more).

After three to four days of injections, your doctor will have you come in to the office visit the clinic for an ultrasound and/or blood work to monitor how your follicles are growing. If your insurance does not cover monitoring, there are ways to decrease costs. Discuss with your doctor the possibility of just checking your estradiol level with blood work in the beginning, and adding in ultrasounds after your E_2 indicates a response. Generally, follicles are growing when your E_2 rises above 100 pg/mL, so sticking with just blood work until that point can save some money (ultrasounds are typically $200 to $400 each, whereas blood work costs about $80 per test).

When you go for your first monitoring appointment of this initial cycle (as we mentioned, usually three to four days after starting injections), expect that there will not be any increase in E_2 or follicular growth. If you started at a very low dose like half a vial, it is common to increase that dose to a full vial at this point. If you started at one vial, we do recommend waiting a full week before increasing your dose (and doing so only if E_2 and follicle sizes have not risen). We also suggest waiting a minimum of four days, preferably a week, before any additional dose increases, especially in this first cycle. When a dose increase is indicated, we strongly recommend adding only half a vial (37.5 IU) at a time. We have seen a number of cycles canceled when the dosage was increased by a full vial—you can go from no response to over-response very quickly! Many HAers respond at 1.5 vials, or 112.5 IU of FSH. If you don't respond at 112.5 units, the next step is to increase your dose to two full vials (150 IU). Be cautious about making this jump, as this seems to be the fine line that delineates over-response for many.

> *Natalie Z*: I had another ultrasound today after the RE increased my Menopur dose to 150 IU. I went from no response to over-stimming! What the heck? I have 13.5, 12, 12, 11, and 10 mm follicles. The RE wanted to cancel, but then suggested just stopping the Menopur and seeing if a couple of follicles take off on their own, and hopefully a couple regress. So I will go back Saturday to see what my body does. Seriously, it is like my body doesn't want to respond AT ALL, or responds too much. I was so happy to see the 13.5 mm, but then the doctor kept measuring and I was like NOOOOO. This is such a difficult journey!

It is not a problem if you are not ready to trigger by CD 14, so it is better not to rush to increase the dose. Once follicles start to respond, they follow a typical pattern of growth to ovulation, so the resulting egg is as healthy as normal. The pregnancy rate is the same for an early ovulation (up to CD 14) versus a late one (CD 23+), or even after CD 30. In addition, as we will describe in chapter 26, miscarriage rates are not affected by the cycle day of ovulation. So, taking it slowly during this first cycle is not going to be detrimental.

Effect of ovulation CD on pregnancy rate in injectable cycles among survey respondents

Cycle day of ovulation	Number of cycles	Pregnancy rate*
<=14	36	36%
15–18	36	44%
19–22	23	35%
23–29	11	27%
>=30	8	38%
Total	114	38%

* There is no difference between pregnancy rates, $p = 0.94$.

> *Monica*: Seventeen days of Menopur (the last seven on 112.5 IU) and five of Pregnyl (hCG, 1500 IU) shots = drum roll, please ... NOTHING! This is like taking a course in patience building. I wonder if I will get a certificate at the end? My lining is around 3.5 mm and I still have no follicles over 7 mm. But I'm fine—I am just a slow responder. I am allowed to increase my dose to the full two vials on Sunday and then I'm back on Monday. Hopefully that will be the ticket. (*Monica got pregnant the cycle after*

> *this one, following a similar dosing scheme. She now has two sons through Menopur injections.)*

Follicles typically hit their growth stride when your E_2 is around 100 pg/mL and follicle size is between 10 and 12 mm, at which point the growth rate is approximately 2 mm per day. If you're starting monitoring with the blood work-only plan, a first ultrasound when your E_2 goes over 100 is a reasonable strategy. If you have just one mature follicle growing, you're golden. You stay at the same dose of meds, then take your trigger shot when the follicle is 17 to 20 mm in diameter[3]*. However, in other cases, this is where the cycle can get particularly dicey; you may have a number of follicles growing at around the same rate, which can lead to overstimulation, as we will discuss in chapter 23.

Oral/injectable combination protocol. For an oral/inject combination cycle, you start with the oral meds from CD 3 to 7, then add a low dose of Menopur, typically 75 IU, from CD 7 or 8 on. The Femara or Clomid has primed your system by dropping the estrogen levels your hypothalamus is detecting, which leads to an increase in FSH and LH as your hypothalamus tries to compensate (chapter 21). Then, in addition to the natural increase in FSH/LH that occurs, you add a bit of external help in the form of the injectables.

> **Sarah G**: I saw my RE yesterday. I'm doing 5 mg Femara for five days, then starting Menopur on Saturday. I'll take 150 IU for two days and then have an ultrasound on Monday to check progress. I'm so excited to get going again. I really hope this works; after eight tries of Clomid or Femara I need to try something else. And I know I have to do everything I can in my power and God will work out the rest.

Priming with the oral meds tends to decrease the number of vials of Menopur that you need, which can be especially helpful if you are on a budget and insurance doesn't cover your medication costs[4]. This protocol has also been shown to help promote growth of a single follicle, reducing the chances of overstimulation, multiples, and canceled cycles[5]. The quicker stimulation, equivalent pregnancy rate, lesser medication, and lower number of mature follicles lead us to suggest the oral/injectable combination

---

* Protocols vary between doctors as far as when to give the trigger shot. Evidence for when to trigger is sparse, however, one group found that follicles 17 mm or greater had an increased likelihood of ovulating.

as the ideal protocol for an HAer or recovered HAer (if oral medications alone do not work).

Step-down protocol. The final protocol that is very rarely used, but has been suggested by a few doctors to HAers on the Board, is the step-down protocol, with two possible implementations. In one study, 29 subjects were started at 300 IU of FSH on CD 3 to get the follicles growing, then took three days off meds[6]. After that, they followed the low and slow protocol described above. In a second study, 19 women with irregular or missing periods but normal gonadotropin levels were started at 150 IU FSH, with the dose dropped by half a vial once they started to respond[7].

The ultimate goal with this protocol, along with the others, is to have one or two mature follicles when you're ready to trigger. Despite promising results in the two studies we mentioned, this protocol is not one we frequently recommend for two reasons: First, as discussed, HAers with low starting FSH and LH often don't have enough of the natural hormones to sustain the response over the few days with no or a lowered dose of medications. Second, there just isn't a lot of experience with step-down protocols among those on the Board, nor any research studies in people with HA, providing little evidence for the protocol's success in this population.

However, the results were promising in both studies, with fewer days of stimulation and similar or better rates of monofollicular development than the standard low and slow protocols. Therefore, if you are struggling with cycle cancellation due to overstimulation, it could potentially be worthwhile to consider these regimens. However, we would only suggest this protocol if your FSH and LH are within the normal range (at least 5 IU) to avoid the problem of insufficient natural hormones to sustain follicular growth after the dose is dropped.

> *Angie*: I started on 150 IU of Menopur for three days and, due to my great response, my RE backed it down to 75 for two days. My ultrasound today showed four follicles between 13 and 15 mm on the left, and three from 14 to 16mm on the right. My lining went from 8.7 to 8 mm. My blood work showed that my E_2 went from 378 to 279 and my LH was under 1. My RE said that I am producing no LH on my own and that is why my E_2 went down when we decreased the Menopur. He is increasing Menopur tonight back to 150 and wants to see me tomorrow for more blood work and an ultrasound. He thinks that a small dose of hCG may help. I am kind of freaked right now! (*Angie did get to trigger this cycle but did not get pregnant. Three cycles later she got pregnant starting at a dose of 112.5 IU.*)

Administering the Injections

We've talked about the dosing plans already, but how about actually administering the injections? This can be really intimidating and scary until you've done it a couple of times, but you will soon get to be a pro, and may even find yourself "shooting up" in random places like the bathroom at a family event or a parking lot.

It is often helpful to actually see what you're going to be doing. Many drug manufacturers provide "how to" diagrams in their patient inserts, and offer additional videos online. You will probably also get training from your doctor or nurse. The biggest points to remember are that the injections are not as bad as you imagine, will be over quickly, and soon will seem like no big deal.

> **Kathleen**: I am taking 150 IU so I have to use two vials. I was OK with the mixing because I watched a video online telling me how to do it. But it was holding the needle near my body and getting up the nerve to actually do the injection that was causing my heart to beat really fast! I think now that I have one under my belt it will be easier.

> **Mary**: My first injection was not bad at all! The only problem is that my hands were shaking so badly when I went to inject it that I thought I wouldn't be able to push the syringe in and that I might hurt myself by bumping it. It was actually no problem, though, and I think tonight it should go even more smoothly. The medicine did burn a little going in, but afterward I couldn't even see where I had injected it and couldn't feel anything.

A couple of tricks to help ease the process include warming the area you will inject (maybe try right after a shower), and warming the diluent up in your hand or by putting it in your pants pocket for a few minutes prior to injecting. Both strategies will help the medication disperse more easily, making you more comfortable. Switch between sides on your belly, and change up the location of the shot (moving up or down, and side to side a bit) so that you're not injecting the same place each time. Other suggestions include pinching your belly fat hard so it hurts, to distract you from the injection, and icing the area afterward. You can also have someone else do the injection if it's intimidating (but over time you will find that you can do it).

Once your follicles are big enough—typically when the largest is somewhere between 17 and 20 mm[8], and your E_2 is around 200 pg/mL per mature follicle—you will be told to trigger. This is when you inject hCG (human chorionic gonadotropin) to cause ovulation, similar to the large LH surge that triggers a natural ovulation (chapter 23).

Some doctors will automatically prescribe some form of progesterone support in an injectable cycle. Others will wait to see if there is a shortened LP before writing the prescription. An analysis of five studies examining effects of progesterone support on pregnancy and live birth rates found a significant improvement in both pregnancy and live birth rates when progesterone was used[9], therefore taking supplemental progesterone seems prudent.

Subsequent Cycles

If you don't get pregnant on your first cycle, it's normal to experience some pretty intense disappointment. But all you can do is keep pressing on. Re-evaluate your eating and exercise habits and take responsibility for the effect those choices may have had, and then try again. At this point you will probably have another CD 3 ultrasound to check if you have any cysts, leftover small follicles that never ovulated during the previous cycle. Cysts sound worse than they actually are; however, they sometimes interfere with another treatment cycle[10], so it is suggested to wait until they are gone to begin injections again. If you do have cysts, one option is to take birth control pills for three weeks to encourage the cysts to resolve. If you prefer not to take birth control, quite a few HAers have had cysts resolve within two to three weeks without using artificial hormones. And who knows? Going without the Pill might give your body the chance to surprise you...

> **Amanda H**: I went to see my doctor today, because something just hasn't felt "right" for the past week. Some cramping mostly, but also sharp, stabbing pains on my right side. Well, I had an ultrasound, and it turns out I have a 50 mm cyst in my right ovary. UGH.
>
> The doctor said it could be one of two things:
> - benign, and it would go away on its own, and won't interfere with this cycle
> - functional, which means it's releasing estrogen and would therefore interfere with the medications and I would have to wait for it to shrink on its own before starting treatment.
>
> So I had blood work done this morning to test for estrogen, LH, and FSH. I'm praying my estrogen isn't high because that will mean the cyst is benign.

> *Three weeks later:* I had an ultrasound this morning to check on the cyst, and it's gone! My doctor said it must have collapsed early this week when I was feeling the most pain. Since Wednesday, I haven't really felt it. I was so happy because it was really worrying me that it would interfere with this cycle.

It stinks to have to take unplanned time off when a cycle gets canceled because of cysts (or any other reason). When you've decided it's time to get pregnant you usually want your baby right now! Try not to get discouraged, and use this time to reconnect with your partner as infertility is tough on you both. Allow yourself to take a break from the all-consuming thoughts about babymaking, and revist your life outside of trying to have a baby. You will feel refreshed when it's time to jump back into treatment.

Once you get the green light to start another cycle, you and your doctor will have a little more information for selecting the dosages in subsequent cycles. In this case, we suggest that the starting dose be half a vial less than what stimulated your follicles to grow during the first attempt. Do not start at the same dose at which you responded in the previous cycle. Remember: the follicular recruitment process starts during the early part of your cycle and is occurring even when it seems like nothing is happening. Frequently, treatment cycles where your starting dose is the one at which your follicles started growing last time end in cancellation due to eventual overstimulation.

For your first cycles, the ideal is to have just one mature follicle. The more follicles you have, the higher your chances of twins or more, with a more challenging pregnancy and higher likelihood of negative outcomes for the babies. After three to four cycles with no pregnancy you can become a little more cavalier about the number of growing follicles (and/or think about moving on to IVF). To give you an idea of how often multiple pregnancies occur, on the Board, 24% of pregnancies resulting from injectable cycles were twins or more. Among those were three triplet pregnancies, one set of quadruplets, and one set of sextuplets.

> *Sarah:* Twins are a blessing in many ways. But coming from someone who spent 10 weeks on bedrest, in and out of the hospital, delivered 10 weeks early and dealt with 8 weeks of the NICU, it is not all fun and games. Twice the blessing but twice the crying, twice the heartache, twice the diapers, twice the sleeplessness, twice the doctor appointments, twice the potty training. Trying to feed twins simultaneously (breastfeed or other), and get them to sleep simultaneously. Twice the cost of daycare.

> Personally, I ended up needing diastasis surgery one year later due to a severe abdominal separation. And now I have six-year-old twins and its twice the tantrums, twice the drama, twice the schoolwork, and twice the cost of clothes, school activities, not to mention twice the worrying. It's definitely not two for the price of one! And this is with healthy twins with no lasting problems even though they were born 10 weeks early.
>
> **Amanda D**: Also, I really believe that having twins takes a greater toll on your marriage. More stress. More for BOTH of you to do, etc.
>
> **Penny**: I had to go off work at 25 weeks for a shortening cervix when I was pregnant with my boys. I was hospitalized for five weeks due to cholestasis of pregnancy (which has an increased incidence with twins) and then had three weeks of bed rest for early labor and a shortened cervix. I had a C-section at 34 weeks because of intra-uterine growth restriction. My twins are doing well now but are very delayed in speech, particularly my growth restricted twin.

Our ultimate recommendation to you and your doctor, when you don't get pregnant on a given cycle, is to err on the side of caution. Start a subsequent cycle with a dose half a vial less than what you responded to in your previous cycle, and remain at that level for about a week before increasing the dose. When you do increase, do so by only half a vial (37.5 IU FSH) at a time. This helps with recruiting just one or two follicles to grow and mature.

It is interesting that, even in the same person, the response during each cycle can be very different. Sometimes you will respond more quickly, and sometimes less so. But it is always better to start with conservative dosing. Remember: it's easy to increase your dose if you need it. It's not so easy to face multiple follicles and a canceled cycle.

When Injectables Don't Work

We are often led to believe hormone injections are a magic bullet and we will get pregnant on our first cycle or two. Unfortunately, there is never a guarantee of pregnancy. Among our survey respondents, the pregnancy rate for injectables was about 35% per cycle. This means that most will get pregnant in the first few cycles, but some will go through three, four, five, or more cycles with no luck. At some point, it makes sense to begin thinking about other options. Choosing whether to continue with injectables or try a different route is an incredibly personal decision, with all sorts of variables coming into play. While we can't tell you what will necessarily work for you, we can provide various options that have worked for our survey respondents to give you an idea of the available alternatives. Among our 240 survey respondents, 115 (48%) used injectables in some form for at least one cycle. Of those 115, an ongoing pregnancy as a result of the injections was achieved by 66 (57%). When pregnancy did not result:

- seventeen (35%) ultimately got pregnant naturally
- seven (14%) used oral medications
- twenty-four (49%) used IVF
- one couple chose to adopt

IVF is a common next step if injectables don't work after some number of cycles, but it is not the only option. In quite a few cases, HAers who were planning on doing IVF but waited for insurance, financial, or timing reasons, got pregnant in the interim. Additionally, if you are still performing high-intensity exercise, or your BMI is not in the fertile range, you may want to think about making some changes before continuing with additional treatment.

> *Andrea*: I have found that every cycle is so different. One injectable cycle took me 16 days, another more than 25. It's so hard to predict or understand what is going on. I always felt like I failed or did something wrong, but in reality, our bodies do things beyond our control. Since most HA ladies like control, this can be so hard for us. But staying positive and trusting your body will do its job in its own time is the key to it all working. Our bodies are amazing and, given love, they will listen and do their thing! Good luck!

Summary

Injectables are a standard treatment for HA when pregnancy is desired. While they can potentially work without making any changes toward natural recovery, they are not a cure-all and often do not work without lifestyle changes. We strongly recommend that you put the Recovery Plan into practice before spending time, money, and emotional effort on trying to get pregnant.

In this chapter, we talked a lot about different protocols you can potentially use to encourage ovulation by injecting FSH and LH. The three options are:

- The low and slow protocol: starting at a dose to which you will most likely not respond, and slowly increasing from there in order to reduce the likelihood of overstimulation.
- Femara or Clomid plus injectables (low and slow): this protocol both reduces the amount of injectables that you need and decreases the chance of a multiple pregnancy—this is our recommendation.
- Step-down protocol: in this case, you start with a high dose of gonadotropins to recruit follicles, then drop the dose so that only a few mature. This is the least common approach and is not recommended unless other protocols have failed, as HAers typically do not respond well to dose decreases.

There are also some additional points to note:

- It is common to experience cysts after an injectable cycle and have to take some time off from fertility treatment for them to decrease in size. Cysts do resolve with time alone, but some doctors will prescribe birth control pills. If you can avoid BCP, you get a chance to see if your body does anything on its own.
- How you responded during your first cycle can guide dosing for your second; we recommend starting at half a vial (37.5 IU) less than the dose you responded to in your previous cycle.
- Progesterone support in the form of vaginal suppositories, gel, or cream after ovulation may result in higher pregnancy and birth rate.

> *Lisa*: No sense in beating you over the head with this take-home message (i.e., a plea for putting in the work before resorting to injectables). I will not even pretend like my head never went to that place of skipping first, second, and third base and sliding directly into home plate, especially when I saw others doing it with success. This is where taking those disordered thoughts captive comes in. When comparison would seep into my mind, I quickly reminded myself that, while the grass may seem greener on the other side, that grass wasn't necessarily best for me. Jumping right into injects would be like receiving a 5K trophy without training for or even running the race. Where's the purpose in that? I knew what I needed to do to reach my overall goal, and you probably do too.

23
Medicated Ovulation and Beyond

WHEN USING FERTILITY MEDICATIONS to encourage the growth of follicles as covered in the last three chapters, there are a few additional steps often recommended by fertility doctors. You might have questions about some of these options, most of which are common among cycles using oral medications, injectables, or IVF:

- When and how might you "trigger" ovulation?
- When and how might you undergo intrauterine insemination?
- Do you need progesterone support?
- When can you test for pregnancy?
- What is overstimulation and what can you expect if it happens?
- How can you deal with a canceled cycle?

When and How You Might "Trigger" Ovulation

Once you are able to grow a follicle (chapters 21 and 22), the next hurdle is getting that follicle to ovulate. Recall that in a natural cycle, as the egg-containing follicle gets bigger, estradiol increases markedly, eventually causing a surge of LH that leads to final maturation of the egg and ovulation. In medicated cycles it is common to use an injection that performs the same function as the natural LH surge. This "trigger shot" usually consists of 5,000 to 10,000 IU of human chorionic gonadotropin (hCG); this is chemically similar to LH, so also initiates the ovulation process. The injection is administered when the follicles containing eggs are large enough, typically 20 to 24 mm (or larger) on a natural or orally medicated cycle, or bigger than 17 mm in an injectable cycle. Ovulation will typically occur about 36 hours after the trigger shot (unless you surge naturally it is extremely unlikely that you will ovulate before this).

Use of trigger shots varies between ob-gyns and REs, and is more common in injectable cycles versus orally medicated cycles. Monitoring of the cycle via ultrasound is required in order to ensure a mature egg. Trigger shots are occasionally used in monitored natural cycles if positive OPKs are not leading to ovulation (this occurs in approximately 10% of cycles[1]).

The trigger shot is generally a subcutaneous injection. Some doctors will administer the shot right in their office; in other cases, you will be sent home with instructions on self-administration.

Occasionally the trigger shot will be an intramuscular (IM) injection that is given in your gluteus maximus (your rear end). Ask your nurse for advice on how to perform this shot, and have her draw a "target" for you. An IM shot is difficult to do yourself, so enlist your partner or a friend. The Z-track method is suggested to be less painful than the traditional method for IM injections. It is difficult to describe, so speak with your nurse or Google to find picture or video instructions. Icing the area afterward can help minimize any potential soreness.

Using a trigger shot allows for optimal timing of sex and/or intrauterine insemination (IUI; see below). Based on the studies we described in chapter 17, sex around the time you trigger is ideal for getting pregnant[2]. If you are taking an intercourse-only approach, an additional session the day after the trigger shot is a good idea. If you are doing IUI, you should have sex around the time of the trigger and then abstain until the IUI.

Intercourse and IUI timing for pregnancy

Method	Time period before trigger shot	Day of trigger shot	One day post-trigger shot	Two days post-trigger*
If using intercourse (IC) only	IC as desired	IC	IC	IC
If using IC with IUI	IC as desired	IC	Abstain	IUI followed by IC if desired

* You will ovulate 36 hours after the trigger shot, typically the morning of the second day after an evening trigger.

It is not common or even necessary to confirm ovulation after the trigger shot; the assumption is that you have ovulated. If you want to know for peace of mind, the best way is to get a progesterone blood test at 6 or 7 DPO. A level above 3 ng/mL indicates ovulation, but ideally it should be 10 ng/mL or more[3]. If your level is lower than 10, you may want to consider progesterone support (chapter 19). You can also potentially confirm ovulation by tracking your temperature as described in chapter 17, but we have found it is mentally easier to simply trust that you have ovulated, because all the external hormones from the medications can cause odd temperature readings. For instance, temperatures can take longer to rise post-ovulation than they do during natural cycles. If you are meticulously temping, these variances can be confusing and needlessly ramp up your anxiety.

Intrauterine Insemination

Intrauterine insemination (IUI) is a procedure whereby sperm are washed and deposited directly into your uterus to bypass some of the initial obstacles they normally face, such as the acidic environment of the vagina or finding their way through the cervix. The bottom line on IUI is that if sperm are normal, there is at best a small (4–6%) increase in pregnancy as compared to well-timed intercourse[4], with many studies finding no difference in pregnancy rates[5]. Therefore, if money is an issue, you can be confident in skipping IUI for at least a few cycles.

It is often suggested that couples have sex two to three days before IUI in order to have optimal sperm concentrations and "freshness." However, because it is impossible to predict when your body will be ready for the trigger and therefore difficult to time intercourse in that two- to three-day window, intercourse shortly before or after the trigger shot is common. This is just the right timing for conception, and also allows sufficient time for sperm to replenish before the IUI.

If you do IUI, you and your partner will be instructed to come to the office about 34 hours after you take the trigger shot. At that time, your mate will be instructed to ejaculate into a cup. Next, technicians will wash the semen and put the sperm into a solution to keep them fresh and viable. At about 36 hours after the trigger shot, the sperm will be placed into a catheter and gently inserted into your uterus.

It is typical to have a single IUI at between 34 and 36 hours after the trigger shot is taken, although some have two IUIs, at 24 and 48 hours after trigger. The pregnancy rates are essentially identical between the two protocols[6], so it is most common to go with the single, 36-hour post-trigger shot IUI.

> *Nico (2005)*: The IUI itself was lots of fun. And I do mean that literally. Doctor T. and my husband had a nice comedy routine going. After a few unsuccessful attempts at getting the catheter in, the doctor said he "didn't like the angle of my cervix," and that I could fix it by coughing. So Mark joked, "It's about time a woman had to 'turn and cough!'" Doctor T. then proceeded to tell us about the first time he had that experience as a sixteen-year-old with a gorgeous female doctor. Meanwhile, I'm having fits of giggles, with the speculum sticking out of me! I was afraid that it was going to fall out or something, but even with it wiggling around down there with every chortle, it seemed to stay in just fine. After I coughed on "three," apparently the angle was perfect, and in the little soldiers went.

Do You Need Progesterone Support?

Approximately 36 hours after the trigger shot, you will most likely ovulate and, if you had intercourse or IUI, you will officially be in the two-week wait! There is one more decision to make at this point: whether to use progesterone support for your luteal phase (LP), the time between when you ovulate and get your period. If you already know you tend to have a short LP, it is helpful to be on some sort of progesterone, which can increase your chance of pregnancy by lengthening your LP. Reviews of a number of clinical studies have found significantly higher pregnancy rates with progesterone support[7]. In addition, as we discussed in chapter 19, people recovering from HA tend to have short LPs anyway, so you should do all you can to stack the deck in your favor for these cycles by using progesterone support. If your doctor is unwilling to prescribe progesterone, review chapter 19 for non-prescription options you can try.

When Can You Test for Pregnancy?

When a trigger shot is given, it is usually hCG, which is the hormone that pregnancy tests measure. It takes anywhere from 7 to 10 (or occasionally more) days for this hCG to be cleared from your system, so early pregnancy tests can give false positives. In other words, hCG from the trigger shot can give you a second line on a pregnancy test if it has not been metabolized (cleared from your blood) yet. Some like to "test out the trigger" by taking cheap home pregnancy tests each day so they can see the second line get fainter as the trigger shot leaves their system. They then keep testing to hopefully see the line get darker again as the hCG from an implanted embryo builds up. Others prefer to wait to test until the trigger shot is almost certainly gone, around 11 or 12 DPO. A line that gets darker at that point is indicative of pregnancy and can be confirmed by a blood test.

Overstimulation

Overstimulation is the term often used when instead of having just one or two follicles ready to ovulate in a cycle using oral meds or injectables, there are three or more. The main reason this is a problem is because of the increased chance of multiples. Even a twin pregnancy is more difficult for both mother and babies; a triplet (or more) pregnancy is best to avoid if possible. Also, many maturing follicles and a high E_2 level can be associated with ovarian hyperstimulation syndrome (OHSS). In essence, what happens with OHSS is that your blood vessels become leaky, resulting in an increase of fluid in your ovaries and abdominal cavity. This is not a pleasant experience. Cases can range from mild, treated by ingesting lots of salt and fluid (beverages like Gatorade are often suggested), to severe, requiring hospitalization to drain the excess abdominal fluid. We'll discuss this further when we cover IVF in chapter 24.

As far as multiples go, this is a top concern when using ovulation induction medications. In some ways, being pregnant with twins or more may seem ideal (two for the price of one!). In reality, a twin or higher multiple pregnancy is taxing on your body, the babies are more likely to be born premature, and dealing with two newborns at the same time is a heck of a lot harder. If you're being monitored during treatment cycles and have multiple follicles, you have a decision to make about whether to continue or cancel the cycle. Most doctors suggest that if the number of follicles is three or less, the cycle can be continued with timed intercourse only, not IUI. More than three follicles, especially on your first cycle when you don't know how fertile you are, can be risky in terms of getting pregnant with multiple babies and therefore cancellation is the usual recommendation.

There are a few options besides cancellation if your cycle is heading toward overstimulation. One simple option is to trigger earlier. In a cycle using oral medications, we have told you that the ideal is to trigger with the dominant follicle(s) between 23 and 27 mm. However, many clinical studies have been performed in which the trigger shot was administered with the lead follicle at 18 mm. Therefore, if you end up with multiple follicles on an oral cycle, triggering when the lead is only 18 mm means that the smaller follicles are less likely to ovulate and you can go ahead with trying to get pregnant.

For guidance in an injectable cycle, we can use information obtained in IVF studies. One research group found that 81% of eggs retrieved from follicles between 13 and 15 mm at trigger were mature and 52% fertilized. Mature eggs were retrieved from even smaller follicles; 80% of eggs from follicles sized 10 to 12 mm at trigger were also mature, with a 47% fertilization rate[8]. So, if you are doing a cycle using injectables and have two or three lead follicles at 14 to 15 mm with smaller follicles at 12 to 13 mm, you and your doctor might consider triggering. It is unlikely that the smaller follicles will rupture and ovulate, but the larger ones probably will, giving you a chance at pregnancy and avoiding cancellation.

You should be aware that if you have a large group of secondary follicles when you trigger, it is likely that some of them will not ovulate, but continue to grow through your luteal phase. If you are not pregnant and want to try another cycle, these non-ruptured follicles ("cysts") can sometimes interfere as we described in chapter 22.

A second possibility if overstimulation seems likely is to convert the cycle to IVF (chapter 24) with reasonable success rates[9].

Another option can be to have some of your larger follicles "aspirated." This is similar to the egg retrieval procedure in IVF. A long needle is used to collect the eggs and follicular cells out of a number of the larger follicles, so that only a few are left behind to ovulate. This is by far the least common option, but can be discussed with your doctor if you do not want to convert to IVF.

Finally, in some injectable cycles, doctors will recommend decreasing the dose of hormones to try and get some of the smaller follicles to drop out of the race. This approach rarely ends well in our experience. Usually what happens is as soon as the dose is dropped, the E_2 falls right along with it and the follicles stop growing. It may be the case that dropping the dose by a very small amount can produce the desired outcome, but because we have no data to support that suggestion, we do not recommend this path.

The ideal scenario is to avoid this question altogether by careful management of dosing, as we discussed in previous chapters.

Nico (2005): I thought I was having a picture perfect, textbook cycle. And I was. Right up until they told me to decrease my dosage. I went in again this morning, and my follicles were pretty much the same size as they were two days ago, as was my lining. The nurse called in the afternoon and said that I might already be ovulating because my estradiol had dropped (yeah, no kidding—what do you think happens when you decrease the meds by 67%?). So I'm supposed to do the trigger shot tonight, and then go in for IUI 12 hours later (instead of the usual 36 hours).

I am really, really angry. With them and with myself. I feel like I should have questioned what they were doing more—I've read too many stories of people's dosages being dropped and cycles getting messed up. I later found out my E_2 levels: 106 on day 7, 271 on day 10, 348 on day 11 (that's when they decided to drop the meds) and then 52 on day 13. I really don't understand why they decided to drop based on the 348. That doesn't seem high to me at all!

Jennifer H: I went through a cycle of Menopur and Bravelle (FSH only) and it took me a few days to show any growth at all. For the first three days, I took 75 IU of both with nothing to show. The next two days I took 150 IU Menopur and 75 IU Bravelle and almost exploded after that increase. My estradiol went through the roof and I developed nearly 50 follicles. However, most of the follicles were between 8 and 12 mm. There were a few at 16 and 17. My RE took away the Bravelle altogether and reduced the Menopur to 75 IU. After that, my estradiol dropped and the follicles began to shrink leading to my cycle being canceled after 14 days.

Dealing with Canceled Cycles

Speaking of canceled cycles, it can be helpful to know what to expect if you are told not to trigger ovulation because there are too many follicles. Some get a period due to the drop in estrogen (this typically happens around a week later); others take birth control pills (BCP) or Provera to induce a bleed; in a few cases, injections can be started a few weeks later with no intervening bleed.

It can feel absolutely soul-crushing to be told that you can't move forward with a cycle you've put so much hope into. But please stay encouraged. The women below experienced cycle cancellations and each now has a baby (or more!).

Becky H: I was absolutely devastated. My husband said he had never heard me cry so hard in my life. I was ready to start kicking and screaming on the floor of the doctor's office when they told me my cycle was canceled. It was such a letdown. So much money... so many precious potential babies gone. I was so excited to finally start injections. Seeing follicles grow was so cool and I thought for sure I would finally be pregnant. Then wham, bam, cancellation, ma'am! Knocked my hopes to the floor.

Belinda: I was gutted and frustrated. I had only ever had one follicle before. My first-ever cycle was one follicle that is now my gorgeous almost three-year-old, and my first cycle to try for baby number two was one follicle but no pregnancy. I couldn't understand how I had suddenly "over-produced"—five follicles bigger than 12 mm. I didn't take BCP but opted to wait three weeks for the cysts to subside. During this time, I found Nico's blog and the Board, gained some weight, upped the fats, and got pregnant with Clomid instead.

Laura: I felt angry and sad that I overstimulated. I also got sick from the large amount of cysts (was throwing up for a day and felt nauseous for a couple days).

Megan E: I took BCP for three weeks. Honestly, I was a bit relieved to have a break. We were able to take a tenth anniversary trip at the last minute and it was great to be able to relax and enjoy wine and beer. The next cycle I got pregnant!

Summary

Whether you are using oral medications or injectables to grow follicles, making sure those follicles ovulate is an important part of the process. A trigger shot, given in the doctor's office or at home, is often used to ensure such an occurrence. This injection should be administered when a follicle is between 17 and 20 mm in a cycle using injectables or between 23 and 27 mm in an oral medication cycle. Other considerations during this time include choosing whether to do IUI, deciding about progesterone support, and the important question of when to take a pregnancy test.

Finally, cycles are sometimes canceled for overstimulation or other reasons; try not to get derailed by expecting each step to happen when it "should." When your plans to get pregnant do not go as anticipated, you may be left with a dark conviction that none of these treatments will ever work for you. However, from what we have seen, there is a way; it just may not be on your timetable.

Nico: The darkest days for me were the time after my fourth failed (as in I didn't get pregnant) injectable cycle. I got my period, heralding the failure,

> while visiting my week-old niece at my sister's house. It stung even worse than the previous negatives because we were supposed to be pregnant together and now she had her baby and I still couldn't even get knocked up. After that, our plan was to move to IVF, but I was utterly convinced that IVF would also fail and we would remain childless (as my husband had expressed that he was not interested in adoption). I'd said in my younger, naïve days, that if we weren't able to get pregnant naturally, I could accept that we were not meant to have children. However, as I stared the possibility of remaining childless in the face, I discovered how wrong I had been. My plans for the future had absolutely included children and grandchildren, and I was not at all ready to give up on those dreams. My husband noticed my despondency and encouraged me to share my fears. As we discussed, he agreed that if IVF were to fail, adoption could be a route to consider. The assurance that I would have children eventually by some path lifted a weight off my mind and I found I was able to breathe again. (And ended up getting pregnant naturally as we waited to start the IVF cycle.)

It is normal to feel like fertility treatments won't ever work and you will never have children after you've experienced even just a few failures. But the odds are overwhelmingly on your side; it really is just a matter of when and which path you will ultimately follow to enlarge your family and your heart.

24
In Vitro Fertilization

IN VITRO FERTILIZATION (IVF) is the pinnacle of reproductive medicine. And just as with the other routes to pregnancy, there are a multitude of paths that might lead you to choose IVF. Perhaps earlier testing showed that your tubes are not clear, or your partner's sperm are unlikely to impregnate you naturally. Maybe you've had a few (or multiple) failed cycles. You might have tried naturally for more than the six months recommended by fertility specialists (12 months if you're under 35), and/or used oral meds with no ovulation or pregnancy. Maybe you tried injectables and miscarried or overstimulated, and you and your doctor feel like IVF, with its higher rate of success, is the way to go.

If your path has led you to the decision to try IVF, you might be feeling like this whole recovery thing was a waste of time and that the weight you've gained or time off exercise was all for nothing.

> *Allison H*: It can be heartbreaking to work so hard to undo HA only to be faced with IVF and the realization that the weight gain and everything else that comes with it has gotten you nowhere. It still upsets me now honestly.

We want to put those uncertainties to rest. There is no loss in having worked toward recovery. Your weight gain, decreased exercise, and change in mindset were absolutely not in vain. While we don't deny that there is a possibility that IVF will work at a low BMI or with continued high-intensity exercise, we can assure you that the time, weight, decreased exercise, and mental growth will only help with IVF. The IVF process is an expensive route (if your insurance doesn't cover it), and time-consuming (most cycles take two to three months, all told). Working toward recovery gives you the best chance of reaching your goal. Unfortunately, there is very little research on the effect of low BMI on IVF success rates. Most studies look only at the upper end of the BMI range. However, one study that did include underweight women found a 30% increase in risk of miscarriage at a BMI of 18 (versus BMI of 24, with the lowest risk)[1].

> *Judith*: I naively thought that by going the IVF route, it would be my magic bullet to a baby. Hmm… after 11 transfers, that clearly was not the case!
>
> I thought that the IVF meds would be so powerful that my lifestyle would not matter, and slid back to HA ways during my first cycle. I wish I had known how important eating, BMI, and rest were, alongside IVF.
>
> It was a really tough time. The best thing I did was take a spontaneous trip with my husband after another IVF miscarriage. It was not a "sensible" thing to do as we couldn't afford the time or expense, but it was SO refreshing, and I still look back on that time as being hard but really important for us as a couple.
>
> Hearing other people's experiences was also really helpful, and the support from my friends on the Board was what really got me though the dark days. I owe sooo so much to them all!! *(Judith got pregnant on her twelfth transfer. Her second child was conceived on an IVF cycle converted to IUI.)*

> *Michelle M*: I jumped right into IVF when I was diagnosed with HA back in 2007. I proceeded to do four unsuccessful IVF rounds. Two of those rounds were when I was underweight. The other two were after I had put on 15 lb. After my fourth failed cycle in 2008 I was told that I had bad eggs since my embryos never developed well beyond day 3. I decided to take a break from treatment because I was just a mess emotionally. It was during that time that I got my first natural period and proceeded to conceive naturally within two months. This is after being told by doctors that my likelihood of having a biological child wasn't great. My point is that if you are not ovulating and your body is not in a good place, IVF is no quick fix. I definitely thought it was a few years ago when the whole infertility nightmare began for me. In retrospect, I wish I had worked on my lifestyle and tried Clomid and injectables rather than putting myself through all of those IVF cycles so quickly. Now, that's not to say that IVF isn't a good option eventually for some. I just think you need to give your body time to recover from HA. I used to wake up every morning thinking about if and when I was going to get pregnant. It was pure torture and

> a terribly sad time in my life. What I can say now is that it forced me to make lifestyle changes that will benefit me for the rest of my life. (*Michelle now has three children, all conceived naturally, when she was 33, 35, and 38.*)

Another reason to put the Recovery Plan into action prior to choosing IVF is that leptin (often decreased with low body fat) might play a role in getting pregnant. Recall from chapter 17 when we mentioned that both leptin and leptin receptors are present in the uterus? The levels of leptin receptors are highest around the time implantation might occur[2]. This, along with experiments performed in mice[3], suggests that leptin plays a part in helping an embryo to implant correctly in your uterus. Implantation is just as important in IVF as in natural or medicated cycles, so having adequate levels of leptin might be important. And as increased body fat leads to an increase in leptin, whatever weight you have gained to this point is not for nothing.

Another benefit of weight gain is that it allows for a healthier pregnancy and baby. Babies born to folks who are underweight are more likely to be "small for gestational age"[4]. Additionally, if you happen to develop the common pregnancy symptom of "morning" (or all day) sickness and are queasy and/or throwing up during your first trimester, having a cushion of weight will be beneficial.

> **Kelly**: I feel obligated to caution you on treatment success at low weights/body fat. Some do fine at lower weights, but many are extremely hindered by not enough weight. I responded wonderfully and it almost worked every time (all four IVFs), but almost doesn't count! We started treatment when I was 29 (I'm now 30) and I was a BMI of 19.4, body fat 14%. The last one ended in miscarriage at seven weeks. The RE told me I would most likely never ovulate naturally. I have since gained 20 lb and am starting to regain my cycles—I have my period right now. Anyway, my point is that when things are really shut down from being underweight or having low body fat, it's really difficult for your body to carry a pregnancy even if you can get pregnant. I feel like we wasted so much time (almost a year), money ($30,000), and tears (buckets full) on something that wasn't necessary if I had only not been so hardheaded and tried gaining the weight to begin with. Just think about it… I know it's SO hard, but if I can do it, anyone can! I was type A, self-critical, a control freak, anorexic, pessimistic, and impatient. Now I'm happy to say I'm basically just self-critical and type A. Hey, it's a step in the right direction! (*Kelly had a successful pregnancy in her eighth IVF cycle; her second child was conceived 18 months later from her first frozen embryo transfer.*)

How about exercise and its influence on IVF success? There aren't many studies answering this question, but we recommend continuing to avoid high-intensity exercise while undergoing these treatments, because of the increased chance of ovarian torsion (twisting) as your ovaries become bigger during your IVF cycle. About half an hour a day of lower-intensity exercise like walking, swimming, and light biking is recommended. Light exercise like this is either associated with improved pregnancy rates, or has no effect[5]. Therefore, it is worthwhile to continue with low-intensity exercise (unless your doctor has advised otherwise), as it will probably help relieve some of the stress you might feel associated with your cycle.

IVF in HA

Once you get to the point of IVF, because you are looking to grow a lot of eggs, there really isn't much that is different for someone with HA from a typical IVF cycle. This is the bread and butter of fertility clinics, with many performing hundreds of cycles a year. It is still worth a few minutes of your time to check your clinic's statistics from the Centers for Disease Control[6]. Look at the success rates for your age group—if you're not comfortable with what you're seeing compared to other clinics in your area, you may want to go elsewhere. Keep in mind that the statistics do not always tell the whole story; some clinics will treat tougher cases such as those with high FSH, whereas others refuse to do so, which will affect success rates—but it's good to have a ballpark idea of how your clinic compares to others. If you've had two to three failed cycles at one clinic, this report can be useful in finding another clinic to get a second opinion and other ideas about steps you can take to help get you pregnant.

Once you're at a clinic you feel comfortable with, you will have to complete pre-treatment testing, some of which we have mentioned in previous chapters:

- A baseline ultrasound to examine your ovaries and get a sense of how you will respond and what medication dosages to use.
- Your partner will do a semen analysis (chapter 20) to determine the best method of inseminating your eggs.
- Tests to check for sexually transmitted diseases/infections (these would be treated prior to starting IVF).
- Genetic testing, including some testing based on your ethnicity to determine if there are any potential mutations or chromosomal issues

that might be of concern and to suggest preimplantation genetic diagnosis (PGD) if necessary, where your embryos are screened to find those without a genetic disease.
- A PAP smear if you haven't had one recently.
- A mock transfer—the doctor practices inserting a catheter into your uterus to place the embryo so that if there are any anomalies they can be noted in your chart. This way the doctor doing the embryo transfer can be prepared for the real event when the procedure is time-sensitive.
- You may have a visit with a social worker to discuss issues such as what to do with any remaining embryos, how you are handling the stress of the procedures and any failures beforehand, and techniques for managing that stress.
- There will be lots of paperwork to fill out—how long to keep any unused embryos, what to do with the embryos in various scenarios, as well as a plethora of consent forms. You can usually take these forms home to discuss the options with your partner and fill them out at your leisure.

Once the testing is complete and the doctor determines your initial protocol, you will be given a calendar telling you what medications to take and when. Then, you will either go to a pharmacy to pick up your meds, or get a big package in the mail. It can be intimidating when you see how many different components there are, but having the calendar with each day's instructions makes the process less overwhelming. There are a number of different protocols that can be used for IVF, so we will just give an overview of the basics here.

The general idea of the IVF process is that you take hormones to encourage growth of many follicles with the goal of collecting around 10 to 20 mature eggs. These eggs are mixed with sperm to create embryos for transfer into your uterus—hopefully the beginning of a successful pregnancy.

Keep in mind that IVF works to ensure that the cycle is as much under the doctor's control as possible, removing natural hormones from the equation. This will increase your rate of success. First, your system is suppressed, often through use of birth control pills. Then, high-dose FSH and LH injections encourage growth of multiple follicles. At the same time, a medication that prevents a natural LH surge is taken so that natural ovulation does not occur (this is important because the egg retrieval procedure needs to be timed precisely). Once the follicles are of adequate size, you are instructed to take a trigger shot. About 34 hours later, after the eggs have undergone final maturation but prior to ovulation, the "egg retrieval" procedure is performed. Under general anesthesia, your doctor will aspirate the eggs and follicular fluid out of each follicle with a hollow needle inserted through your vagina (hence the anesthesia). The eggs then go to the lab where they are either mixed or injected with sperm. Eggs that are mature have a good chance of fertilizing, creating embryos that are grown in the lab for the next two to five days. At that point, you return to the clinic and a growing embryo is transferred into your uterus.

> *Nico (2011)*: Monday morning before my day 5 embryo transfer, I was so nervous I wasn't hungry, which NEVER happens. I managed to force down some cereal as that was the only thing that seemed remotely appetizing. I had doubts about the Valium prescribed to be taken before my transfer, but I found myself counting down the minutes until I could pop one in my mouth! When I finally did take the pill, I felt much more Zen within 15 minutes or so, which was great. I took the second when we arrived at the clinic, and had a full bladder as instructed. We didn't wait long before we were called back for the procedure. Of course they had me change into my hospital gown in a room with a toilet—such a tease!
>
> After my husband and I gowned up, we headed in for the transfer. I lay down on a table with strange stirrups that held my whole legs up. After I was in position, the entire table was tilted backward so I felt like I was at maybe a 30-degree angle. Bizarre! I suppose it helps with getting the catheter into the cervix. I tried as best I could to just relax, but I found myself tensing my legs as if to hold them up myself. Basically all I could think about though was how my bladder felt like it was going to explode every time the doctor pressed on the ultrasound probe. They did a practice run first with just the catheter, then got the embryo, claimed they could see a little flash on the ultrasound as the embryo was deposited (I could see where the catheter was but did not see the "flash"), checked that the catheter was empty, and then we were done. So now I'm pregnant until proven otherwise!

Questions About IVF and HA

There are some questions related to IVF in HAers that often crop up. First, it is common to wonder whether suppression (also called down-regulation) by birth control pills (BCP) at the start of an IVF cycle is needed. The answer is that it depends.

- Studies that collect data from a number of clinical trials and look at the pooled results (meta-analyses) indicate that there is no negative effect of BCP on IVF success rates[7], but the vast number of choices of BCP complicates this conclusion.
- If you try BCP in one cycle and do not respond well to the injections, it is reasonable to try without down-regulation by BCP on your next cycle.
- A case in which taking BCP might be advantageous is if you have a high AMH level (hormone associated with follicles that are ready to grow) or lots of antral follicles. A study that looked at how many eggs were retrieved in cycles using a young (average age 24) egg donor found that using more androgenic* BCP (levonorgestrel, e.g. Norethindrone) resulted in fewer eggs retrieved (average 11.3) than not using BCP (16.6) or using anti-androgenic BCP (drospirenone, e.g. Yasmin) with an average of 19.0 eggs[8].
    - We mention this as something to think about in order to avoid ovarian hyperstimulation syndrome (OHSS), although the study in question did not mention the incidence of OHSS.
- On the flip side, if you do have a lower AMH or follicle count, you should avoid the high androgen BCP, and perhaps consider the anti-androgenic ones (e.g., drospirenone) instead.

Whew, that ended up being a long answer to a short question!

Getting back on track, there is also the question of whether it is necessary to prevent a natural LH surge (e.g., by injecting a GnRH agonist such as Lupron), because HAers typically have low natural LH. Even with low baseline LH a surge is possible, so some form of surge prevention is standard because a premature increase in LH could cancel the whole cycle. There are two ways to do this: either a GnRH agonist (e.g., Lupron) is taken before you start stimulation, or GnRH antagonists like Ganirelix are taken during stimulation. The question of what would be recommended to prevent a natural LH surge in your case is a great query for your RE.

Finally, some wonder about egg quantity and quality. HAers usually have a lot of eggs that mature (and have to be careful of OHSS, as we will describe shortly); therefore, there are no HA-specific concerns about number of eggs. In addition, typical fertilization and pregnancy rates suggest that the eggs are normal.

---

* Androgenic means that the pills affect you in the same way as your naturally occurring male hormones; anti-androgenic suggests that activity of those male hormones is blocked.

What Else Should I Do?

As with oral meds and injectables, you can find all sorts of advice on foods you should eat, supplements you can take, using acupuncture, being on bed rest for a few minutes or sometimes even days, etc., for a "more successful IVF cycle." It is so hard to know what is reasonable and what is a myth. For example, you might read that eating pineapple core can help with implantation because it has anti-inflammatory and anti-coagulation effects. It is true that bromelain, the enzyme contained in pineapple, has anti-inflammatory effects[9], but no studies have been performed to assess the claims of its effect on implantation, and certainly people get pregnant all the time without gorging on pineapple. As far as other supplements go, there is not enough well-controlled evidence to support any specific recommendations other than increased folic acid to prevent spina bifida, which everyone trying to conceive should be taking[10], and DHEA supplements if you have low AMH[11].

Acupuncture is often recommended during IVF cycles, and some studies do show a positive effect, but analyses that combine data across studies find that, overall, acupuncture makes no difference to pregnancy rates[12]. However, other more detailed analyses find that pregnancy rates may increase under certain circumstances[13]. One well-controlled study found an increase in pregnancy rates from 10% to 35% after two or more failed IVF cycles, with the addition of four acupuncture sessions[14]. We conclude, from these data, that acupuncture probably doesn't make a difference when you initially try IVF (although it won't have negative effects). But, if you experience a few failed cycles, you might as well change something up, and adding acupuncture following the protocol described in the Villahermosa study[15] seems like a reasonable route to try.

Some clinics recommend bed rest for a few minutes or even a day or two after transfer; others say you can get up and go right away (however, as we mentioned, high-intensity exercise is not recommended due to possible damage to enlarged ovaries). Analyses of multiple studies suggest there is no difference in pregnancy rates based on bed rest[16].

What it all boils down to is that some options work for some people, and different alternatives for others. If you feel like doing research, as well as implementing some of the suggestions you find, go ahead—it is unlikely to do any harm. But if you don't feel like doing that, your chances of pregnancy as far as science can determine are equally as likely. So do what makes YOU feel best about your cycle, because the positive thinking quite possibly will help.

Ovarian Hyperstimulation Syndrome

One potential problem we can face as HAers doing IVF is ovarian hyperstimulation syndrome (OHSS). People with HA tend to have a lot of antral follicles, which means that a large number will grow with the high doses of drugs you are typically given for an IVF cycle. As we've mentioned before, this syndrome occurs when your ovaries are overstimulated (producing too many follicles). This leads to production of proteins such as vascular endothelial growth factor (VEGF) that cause your blood vessels to leak fluid into your ovaries and sometimes your abdominal cavity. Early OHSS starts shortly after your trigger shot and will resolve within a couple of weeks if there is no pregnancy. Late OHSS can commence if a pregnancy occurs. With both early and late OHSS, hCG from the embryo sustains the hormonal changes, and OHSS can worsen and persist for up to three months.

There has been extensive research into ways to reduce the likelihood of OHSS and how to treat the symptoms, as it can be life-threatening. In the extreme, OHSS can cause severe pain and/or the shutdown of various organs, and require hospitalization. Before your IVF cycle starts, you should talk to your doctor about the likelihood of OHSS in your particular case, and ask what protocol you should follow to reduce the chances of experiencing the syndrome.

In order to understand the most common method for OHSS prevention, you need to know about the two major types of IVF cycles, which differ in how a natural LH surge is prevented in order to control ovulation timing. The majority of cycles use a GnRH agonist (like Lupron) that binds the GnRH receptors in your pituitary, causing the release of all stored FSH and LH. The agonist then prevents any further discharge of either molecule, and a shot of hCG is given to cause egg maturation prior to retrieval. On the other hand, the antagonists (such as Ganirelix or Cetrotide) block the binding of your natural GnRH and prevent release of any FSH or LH. This means that an agonist can then be used to trigger a large surge of LH that has been stored, beginning the egg maturation process.

Here are some options for preventing/treating OHSS:

- Using an antagonist protocol, with the LH surge prevented by Ganirelix or Cetrotide, then triggering with a GnRH agonist (Lupron), which causes a natural LH surge. This protocol has a very low rate of OHSS[17].
    - Some HAers do not respond to a Lupron trigger as it requires natural LH. If your doctor is considering this, it might be worth doing a trial Lupron shot to see if you respond prior to your treatment cycle.
    - Luteal phase support is very important with this protocol. Options include[18]:
        - Estradiol (0.3 mg in patches every second day) with progesterone (50 mg intramuscular), with blood levels tested a few times to ensure adequate progesterone (not the best pregnancy rates)
        - 1500 IU hCG at egg retrieval (some incidence of OHSS)
        - 1500 IU hCG three days after retrieval if not showing OHSS signs[19]
        - 500 IU hCG at days one, four, and seven after retrieval (low rate of OHSS)
        - 300 IU LH on day of retrieval then every second day after that
- Freezing all embryos (preferably through vitrification, a quick-freeze process) reduces OHSS due to no ongoing hCG stimulation of VEGF production[20]. Ongoing pregnancy rates after a subsequent frozen embryo transfer (FET) are similar or better than fresh IVF pregnancy rates[21].
- Using an hCG trigger followed by the dopamine agonist cabergoline at 0.5mg/day for eight days after the trigger[22]. Cabergoline has been shown to reduce vascular permeability (responsible for fluid leakage into the abdominal cavity) by decreasing VEGF signaling[23].
- Intravenous (IV) fluids with various additives have been shown to decrease OHSS rates, although a recent review recommended not using these methods[24]
- "Coasting" (no gonadotropins administered a few days before the trigger shot) was shown in a meta-analysis not to decrease the OHSS rate, and to cause fewer eggs to be retrieved[25]. Therefore, it is probably not advisable, especially for HAers.

Celena: I had moderate OHSS in October 2009. I was told to eat protein and drink Gatorade. It didn't help much. My ovaries were enlarged, and my estrogen skyrocketed. I injected with Ganirelix before I triggered with a half dose of hCG. The Ganirelix brought my E_2 levels down to 3,800 and then to around 1,800. They collected 45 eggs, and prescribed Dostinex (cabergoline) in an attempt to prevent OHSS. On transfer day,

> my estrogen was still quite high and my ovaries were enlarged. The RE refused to transfer. They froze the embryos, and I had my first frozen embryo transfer (FET) in January 2010. It was unsuccessful. I had another FET in March 2010 and conceived my daughter.

OHSS Symptoms and Treatment

If you do get OHSS, a few symptoms you might notice include quick, unusual weight gain (5 lb in a day or 10 lb over three days), bloating, reduced urine output, nausea and vomiting, and/or abdominal pain[26] (sounds lovely, right?). You should absolutely be in contact with your doctor; depending on the severity of your fluid buildup you may need to be hospitalized to have the fluid drained. Even if your case is not severe, there are a few recommendations that can theoretically help any symptoms subside. Remember that the problems occur because fluid (that is supposed to be in your blood) leaks out into other places, so you need to help get fluid back where it belongs. Think back to learning about osmosis in high school. If your blood has a higher concentration of salts and proteins than that wayward fluid, the fluid will move toward the higher concentration: back into your blood. Common recommendations are that you should NOT drink plain water, but rather lots of Gatorade, similar electrolyte-containing beverages (Gatorade Recover, with whey protein, is particularly recommended if you can find it), and protein shakes, and eat plenty of salty and protein-rich foods. However, even these measures can sometimes prove futile, and drainage is required. Be aware that regardless of the severity, OHSS symptoms often take many weeks to subside. Please contact your doctor if you experience any of these symptoms, or are not feeling well at any point after you take the trigger shot.

> *Robin*: I had awful OHSS three times. The first time I didn't even do a transfer; onset was at retrieval (40+ eggs retrieved) and I scared everybody by having a hard time waking after the procedure. I knew it would resolve 14 days after the trigger, but I remember telling my husband that I wanted to die; it was unlike anything I've ever experienced. I was on Zofran to reduce the nausea and God knows what painkillers, but I basically was in bed all day crying and family members would take turns sitting downstairs in case I needed anything. My abdomen was so stretched out, I weighed more than I did full-term pregnant.
>
> Second time was when I got pregnant but miscarried; onset was before the transfer. I had around 20 eggs retrieved.

> Third time I was pregnant with twins (lost one late in the first trimester) and had late-onset OHSS. I had to get drained and looked nine months pregnant until I was about two months along. I ate lots of salt, no carbs, and high protein. I would salt my Powerade.
>
> As to what I wish I'd known? Every case is different, but freezing all embryos with a delayed transfer to avoid OHSS can have good results.
>
> *Jill:* It truly was the most miserably sick and painful I ever felt. I could hardly breathe, and only slept sitting up. I was almost at my RE's cutoff estrogen level to transfer but went ahead with it. I felt OK until after my embryo transfer. I started getting really sick later that day. My RE did nothing to help or treat the OHSS. Robin was my personal coach through this and had me on the salt/protein/Powerade diet. After this mess I went to a new RE (for many reasons) and he said he wanted me to trigger with Lupron on my next cycle. I ended up getting pregnant naturally, though.
>
> *Leslie E:* I had OHSS mildly, both times after my egg retrieval and day three transfer with IVF. I didn't even have that many eggs—only 20 follicles each time. My RE said my ovaries were the size of large oranges, and I looked like I was in my second trimester from the bloat. I was advised to drink Gatorade and eat high protein and high salt to try and get rid of the water retention. Nothing really worked. My RE said it just takes time and luckily it wasn't bad enough to need drainage. I felt much better by the second trimester both times; that was when the bloat finally went away and my ovaries got smaller.

When IVF Doesn't Work

Hopefully you will not get OHSS (it happens in about 1% to 4% of IVF attempts in the normal population), and your first IVF cycle will get you pregnant. But if pregnancy is not achieved, the despair can be overwhelming. There is often a fear that you will never get to experience pregnancy and having children. And it's even worse if you end up with no frozen embryos. There have been a few on the Board who have experienced this; most of them found it helpful to talk to others who had been through similar experiences and could empathize. If you don't participate in an infertility support group (online or in real life) or have a friend to lean on, find a group or someone you feel comfortable reaching out to. Just as with miscarriage, it can be a huge relief to connect with another person who can understand your anger, despair, and all the other huge emotions you have swirling around in your heart. Always remember that you can try again (typically with a month off in between cycles), and that even though it probably doesn't feel like it right now, the odds are on your side.

> *Allison H*: Failing IVF is the worst. The worst worst worst worst worst. I think knowing that everyone who has failed an IVF cycle feels this way is helpful—that everyone thinks, "This is it, I'll never get pregnant." My doctor told me that even when you have a good embryo and a good environment, it truly is just a numbers game. Sometimes it works and sometimes it doesn't. The fact that it didn't work now has no bearing on the next try.
>
> I tried to take that month between cycles to just do whatever I wanted and enjoy myself, but it was a worthless cause. Every time I went out with friends I ended up crying... at a table in a restaurant, at a bar, in a bathroom... I had to just stop.
>
> I talked to a couple of people who went through multiple failed cycles before they got pregnant, and that did help. I also went home to visit family for a few days (500 miles away), and that was probably the best thing I could have done.
>
> Afterward, I put together a very concrete plan and timeline of what we were going to do if the next try didn't work. There were three embryos from my first IVF; I had transferred one that didn't implant. I did a frozen embryo transfer (FET) with the last two (I now have twins) but that was it; we had no embryos after that so I needed to know what we would do next if the FET failed. My plan was to do one more IVF at a different clinic (I had to change something to feel like we weren't just doing the same thing but expecting a different result). We would transfer all of those embryos but if that didn't work, I needed to move on; adoption would have been next.
>
> *Becky H*: The dark times... well, those were pretty lonely and sad. The Board helped, but sometimes it was a burden. Seeing other people get pregnant after my failed cycle was always hard—especially when it was someone's first attempt. And to even get another try with IVF was not guaranteed. I read about women having cycles canceled because of lining issues, or an embryo not surviving the thaw. That didn't happen to me, but I knew it was a possibility, which scared me.
>
> *Celena*: What got me through was support from my husband, the Board, and hearing others' experiences with IVF. I just kept my eyes on the prize: baby! I knew IVF would increase my chances, but that I could still go through it without conceiving. I also had 12 embryos frozen. That assurance helped me come to terms with my canceled cycle. I was also told that

an FET cycle wasn't nearly as daunting. During this time, I joined another online support thread that consisted of women going through IVF or FET cycles. The women on that thread didn't have HA but having them as cycle buddies helped boost my morale.

Jaclyn: I tried IVF in October 2011 and ended up with a chemical pregnancy and no frozen embryos, which devastated me. From there, already at a healthy BMI, I decided to try Clomid and Femara again as I did not want the stress and pressure of IVF for a second time (plus, I learned the hard way that bigger guns do not always mean better success). I ended up conceiving on my third round of a Clomid/Femara extended protocol. I now have a 13-month-old son and have had one natural period since I stopped nursing him at 12 months. I also believe I just ovulated again, naturally! The difference? My attitude to life—letting go of striving, controlling, worrying, and being overly responsible and perfectionist; opening myself to love and life; being more flexible, doing activities for the enjoyment, eating for the enjoyment, having strong social ties, believing in myself, and forgiving myself daily. Looking back on everything with what I know now, I wish I could have spared myself the stress and pressure (and money) of IVF when it wasn't what I needed. However, if you are already invested in another cycle, then I would say that letting go of the need to control every aspect of it is important. Just be as much as possible. Be mindful of where you are emotionally every day and be really, really good to yourself. If you do, you will be doing nothing but wonderful things for your body. I'm not sure if that will help with conception, but it will help your entire system to flow and not be stuck, which can dramatically improve all aspects of life. I am living that truth out! Be easy on yourself as much as possible. Know that the pressure we put on ourselves to go-go-go and be perfect all the time, just because it seems "normal" (as in everyone else on the planet seems to be doing it), does not have to be so. Peace starts first in your mind; quiet it and let it be.

Parting Thoughts

As we mentioned, HA does not usually impact response to IVF, so we don't have much specific advice as far as protocols go. A bright side is that HAers tend to have lots of follicles that just need a bit of FSH to take off. This also means a greater potential for OHSS, so it is important to talk to your doctor before your cycle about what can be done to minimize your likelihood of your getting it (because as you read, it is pretty awful).

IVF isn't a sure thing, but there is always hope. Putting 100% into your recovery before beginning down this path (and during your cycle as well) will only increase your odds of a successful IVF experience.

> **Lisa**: If you have journeyed your way to the point of IVF, then you have had plenty of opportunities to practice patience. Whether it was waiting for your body to recover via decreased exercise and increased weight, or a few months of oral meds, injectable cycles, or taking a break from the whole trying-to-conceive scene—you've probably had a good dose of challenges requiring patience. Boy, will that virtue come in handy now. While IVF is an incredible and exciting opportunity to help you reach your goal, there are many steps that happen slowly during the process (like most things in life that are really worth having). And because of the time, money, and emotion you will continue to invest toward baby making, the "patience tool" needs to be your new best friend. When and if doubt starts to seep in, take a few deep breaths, and focus on what is good, lovely, and true.

Part 4:
What Comes Next?

Nico: After I'd been on the Board for about a year, I noticed that there were a lot of questions that came up in newly pregnant HAers that weren't really appropriate for a thread where most were still trying to conceive. So I started some "vets" threads for veterans of the Board, who had successfully conceived, each of which acquired thousands of posts over time. We discussed everything from pregnancy symptoms and concerns to naps, feeding, and even discipline after our babies were born. Through these threads, just as with the main HA thread, there are common concerns and questions, which we have captured here for you.

This section of the book contains more data collected from our survey respondents. We will devote a chapter to pregnancy, including eating and exercise in ongoing pregnancies. After that, we provide information and support for those who have experienced or are experiencing a miscarriage. Next will come data about postpartum recovery, regaining natural cycles after having a baby, and conceiving again. Finally, we end with discussion on maintaining your new lifestyle for the long term.

25
I'm Pregnant—Now What??

Nico: I WAS SO SURE I wasn't pregnant that I took my test after staying overnight at my sister's house, with my husband not even around. I walked out of the bathroom astounded, but grinning like the Cheshire Cat, and my sister knew right away.

Steph: I was having an ultrasound at my RE's office when we found out. We all believed that the first round of Clomid had not worked, so I had already started the second round. I waited nervously hoping to hear we had some growing follicles. As the picture of my uterus appeared Aaron commented, "What is that, we haven't seen that before?" The sonographer gasped and then informed us that we were looking at our almost 5-week-old baby. I will never forget Aaron's face of joy and surprise. I, myself, was beyond shocked and excited. Clomid round 1 for the win!

There is nothing like the feeling you experience when your pregnancy test is finally positive. Elation, anticipation, relief, and pure joy spread through you from the fingers clutching that urine-soaked stick to the heart that has so longed for this potential addition to your family.

After the fact that you are finally, finally pregnant has had a chance to sink in, you start to realize you really have no idea what comes next. You have spent so much time learning about how to get pregnant, but next to none on what comes after. For most HAers that comes as a bit of a surprise because we are generally good planners with our paths mapped out well in advance. Realizing you know very little about what's next can be scary. Fear not, the HA crew has your back!

> *Nikki*: I feel like I know so much about getting pregnant, but now that I'm here, it's a whole new ball game… nay, it's a whole different sport!

The first thing to know is that by the time you get your positive test, you're almost four weeks pregnant. A pregnancy is normally dated from the first day of the last menstrual period (LMP), so you are considered two weeks "pregnant" when you ovulate. If you didn't ovulate on CD 14, you will find it easiest to count back 13 days from when you did ovulate and give that date whenever you are asked for your LMP. It will save having to explain over and over again that you ovulated later than normal, because you will get the question a lot throughout your pregnancy. It also can mean that even if your pregnancy is proceeding exactly as it should based on your ovulation date (the most accurate way to date your pregnancy), you might be told the embryo is not growing as expected because your testing does not line up with your LMP.

> *Nico*: For my first pregnancy, I ovulated on CD 42—December 10, 2005 (a date I will never forget). At my first few appointments when I was asked my LMP I would say, "My last period started October 31, but I ovulated later than normal, on December 10." This apparently novel event—ovulation not on CD 14—did nothing but create confusion. So, assuming December 10 was CD 14, I counted back (yes, on my fingers), which got me to November 27 for "CD 1." That's the LMP date I gave from then on out. The revision made appointments go much more smoothly.

There isn't much that needs to change from recovery to pregnancy in terms of eating, and in fact, once you have a positive pregnancy test, a bit more exercise is totally fine (read more about this later in the chapter!). There are a few small recommendations we do have. If you have been taking supplements to support HA recovery or your luteal phase, we suggest stopping most of these. There is no evidence to support benefit of acetyl-l-carnitine, high dose vitamin C, or flax seed during pregnancy. Occasional intake is not an issue, but there is no need to be taking these daily any longer.

Additionally, if you have been taking progesterone, please talk to your physician about whether to stop a few days after your positive pregnancy test or continue. As we discussed at the end of chapter 19, a couple of recent studies raise some concerns about continued use of progesterone through the first trimester[1] as has been standard practice to this point. Additional studies find that because the hCG from the embryo takes over support of the corpus luteum[2], even in cases of IVF where the corpus luteum has not developed properly, there is no change in the rates of ongoing pregnancy whether progesterone is stopped at 16 DPO versus eight weeks[3]. While it is the case that low progesterone levels are associated with a higher risk of miscarriage, that low progesterone is in the context of many other hormonal abnormalities like estradiol, hCG, and placental lactogen[4], and thus much more likely a result of an already failing pregnancy rather than the cause. If you are concerned about stopping progesterone support, you could ask for an assessment of progesterone levels before making a decision.

Medical appointments

In a typical natural pregnancy, your first ob-gyn or midwife appointment is around the 9- to 10-week mark. At that point, your provider will take your medical history, talk to you about what you should and shouldn't eat, discuss various other habits that are helpful for a healthy pregnancy, give you some information packets about various genetic screening tests you can have done, and tell you they'll see you in another month. Following appointments will be fairly standard: first you will be weighed, your urine will be tested for pH and protein content, and your blood pressure will be checked. Next, you will often get a chance to "listen" to the baby's heartbeat using a Doppler ultrasound. This small machine has a probe that is lightly passed over your lower stomach so you can hear your baby's heartbeat. After that, your obstetrical practitioner will feel and/or measure your abdomen to confirm your uterus is growing appropriately, and you will address any upcoming testing and questions you may have.

On the other hand, if you are seeing an RE (or have been doing fertility treatments through your OB), you will have a lot more hand holding at the beginning of the pregnancy. To start, you will most likely have a blood test termed a "beta" scheduled when you report a positive pregnancy test. "Beta" is short for human chorionic gonadotropin (hCG) beta. The hCG protein, which is produced only by a growing embryo, has two parts, labeled alpha and beta subunits. The alpha portion is used in other proteins like LH, which is why you can detect hCG on an OPK after levels get high enough. The beta subunit is unique to the pregnancy hormone, and is detected on home pregnancy tests when present in your urine. A blood test will tell you what the hormone level is, which correlates to some degree with how far along the pregnancy is. The amount of hCG beta in your blood and the rate at which it increases can give you an idea of whether your pregnancy is proceeding normally.

We have mixed feelings about these blood tests. On one hand, if you get a good, strong number, it can be reassuring. However, if the number is on the lower end, it can lead to a great deal of worry—and the thing is, there is nothing you can do at this stage to affect the outcome of your pregnancy. But you know yourself best. Will knowing the number, whatever it is, make you worry less or more? Unless you've done IVF, there is no requirement to have this test (IVF clinics need the results for reporting to the Centers for Disease Control), so decide what would be mentally healthiest for you.

> *Lindsay*: Well, this completely, totally stinks… Woke up early to get a beta; today is 11 DPO. They wouldn't let me! Even though every other cycle they did. They actually said I have to wait two weeks PLUS two days (what the heck is this "plus" stuff?). The nurse said, "Please don't test until two weeks after your missed period. Then if it's a positive call us." They're worried about false positives. I felt like I had been scolded—I mean, it's my money paying for it… geez! So now they're saying to wait until Thursday, six more days! Ugh. Now what? How do I just wait? You know what I mean? I really don't want to be walking around for six days thinking I'm pregnant and that I'm going to have a baby come December if I'm not (if my beta is too low, not doubling appropriately, etc.)! Ack!!!!!

Clinics typically look for a beta around 100 at 14 DPO, with that number doubling about 48 to 72 hours later. However, there is a huge range of betas that result in a baby, and also a large range of doubling times. The BetaBase[5] has collected beta information from over 180,000 pregnancies and is a good resource for comparing your numbers to get an idea of the potential your pregnancy has to continue on to where a heartbeat can be detected.

There is some correlation between high beta numbers and twins, although it's not absolute by any means. By far the better way to diagnose twins is with an ultrasound, which is often the next step when you're seeing an RE. Around the six-week mark, a vaginal ultrasound will be performed, during which the sonographer will examine different parts of the pregnancy. If you're not seeing an RE, you may have an ultrasound around the 9- to 12-week mark. This ultrasound is typically abdominal, and can confirm the pregnancy and dating, as well as screen for genetic anomalies like Down syndrome or spina bifida if performed between 11 and 13 weeks. At 18 to 20 weeks you will typically have an "anatomy scan" to examine the baby's growth and organs and detect potential problems that may need extra care or treatment. This is also when you can find out the gender if you are so inclined or have not found out earlier!

What you typically see at six weeks, if you get to look at the ultrasound screen, is a little black circle inside a larger area of gray and white stripes (your uterus). The black blob is the gestational sac, a fluid-filled structure surrounding the developing fetus. Inside that, you may see a "yolk sac," which in a few days will develop into the "fetal pole." This is the collection of cells that will divide and differentiate to become a full-sized baby. The sonographer or your doctor will measure the gestational sac, yolk sac, and fetal pole to make sure they are growing appropriately. At this stage the size does not vary much between babies, so a measurement will tell you (within ±5 days) how far along you are. If the ultrasound is zoomed in more, you may be able to see a little flicker that is the baby's heart beating. It is absolutely incredible that there is a heart doing its work in an embryo not even a centimeter long, and even more surreal to think of this miracle developing inside you. If you have an early ultrasound like this, it can be terrifying to not see the heartbeat, but it is not expected until you are about six weeks and two or three days (which we abbreviate as "6w2d"), so try your best not to fret. If no heartbeat is seen, your doctor should have you return about a week later, and hopefully you will get to see the heartbeat then. Among our survey respondents, 45 had ultrasounds before six weeks in which no heartbeat was seen, and went on to see the heartbeat later.

> *Amy:* So after three LONG years of trying to conceive and more complications than I could ever imagine, I can finally say I'm PREGNANT!!! I had my first beta on Friday and it was 450, second beta on Sunday that was over 1200, and then I had an ultrasound today to make sure the sac was in the uterus. We saw one sac measuring four weeks, six days and another smaller sac, which is probably just fluid, but there's a slight chance that it's a late implanter (and I stress slight chance). So I am cautiously optimistic. It just seems unreal at this point. The doctor wants me to come in for another scan next week but I think that's way too soon—I wouldn't even be six weeks yet, so I think I'm going to wait until the following week. I'd rather have a chance to see the fetal pole and heartbeat than go too early and still just see a sac.
>
> *Two weeks later:* I had my second ultrasound today and we saw one peanut and the heartbeat!!! It looks like that second sac was just fluid. I am still in shock and can't believe it. I am around seven weeks and due early December!

> *Suzie*: I went to the RE on Thursday; she did an ultrasound and said everything looks fine. I can't tell you how excited I was to see the little sac! She's now on holiday for three weeks so I have to wait until March to see her again. Then I'll get another scan and hopefully see the heartbeat. But I'm so scared it's not going to work out that I don't want to tell anyone yet.
>
> *Three weeks later*: I had my second ultrasound yesterday and saw the heartbeat and even the little bean waving its arms and legs around… it was mad! Celebrated with a big lunch at the Gourmet Burger Kitchen, mmmm…

Usually once you have seen the heartbeat with your RE, or perhaps after one or two more ultrasounds (the number depends on the clinic), you will be released to your OB, and then you are on the same plan as everyone else (unless you have twins, in which case you should expect more monitoring as your pregnancy is higher risk).

The best piece of advice we can give you once you're pregnant is to take it one day at a time. Try your best not to consider negative possibilities, but rather celebrate that today you're pregnant!! As much as HAers like to be in control, at this point the outcome is out of your hands, which is why we encourage new mothers to focus on the joy until proven otherwise. Let yourself enjoy the amazing baby that is growing inside you.

Despite having a positive pregnancy test and no period as confirmation of your pregnancy, it is often hard to believe that anything is actually happening. In the early weeks, there are no visible signs of the incredible process taking place inside you. Some feel cramping starting around the time of implantation (7 to 10 DPO); some have sore or enlarged breasts or feel warmer at night; some start to feel nauseous, while others feel completely normal. Many symptoms don't start until around the six-week mark, so it is common to not feel pregnant until then. Sometimes it's hard to fathom that you're actually pregnant until much later, when you can start to feel the baby move.

> *Vanessa*: It is totally normal not to have symptoms, especially so early. I was told symptoms often don't start until after the beta is above 600, but everyone is different and it depends on how sensitive your body is to the hCG and progesterone. It's so hard, I know, but try to enjoy these initial feelings of knowing you are pregnant!

Concerns About Pregnancy After HA

There are a few common worries about lingering effects of HA among those who become pregnant during or after recovery. These include fears about an increased rate of miscarriage, other pregnancy complications, and trepidation about the ability to breastfeed a baby.

Please set your mind at ease! There are no data that suggest that a pregnancy in a recovered HAer is any different from a typical pregnancy. The miscarriage rate is very similar to that seen in other populations (and is not affected by late ovulations, which are common with HA—we will discuss this more in the next chapter). There have been no other pregnancy complications that have occurred frequently enough to be notable. Getting pregnant seems to be the only part of the process that is a common struggle with HA. That's not to say there haven't been individuals with various issues like preterm delivery, subchorionic hematomas, or placenta previa, but these are no more common in HAers than in standard pregnancies.

Finally, the concern about breastfeeding among HAers is just that—a concern but not a reality. Having had HA does not seem to affect the ability to breastfeed. Most HAers have no issues with breastfeeding, aside from normal early feeding struggles experienced by many new mothers. There is no correlation between having had HA and having low milk supply or other breastfeeding problems. Again, that is not to say that breastfeeding is easy for everyone, but the rate of difficulties is no different from the normal population.

Eating and Weight Gain

We mentioned that your OB (or midwife or nurse) will talk to you early in pregnancy about what to eat and what not to eat. They may counsel you that you need about 300 additional calories per day while pregnant since that is the typical recommendation (perhaps more if you are starting your pregnancy underweight, i.e., BMI less than 19.8[6]). However, please don't get hung up on this number, just as we're encouraging you to stop counting calories overall. Listen to and satisfy your hunger cues. You may feel like a bottomless pit at various points during your pregnancy. That is normal; your body needs more energy for the incredible work it is undertaking. Some days you may eat an additional 500 or 600 calories, or more; other days you will find you don't feel like eating much extra at all. If you find that you are not gaining enough weight (we'll discuss this in more detail shortly), you may need to override these signals and eat even when your appetite is low. No matter what, most certainly eat when you are hungry—even if your mind thinks you've had enough already, or you question if you're gaining too quickly, your body needs that food!

On the flip side, usually during the first trimester and sometimes beyond, you may feel too sick to eat much at all. This is a common occurrence. Once again, listen to your body. Do what you can do. Eat what you can, when you can. Do not worry if all you eat is chips, crackers, or peanut butter, for example. You may find it easier to just sip fluids (try for those with calories like Gatorade or juice). While you are listening to your body, you may need to distract your mind. Old thoughts about eating less can easily creep up when you go through a period of time where it is difficult to eat. Instead, think of that little baby you worked so hard for and push through. When you can, add more calories back in. Don't let old habits hold you back. If you can do this, it will balance out in the end.

> **Lea**: My eating routine while pregnant goes like this: I usually eat breakfast before I head to work (teaching), a snack with the kids, then a big lunch, and another snack with the kids. Yesterday I decided to just eat a very big lunch and see if it held me over because sometimes it's hard to eat with all the kids going crazy. Well, it didn't work—I was so full and felt like nothing was digesting so I had indigestion and felt nauseous. Not cool! Small frequent meals, like they say, is best. Funny, though, that my "small" isn't small to the women I work with who eat next to nothing at all. I love eating lots!!

At your visit, the clinician will probably suggest avoiding various foods that could potentially cause illness in your baby if they are contaminated; deli turkey, for example, because of the potential of getting a bacterial disease called listeriosis. Fish that is high in mercury, like tuna or swordfish, should also be limited to around one serving per week. A quick Internet search will provide you with a comprehensive list of what not to eat (which varies by country; in the US we are told not to eat sushi, however people in Japan eat sushi throughout pregnancy); the book *Expecting Better*[7] is another good resource.

Besides the foods you are asked to avoid when pregnant, remember to listen to your body as you have learned during HA recovery when making meal choices. Your body is smart and knows what it needs; this is never so clear as during pregnancy. If your body wants three nights of red meat, maybe your iron is low. If it wants lots of milk, perhaps you require calcium. An egg craving suggests protein is needed. And if all you can do is think about chips, pizza, almond butter or ice cream, maybe you could use more fat. Whatever the need may be, go for it.

> **Steph**: When I was first pregnant with Lee, I used to joke that my body was making up for the ten years I neglected to feed it fats and forced only fruits, vegetables, and granola. During those first months, I couldn't even look at a piece of fruit. I wanted pies, cookies, anything fried, and McDonald's (yes, I had McDonald's, milkshakes and all)! One week, I remember having three different dinners of tempura vegetables followed by tempura ice cream for dessert! The extra fat felt like it coated my stomach and took away the nausea, which was enough of a reason for me to listen to what my body wanted. As my pregnancy progressed, I was able to eat more fruits and veggies, but it wasn't truly until post-pregnancy that my diet began to even out a bit more. Even then I wanted things I hadn't thought of in years—ginger ale and M&Ms became a nightly habit. Bottom line: your body knows what it needs; it's time to trust it!

We have found through conversations on the Board that medical practitioners often don't talk about how important it is to gain weight while you're pregnant. This is probably because under-gaining is rarely an issue among the general population. The recommended range for weight gain when commencing a pregnancy at a "normal" BMI is between 25 and 35 lb according to the Institute of Medicine[8]. That weight comes from the extra food you're eating each day, but also water your body is retaining. For some, the gain should be higher, and that is perfectly healthy. For example, if you started your pregnancy underweight, then a 28 to 40 lb gain is recommended, or if you are pregnant with multiples, then 37 to 54 lb[9]. Whatever the case, do not fret about going over 35 pounds (however, we would recommend examining your diet if you are not getting to 25). There are good reasons for the weight you gain. Here's the breakdown of where that weight goes in a singleton pregnancy, for a 30 lb gain, right in the middle of the recommended range[10]:

- Baby: 7.5 lb
- Placenta: 1.5 lb
- Amniotic fluid: 2 lb
- Uterine enlargement: 2 lb
- Maternal breast tissue: 2 lb
- Maternal blood volume: 4 lb

- Fluids in maternal tissues: 4 lb
- Maternal fat stores: 7 lb

The "normal" pattern of weight gain is around 5 lb in the first trimester (through week 14), followed by a pound a week after that. This gets you to a total of 31 lb. By now you should have a good sense of whether knowing your weight will be helpful or harmful for you; we continue to recommend no more than weekly weight checks. If you choose to step on the scale (or find out your weight at the doctor's office), keep in mind that weight gain is rarely steady; some weeks you won't much change, while others you might have a 2 or 3 lb increase or more. Some might gain 10 lb or more in the first trimester, but less toward the end of the pregnancy. It all evens out. But, if you are not gaining at approximately this rate, you should examine your eating habits and think about how you can add in more calories. Just as when you were trying to gain weight during recovery, if you are not gaining appropriately during pregnancy you may want to consider decreasing the number of fruits and vegetables you're eating as they are filling without providing many calories. In place, you can increase your intake of calorie-dense foods or drink caloric beverages. Liquids are less filling and can be particularly helpful when the growing baby starts to squash your stomach.

> **Maura**: Just wanted to pop in to tell you not to worry about the weight gain! There were a few weeks in the second trimester when I gained two pounds a week, but my weight gain has slowed down since then. I didn't change anything other than drinking more water, and I'm actually now stuffing my face because I'm worried about not making it to 25 lb! I'm wondering if maybe my HA-induced slow metabolism may have finally picked itself up now that I'm eating a lot more and that's why the gain has slowed. Who knows? Anyway, put the scale away and try not to stress about it!

Take a good look again at the breakdown of the weight you gain during pregnancy. Let's say you don't gain any fat, which, as we will describe, may make postpartum life more difficult for you. That gets you down to 23 lb total gain. Which other components on the list do you think will get skimped on if you don't gain at least that amount?

It seems that ob-gyns are only concerned about weight gain if someone is gaining more than expected. If weight gain is low, the doctor might do an ultrasound to check the baby's growth. If all is normal, the ob-gyn often comments that the mother's weight gain is sufficient. And perhaps the baby is perfectly healthy; however, studies show links between low maternal weight gain and premature delivery, and babies that are small for their gestational age[11]. Another issue that has been found in babies after low pregnancy weight gain is called the "thrifty phenotype[12]." Alterations in metabolic functions, such as insulin sensitivity, can be found in a baby whose mother underate during gestation. This occurs in order for the baby to capture and retain every last bit of available energy in utero. After birth, if nutrients are plentiful because of readily available breast milk, formula, and solid food, the ability to hold onto every calorie may continue, but at a cost. In the long term, rates of type 2 diabetes and cardiovascular disease are higher in affected individuals[13].

Weight gain is particularly important in a multiple pregnancy. Many studies have found that low maternal weight gain is associated with preterm birth and small for gestational age babies[14]. A recent study[15] found that inadequate maternal weight gain from weeks 20 to 28 was most highly correlated with preterm birth; 37.6% of those with inadequate gain delivered prior to 32 weeks versus 15.2% of those with normal weight gain. The size of babies is also strongly associated with maternal gain.

> **Michelle S**: I started off 10 lb lighter with my second pregnancy than my first, but still watched everything I ate while I was pregnant and ended up not gaining as much as I should have. I took pride when the doctor complimented me on my low weight gain, but then my son ended up coming two weeks early. I don't know if my low weight gain contributed to that, but I still felt guilty.

In addition to potential negative effects for your baby, low weight gain is not healthy for you. If your pre-pregnancy BMI is less than 25 and you don't gain at least 23 lb through your pregnancy (the sum of all pregnancy-related gains not including your fat stores), you are essentially on a diet while you are pregnant. And no, weight gained prior to pregnancy does not count toward this. The weight you gained during recovery was to get you to a healthy starting point for your pregnancy—not gaining sufficient weight while pregnant has the potential to undo all that hard work. It may make postpartum breastfeeding more challenging due to lower supply. It also means you might experience effects of under-nourishment after birth—at the same you're coping with little sleep, adjusting to life with a new baby, and undergoing significant hormonal changes. Breastfeeding burns a lot of calories, so having a few pounds of extra fat stores at this time will give you the energy to bounce back to your pre-pregnancy self much quicker.

Among our survey respondents with weight gain between 25 and 35 lb, the average gain was 6 lb in the first trimester, 13 lb in the second, and 9 lb in the third. Many don't gain at all in the last month or so of pregnancy (it gets hard to eat enough volume when there's not much room left for your stomach). Among respondents who gained 20 lb or less, average gain was 3 lb in the first trimester, 6 lb in the second, and 6 lb in the third. The best time to gain weight is in the second trimester—you're probably feeling better than you did in the first trimester, yet not so big that your stomach feels squashed to the point you can't eat much. Don't deceive yourself by thinking you will catch up in the third trimester. Less than half of low gainers were able to gain more during the third trimester than they did in the second, and then only gained a median of 3.5 lb, still keeping them well below minimum gain recommendations.

Worrying about losing your pregnancy weight after birth is not a healthy reason to limit your gain while pregnant. Among our survey respondents, it made no difference what the total pregnancy gain was; the weight was lost afterward, unless people were underweight to begin with. In those cases, some made a conscious decision not to return to their starting weight. For those who did not gain the recommended minimum of 25 lb, postpartum weights were often quite low, requiring HA recovery all over again. If you take care of yourself while pregnant by gaining the recommended weight for your body, your potential for postpartum health will be much increased.

> *Kathryn*: I'm struggling because I'm back in HA-land after my baby was born (weight-wise). I didn't gain enough while pregnant and now I'm almost done breastfeeding and want to try to conceive again in a few months, but I have to start from scratch—I need to gain and fast!
>
> *Becky*: I only gained about 15 lb during pregnancy. It was not enough. I ate a ton but I was running quite a bit. My son was tiny and it's been a mission to get him up to a healthy weight. Did that have to do with my low weight gain? Maybe. And I lost too much weight too quickly postpartum. I was scared of gaining weight—I learned the hard way and really wish I would have worked harder to gain more. I'll know for next time (God willing) to take it easy. Please, for the health of your baby and postpartum health, stack on the pounds now and enjoy your pregnancy.

For folks who have struggled with body image, disordered eating and/or overexercise, anxiety over weight gain seems to heighten during pregnancy.

While some may use being pregnant as an opportunity to finally let go as "you have to gain weight anyway," others find old thoughts resurfacing: "I am only going to gain X pounds"; "I don't need too much extra food"; "I want to be slim and trim when I'm pregnant." These are thoughts many experience whether they have suffered from HA or not. But you are at an advantage: you have recovered and know how to fend off society's warped ideals to do what is best for your body and baby. Listen to your hunger cues (and/or eat more if you are not gaining sufficient weight) and the rest will fall into place.

Exercise During Pregnancy

The next question is, what to do about exercise now that you're pregnant? If you stopped all high-intensity exercise while trying to recover from HA, you might be yearning to add physical activity back into your routine. Discuss with your OB what you are used to doing, and get clearance for re-starting or continuing. If you've taken some time off from exercise, you should add it back in slowly to allow your body to adapt to the intensities and movements. Moderate and even occasional high-intensity exercise while pregnant is unequivocally healthy for both you and your baby, as long as your pregnancy is not high-risk. But overexercising (no rest days, or exercising for hours on end) can burn calories your baby needs, and cause problems for him or her down the line. Some HAers choose to continue with only low-intensity exercise such as walking or yoga during the first trimester, or for the whole pregnancy (often recommended if you are pregnant with twins or more). Others resume a somewhat more strenuous exercise program. If you are exercising, make sure that you are eating enough to support your activity. If your weight gain is not on target, you should seriously consider reducing or stopping your exercise so nutrients can go to your body and baby.

> *Emily*: As far as activity is concerned, I was nervous about changing any part of my routine so I did nothing, not even walking, until my six-week appointment. Then the nurse practitioner I saw recommended 30 minutes a day. I still barely do that much. I walk for maybe 40 minutes and then do very easy elliptical for about 20 minutes. Then I take the next day off. But some HAers have run throughout their pregnancies with no problems, so I think it's whatever you're comfortable with that doesn't feel like too much.

Some healthcare professionals will tell you to limit your heart rate to 140 beats per minute, but a fairly substantial body of evidence suggests that this limit is unnecessary. The book *Exercising Through Your Pregnancy* by Dr. James Clapp[16] details a number of clinical studies that were performed examining the supposed negative effects of getting your heart rate too high and other commonly recommended exercise restrictions. The studies found that the placenta is larger in people who exercise regularly during pregnancy to adapt to times when placental blood flow is lowered due to exercise. Dr. Clapp advises against exercise that is so strenuous you can't talk through it, but otherwise endorses activity as long as you listen to your body and follow your instincts[17].

There is no evidence suggesting exercise causes problems in typical pregnancy. However, there are some potential complications for which limits on exercise are often suggested. These include:

- Subchorionic hematomas; a small bleed behind the placenta. This can cause some bleeding or spotting (frightening, but rarely indicating a miscarriage). In such instances, your doctor will likely recommend avoiding exercise and pelvic activity (i.e., anything to cause an orgasm). However, there is no evidence that exercise causes these hematomas.
- Placenta previa; your baby's placenta is lower in the uterus than normal. Placenta previa can also cause bleeding or spotting, particularly if the placenta is covering the cervix, and again, exercise and pelvic activity should be avoided.
- Braxton Hicks contractions; normal "practice" contractions typically not felt until late in the third trimester in first pregnancies, possibly earlier in subsequent ones. These are generally not a problem, but in some the contractions can be frequent and exacerbated by exercise—in these cases exercise should be avoided so as to prevent possible preterm labor.
- Multiple pregnancy; there is a much higher chance of preterm labor when you are pregnant with twins or more, so discuss any exercise plan with your doctor.

Julie: I looked through my packet from the OB today and saw it recommends not getting your heart rate over 140... I wonder if that advice is ever going to go away. I don't track my heart rate when I work out; I just listen to my body. If something starts to hurt or feel funny, I'll stop.

Nico: I continued with much of my activity while pregnant. I biked, lifted my normal weights, used the elliptical, and swam. I exercised around four days a week, for about 45 minutes at a time. I felt great. And when I didn't feel energetic, I skipped my workout. In my last pregnancy I was commuting to work by bike, but toward the end of the third trimester found I was getting tired on my way home. Rather than forcing myself to continue, I started taking the subway halfway. Then for the last few weeks I limited myself to shorter rides close to home. I listened to my body, and I didn't force the exercise when I wasn't feeling up to it. I didn't push myself to do more because my conscious mind told me I should. I also wasn't using exercise to keep from gaining weight; I was in the recommended range for each pregnancy, and if my weight gain had been low I would have cut down on exercise.

Parting Thoughts

There are entire books devoted to pregnancy, so we cannot possibly cover everything you need to know here. Some of our favorite books are *What to Expect When You're Expecting*[18], *Expecting 411*[19], and *Your Pregnancy Week by Week*[20]. Many also sign up for weekly emails from various websites; these digests give you a weekly summary of how your baby is developing and can be fun to share with family members. The emails continue after your baby's birth to help you know what to expect as your child grows. An excellent resource for what to anticipate during labor and delivery is *Natural Childbirth the Bradley Way*[21], whether you're planning a natural birth or not (as long as you can get past the 1970s era pictures!). Your OB and nurse are good resources for what medications are safe to take while pregnant, along with the NIH drug reference website[22] if you want to view the drug label information for yourself.

> *Lisa*: It is a humbling experience to go from your body being so stressed that it has shut down your ability to conceive, to having it trust you enough to become pregnant with your future baby/ies. At the moment of conception, you become a mother; your life is forever changed. It is a privilege and responsibility you have earned and been entrusted with. Just as you have sacrificed your comfort to have this miracle bundle, it is also a wonderful revelation to know that the choices you make during your pregnancy can benefit your baby. Continue to nourish yourself properly and listen to your body when it needs rest. If being able to conceive and have children isn't a reason to love and care for your body, I don't know what is!
>
> Yeah … it's a pretty big deal. Enjoy it!

26
Pregnancy Loss

THIS CHAPTER CONTAINS *information, hope, and solace for those who are experiencing or have experienced the loss of a pregnancy/baby. In particular, we describe what happens during a miscarriage, as knowing what to expect can make the process less scary. However, if you are currently pregnant, you may not want to read about these losses, as the awareness might result in unnecessary worry. Hopefully you will never need the material, but if you do, it is here to return to.*

> *Nico*: With my third pregnancy I wasn't under the care of an RE (it was a natural pregnancy on our first cycle "trying") so I was treated just like any normal pregnant person. My first OB appointment was at nine weeks, and I was hoping we'd be able to hear the baby's heartbeat with the Doppler. But the nurse couldn't find it. I was a little nervous, but figured maybe it was just too early. Then they sent me for an ultrasound. The tech checked my ovaries first, then my uterus. I saw the baby on the screen, but there was no flicker of a heartbeat—I knew what to look for after my previous two pregnancies. I also realized that the baby, whom we had nicknamed "Schweffel," was not moving. So still. After finishing, the ultrasound technician said she had to get the doctor. I choked up a little, hoping against hope that I had missed something, and said, "I didn't see a heartbeat, did you?" She responded, "No, I'm sorry," handing me a box of tissues. I called my husband. It was so hard to get the words out, to say out loud that Schweffel hadn't made it—waterworks all the way. He asked if he should come to get me; I said I didn't know. He responded that he was heading to his car, which was exactly what I needed.

> Through my time posting on the Board and blogging, I had known many people who had experienced losses, from chemical pregnancies to second trimester miscarriages, so not seeing a heartbeat wasn't a complete shock—but it was devastating nonetheless.

Unfortunately, miscarriages are much more common than any of us would like, making this chapter necessary. Among pregnancies conceived in our survey respondents, 28.9% ended in loss (148 out of 513 pregnancies). Some had miscarriages prior to their first child, others in trying to conceive a second or third time, so all in all, 37% of our survey respondents had at least one loss. That's more than one out of every three women, sadly. These losses occurred almost immediately (chemical pregnancy; before a heartbeat had started), later in the first trimester, and, even more heartbreakingly, well into the second trimester or beyond. To counterbalance this sadness, it may set your mind at ease to know that everyone who tried again to get pregnant after her loss did subsequently have a successful pregnancy.

If you are concerned that there is an increased risk of miscarriage because of HA, you can set your mind at ease. The chance of miscarriage in our survey respondents is right on par with that experienced by the general population. A few sources of data support this assertion:

- A systematic review of miscarriage studies undertaken in 2009 found that the rate of pregnancy loss from weeks 5 to 20 was between 11% and 22%[1].
    - A study that recruited 9,055 women found to be pregnant in Northern California between 1981 and 1982 determined that 13% of pregnancies were lost after the fifth week[2].
    - A prospective study of 4,887 women found that 21.3% miscarried between weeks 5 and 20[3].
- A smaller study of 221 women trying to conceive measured hCG levels in 707 menstrual cycles, and detected 198 pregnancies. Of these, 22% were chemical pregnancies[4]. The overall rate of miscarriage in this study, from conception, was 31%.
- Taken together, these studies suggest that 30% to 40% of known conceptions end in miscarriage.

What these statistics tell us is that HA does not increase the chance of miscarriage, but that pregnancy loss is way more common than we think. We often have no idea about the prevalence of miscarriage until we experience it ourselves because, as a society, we have an unspoken "rule" about not revealing a pregnancy before the second trimester. However, what that does is cause those who do experience a loss to suffer in silence, often without the support of friends, family, and others who have experienced similar bereavement.

> *Stefanie*: I've had five miscarriages and the worst part is how I feel like it is something you shouldn't talk about. It is devastating, but having to internalize it and carry on like nothing happened is unnatural and wrong. I think people should openly grieve as they need to. I remember having one of my miscarriages at work in the bathroom stall. To this day I'm horrified by the experience, but I didn't feel like I could talk to anyone. I still feel like I'm disclosing a secret when I tell people I've had six pregnancies and only one child. I don't care though. It's part of my story and who I am, and all the more a miracle my daughter is.
>
> *Sarah R*: Even now I don't feel comfortable telling people that I am in my fifth pregnancy. It's even harder telling them I have two other children, only one of whom is living. I feel like I'm doing them a favor if I don't mention all of the heartache, but it only makes me feel worse. And who really knows, they could be dealing with a similar situation and by us internalizing we aren't helping. I've really been struggling with this lately and I'm just not sure how to deal with it. I wish it were more socially acceptable to talk about our losses and how we feel about them.
>
> *Nico*: When I was pregnant the first time I struggled with whom to tell. I was ecstatic to finally be knocked up. I wanted to shout it from the rooftops—but you're not "supposed" to. I could understand not wanting to share with acquaintances in case something went wrong and I then had to "untell," but not sharing with friends and family? No way. In the end I decided to tell those whose support I would want if something did go wrong. And in my third pregnancy, when I did lose the baby, I was glad to have those people in my corner. Although my biggest source of consolation was a friend whose due date was very close to mine who had lost her baby a few weeks before. We leaned on each other a lot.

It's important to realize, if you do have a miscarriage, that you are not alone. Millions of healthy people have had a miscarriage. But of course we all have different experiences based on a wide variety of factors from whether the miscarriage is natural, medically induced, or surgical, to how we process and cope with adversity. Just as with other forms of grief, there is no right or wrong way to deal with this loss. Some parents are able to move through it freely, while others feel crushed and in deep despair. Talking to those who have experienced a similar bereavement, and who understand both the anguish and the myriad other thoughts and emotions is helpful for many. Partners can also be a source of solace and comfort, although many of us have found that men can move on more quickly than we can, which can cause some strife and difficult feelings in the marriage. If you feel like you're drowning in sorrow and can't escape, please seek out some help, whether from a friend, family member, or professional.

> *Cat*: I remember sitting watching TV and then all of sudden bursting out in tears... and waking up in the middle of the night crying the hardest I have ever cried and asking God, "Why?" But, He had a plan. I got pregnant seven months after I miscarried and have a perfect, healthy, happy baby girl now.

> *Erica*: It straight up sucks. It's awful. It hurts so badly, especially after trying so hard for so long. It's OK to cry and be angry!

> *Nico (2010)*: Emotionally I'm doing all right. But despite the fact that I feel OK most of the time, I have a really hard time telling anyone who doesn't know already. And I also am feeling really crappy in general because I totally still look like I'm pregnant (I have an abdominal muscle separation from my first two pregnancies so I showed really early)—I have never had a small waist, but I was already busting out of my pants and now I just feel gross. It's very different when you can rationalize it because you have a baby in there. And on top of that my skin is being really crappy now, so in general I'm just feeling really unattractive. Again, not that anyone really cares, but it's just one more thing to add to the pile of you-know-what. It stinks. And of course, I'm worried that it's going to take me forever to start cycling again. Also stupid, I know, but I can't help it. Sigh.

> *Amanda T*: I had my D&C two days ago and I had some relief feeling that I could now move forward, grieve, mourn my loss, cry and cry and cry. The sadness is so overwhelming and takes over me so unexpectedly. I am so taken aback by how something that I never met, saw, or held in my arms has permanently scarred me. None of my friends have experienced this, and surprisingly, my mother, who had two miscarriages, is telling me to move on, not be sad, and keep my husband happy and my marriage going—so basically to act like nothing happened. I am so angry at her for being so insensitive, for not validating the hurt, pain, loss, and devastation that I am experiencing.
>
> To further compound things, my ob-gyn is telling me to return to my RE so we can have a game plan to maximize my chances of a successful

pregnancy. I understand this because I am 37, and time is not on my side if I want to have more than one child. I just feel like it's too soon for me to be thinking about getting pregnant again, but the doctor has planted the seed, so now I worry about taking too much time to grieve before trying again. This pregnancy was spontaneous—something I never thought would happen for me. I can't help but wonder if trying again naturally is a bad or good idea. I just don't know.

Meg: One thing that you can do is make a little remembrance-corner type thing to come home to. After my third loss, I bought myself a big bouquet of flowers and put it out with a few sweet cards that people who knew about the loss had sent. I'd go out in the world with my secret funeral going on inside, but when I'd come home, there was this physical thing to remind me that the loss was real, and a big deal, and that it was OK to be sad. It was so helpful.

Sarah R: I have one friend in particular who has made it a point to sit down and talk with me on a regular basis and never avoids the topic. She had a couple of miscarriages herself, so she really gets it. There's nothing in particular she has said, but to know that she still thinks of my Benjamin and how that loss has changed me shows me that she really cares.

Another thing to be aware of is how normal it is for emotions to come from out of the blue. Even if you feel mostly OK after a few days, weeks, or months, there will probably be times when the feelings all come crashing back in on you. When you would have been reaching the second trimester can be particularly difficult—everyone else due around the same time as you is now announcing their pregnancy, sharing the joy of their baby here on earth—while you are left with no announcement to make. Then a couple of months later come the anatomy ultrasound pictures; all you have is maybe a photo of a positive pregnancy test. Or when you reach your due date, a particularly sensitive time, and the other babies are born, while yours is nothing but a hole in your heart. It will probably be easier to deal with these emotions if you're fortunate enough to be pregnant again by the time those dates roll around, but even still, they can bring back or create feelings of sadness, hurt, and anger. Even later, birthday celebrations at the times when you "should have been" celebrating too can bring up some sadness and jealousy.

Jessica W: The milestones are hard… last week would've been my first scan, and I was very aware of that. My stepmom gave me the most beautiful bracelet to commemorate my baby a few days ago, and it was beautiful

> and means so much, but I still had the thought that man, I would way rather be getting a baby than a consolation prize.
>
> *Nico (2010)*: I would have been 13 weeks tomorrow. Which means that everyone who is due around when I was is now announcing their pregnancies. I absolutely do not begrudge a single one of them. But I'm finding it a lot harder than I thought to say congratulations. I want to say that I was supposed to have a baby then too. But then I don't know if that's raining on their parade and I should just say congrats and be done with it.
> In many ways I'm sadder now than I was when we first found out. Then we had to deal with the logistics. Now I'm just waiting. And thinking.

Is It My Fault?

Many of us spend time and a lot of mental energy thinking back through everything we did during the pregnancy and before to figure out why we lost the baby. Probably because we want there to be something we can change to avoid going through the heartbreak again. Please know, however, that it is highly unlikely this miscarriage or loss is your fault. Instead of being consumed by guilt and worry over what you might have done wrong, be as kind to yourself as you would to a friend struggling with similar questions and "what ifs."

The most common reason for miscarriage is embryonic chromosomal abnormalities that are incompatible with life. A five-year study examined 5,555 samples of unknown gestational age—52% of the 3,361 amenable to chromosome analysis were found to have abnormalities[5]. In a more recent study in Germany in which genetic testing was performed after 534 spontaneous miscarriages between weeks 7 and 34, chromosomal abnormalities were detected in 61%[6]—these included an extra copy of one chromosome (trisomy, 53%), extra copies of all chromosomes (triploidy or tetraploidy, 22%), missing chromosomes (aneuploidy, 7%), and other abnormalities (18%). And those are the abnormalities that can be detected using current technology examining entire chromosomes; it is certainly plausible that there are smaller abnormalities that could also be incompatible with life but are not detectable by current methods. Unfortunately, the DNA of embryos lost before week seven cannot be tested due to insufficient tissue amounts, but the hypothesis is that losses this early are even more likely to be caused by chromosomal abnormalities.

Many who have conceived during or after recovery from HA have expressed concerns about whether common issues related to HA or recovering from HA played a part in their miscarriage. One frequent occurrence in HAers is late ovulation (i.e., after CD 21). Internet research sometimes suggests that late ovulation is associated with a higher rate of miscarriage. However, while it may be the case in other conditions that cause later ovulation, in someone with HA, hormones remain in a baseline state for longer than normal, but then the follicle develops and ovulates at a standard rate, so the egg is not over-mature or of poor quality. This is supported by our data, where we found the same rate of miscarriage in our survey respondents irrespective of ovulation timeframe: in first pregnancies the miscarriage rates by day of ovulation were (differences were not statistically significant):

- 27% for those who ovulated before CD 21
- 34% in those who ovulated between CD 21 and 45
- 28% in those who ovulated after CD 45

We also examined a second factor sometimes seen in those with HA: low BMI. Even if some steps have been taken toward recovery, many remain underweight or at the low end of normal, with a BMI under 21. While we did see small differences in miscarriage rate when we looked at various BMI ranges, the results were not statistically significant. However, there were a few other studies[7] that did find an increased rate of miscarriage among those who are underweight. Keeping these results and studies in mind, we would suggest if your BMI is still less than 21, you should consider gaining a few more pounds—it's not going to hurt, and perhaps it will help. Remember though that it is *current* size potentially associated with an elevation in miscarriage risk. A few of our Board members were worried that former very low weights during the time they were anorexic could cause miscarriages down the line even if they were at a healthy weight now. There is no evidence to support an increased rate of miscarriage in those formerly anorexic, and it doesn't make sense from an evolutionary perspective either. In the past there would certainly have been times when resources were scarce and people were starving and therefore unable to reproduce (hello HA); once food was more plentiful, it makes much more sense that fertility would be high and miscarriage rates low in order to allow for reproduction. Having a permanently high rate of miscarriage would mean fewer babies during plentiful times, which would be counterproductive for the species.

The final factor we examined in our data was whether the method by which the pregnancy was achieved made a difference in miscarriage rates. For this question as well, we found that the differences in miscarriage rates between pregnancies achieved naturally or through use of oral meds, injectables, or IVF were not significantly different.

There are other issues that can cause miscarriage, such as[8]:

1) Low progesterone due to premature corpus luteum degradation that is often seen when late implantation occurs; the late increase in hCG is not sufficient to rescue the corpus luteum. This would cause an early miscarriage, around four to five weeks.

2) A failure to block the spiral arteries that supply blood to the uterus; early embryogenesis (weeks five to six) takes place in a low oxygen environment, and failure of the trophoblast cells to migrate to block the spiral arteries can cause developmental defects because of too much oxygen.

3) Around weeks seven to eight the placenta starts to produce progesterone and the corpus luteum phases out. It is theorized that incorrect synchronization of these two events might be responsible for an increase in miscarriages seen around this time.

4) During the early part of the second trimester (weeks 10 to 12) the oxygen requirements of the fetus increase and the spiral artery blockage is broken down. Failure of this step to occur correctly or for the fetus to adjust to the new oxygen environment can also lead to pregnancy loss.

These four points require much further study, but it is theorized that each of these is a checkpoint that evolved to prevent pregnancies that could cause maternal death due to excess bleeding, infection, or obstructed labor[9]. It may be the case that issues involving the corpus luteum (i.e., types 1 and 3) can be prevented with progesterone supplementation. So if you did not use progesterone support in the past and miscarried, it could be something to discuss with your doctor for a subsequent pregnancy (see chapter 19 for more information on possible options).

Other factors that can affect the viability of a pregnancy include maternal clotting disorders, maternal or paternal genetics, and sexually transmitted diseases. It is not standard to test for these issues after a single miscarriage, but if you have more than one miscarriage, testing may prove helpful. Some of the tests performed, and potential options based upon results, are shown on the next page. This list is far from comprehensive as there are many ongoing studies into recurrent pregnancy loss prevention.

Factors potentially affecting pregnancy viability

Factor	Testing	Potential Treatment
Abnormal blood clotting	Genetic screen, antibody panel	Injections of anti-clotting medications
Uterine abnormality	HSG, hysteroscopy, laparoscopy	Dependent on condition; potentially surgery
Genetics	Genetic testing for male and female parents	Discussion of options with genetic counselor; potentially IVF with pre-implantation genetic testing
Sexually transmitted disease	Cultures	Treatment of STD with appropriate medications prior to attempting subsequent pregnancy

With all of that said, there are a few factors known to increase the chance of miscarriage that are within your control. The biggest risk is seen with smoking, where every cigarette smoked per day during pregnancy increases the risk of miscarriage[10] by approximately 1%. Secondhand smoke is also associated with an increase in miscarriage[11]. Drinking alcohol while pregnant is another behavior that increases miscarriage risk. Estimates of that risk vary from 46% per drink per day (so seven drinks per week has a 46% increase in risk of miscarriage[12]) to more than twice the risk of a non-drinker for only four drinks per week[13]. Finally, caffeine intake has also been found to increase risk of miscarriage, with an increase of 14% in likelihood of miscarriage for 100 mg of caffeine per day. This was the result of a meta-analysis that combined data from 53 studies[14]. The authors of that study recommend limiting caffeine intake while pregnant to 200 mg per day at a maximum. However, there is also evidence that points to no effect of caffeine on miscarriage rates[15], which is why the American College of Obstetricians and Gynecologists has not made a firm statement on the point[16]. As many of us are already aware of the negative effects of smoking, alcohol, and caffeine and do not consume those substances while pregnant (aside from a minimal coffee intake), these factors are not in play for most of us. Even if you did engage in such behaviors, there are still many other possible causes of your miscarriage. You can't change what has already happened; all you can do is learn from it and alter your future behavior.

The Actual Miscarriage

No matter what the reason for it, when you find out your baby is not going to end up in your arms, it's heartbreaking. Sometimes it's the repeated beta blood tests that let you know all is not well; either they are decreasing, or rising too slowly. Sometimes, a miscarriage starts with bleeding. In other cases, there is just an empty sac seen in an ultrasound exam, or there's a baby but no movement or heartbeat. Later losses can be discovered because you suddenly notice the baby isn't moving any longer. No matter what the situation, there are few words to explain the despair you might experience while attempting to understand this type of loss.

And then you have to decide what you want to do. If the miscarriage happens naturally, or you are within a few weeks of conception and your betas are falling, your doctor might give you some pain medication and tell you to go home to undergo the experience in private. If the miscarriage is discovered through an ultrasound and there are no signs of nature taking its course soon, the options are:

- Expectant management: wait some amount of time (one study found that 58% miscarried naturally within two weeks[17]; a separate study found that 60% miscarried within two weeks and 81% within four weeks[18]) and see if the miscarriage happens without intervention.
- Medical management: take oral medications (misoprostol and/or mifepristone) that will cause delivery of the baby within a few hours. In the first trimester, this can occur at home; second trimester or later will likely be at a hospital.
- Surgical management: have the pregnancy surgically removed, typically through a procedure called dilation and curettage (D&C). In this procedure your cervix is dilated to about a centimeter, and a vacuum and/or scraping tool is used to remove the pregnancy.
    - o   For second trimester losses, surgical removal would entail a dilation and evacuation (D&E). This is somewhat more involved than a D&C because of the larger size of the fetus.

We thought the best way to describe different miscarriage experiences to you would be to let some of our contributors share in their own words. Our hope is to prepare you for different possibilities, which is why no details have been spared; however, please keep in mind that the following accounts may be emotionally difficult to read.

Clover (natural miscarriage, 12 weeks): I started to have light spotting almost two weeks after finding out our baby had no heartbeat. The next morning, I woke up and saw darker blood and felt crampy. I thought, OK, this is no biggie (the pain), though a couple of times the cramps were intense. I'd bend over at the waist and wait for them to pass as I continued morning chores, getting ready for work, and other stuff. My husband asked if he should stay home but I was pretty confident and replied, "No, lots of people go through this on their own. I will be fine." He then gathered his stuff and I mentioned to him that I was going to take the dogs on a walk. Walking out the door, I felt dizzy but just told myself to make it quick. When I got to the corner with the dogs, I was suddenly in significant pain and lightheaded. I thought, oh, God... please let me make it back home with the dogs. The cramping was intense. My biggest concern at this point was passing out while walking my over-protective dog Buster and him chasing someone. My husband was getting into his car and saw me all hunched over; he got a bit aggravated because he *knew* I wasn't OK despite my protestations that "I'm fine... go ahead and go." He helped me back to the house, where all I could do was curl up in a ball on the bed and run back and forth from there to the bathroom.

There were a lot of clots being expelled. At first a clot the size of an egg passed. It felt weird. I wondered what was coming out. When I looked down I questioned if that was the baby but now I am certain it was not because lots of the same matter came out. At one point my husband asked if I was peeing and I responded, "No, that's blood." It was so intense. I would go back to the bed... my uterus would cramp big time trying to expel what was in there. I would run back to the toilet and more blood would come out. I was both in pain and scared but in an odd way very thankful for the experience (even if the outcome was not what I had planned). I had NO idea that my body was strong enough to pull this off. I was texting Stephanie from the Board throughout because I knew she had a similar experience and she told me that she was scared too. She was able to prepare me with what would happen and what was normal which helped ease my fears. After about two-ish hours of on and off pain at pretty regular intervals I had a SUPER KILLER uterine cramp, went to the toilet, and out came the baby and placenta. After that, the cramping ceased immediately and I felt better physically. I was still lightheaded, but felt very relaxed as if I had indeed passed everything the way I was supposed to. As the day progressed I didn't experience any more pain and the bleeding continued to decrease.

How did I feel emotionally? It was hard to pinpoint. I was mostly OK. When we first learned the baby stopped growing I allowed myself to mourn. Then I chose to focus on what was ahead (though it was confusing because I couldn't really move ahead while waiting to miscarry). The night after I miscarried, I cried when I went to bed, asking, "Why?" But I have a great faith that my baby is in Heaven and that something was not right; otherwise my pregnancy would not have ended early. Both of those things bring me peace.

Sarah R. (natural miscarriage, 11 weeks): With my first miscarriage, the baby stopped growing at 9.5 weeks. We found out at almost 11 weeks and scheduled a D&C for the following Monday. That weekend was a bit of a blur. I had some cramping off and on and really felt pretty miserable for most of the weekend. I was sad and angry. I was confused and mopey. I didn't know where to go from here. Monday morning rolled around and I started having some pretty painful cramping. Thank goodness the procedure was just a few hours away and this would soon be over with. My cramps seemed to be getting worse on the drive to the surgery center and by the time we arrived I felt awful. As I walked to the front door I felt a gush and I knew that I was beginning to miscarry on my own. I stayed longer for my OB to check things out via ultrasound and for the bleeding to slow enough that I could make it home. Then they sent me on my way. Every time a contraction would come I would gush. I found it easiest to just sit on the toilet for the first hour or so after I got home. I was glad that I got to see my OB and that she seemed to think all was normal. I think I would have been really freaked out by the amount of blood if I hadn't seen her. I had heavy bleeding like this for about four hours, at which point I quit having gushes and it was more like a very heavy period. I bled for a little over a week, slowly tapering, similar to my menstrual cycles.

My second miscarriage was a confirmed chemical pregnancy at four weeks. I miscarried naturally at 5.5 weeks. This one was very similar to a heavy period with cramping and heavy flow, which lasted about six or seven days. (*Sarah went on to get pregnant two months after her chemical pregnancy; but sadly her son Benjamin was born still at 21 weeks. Her next pregnancy, conceived three months after the loss, resulted in a healthy baby girl.*)

Becky (induced miscarriage, 6.5 weeks): Although I felt very pregnant and nauseous, the day I went for my first ultrasound at 6.5 weeks, not only was there no heartbeat, but there was no fetal pole and only a gestational sac. My RE explained that the embryo was absorbed, but my body still recognized the sac as a healthy pregnancy which is why the hCG levels continued to rise and I still felt pregnant. With my beta still rising I might not miscarry naturally until possibly 12 weeks, and I couldn't take the uncertainty of waiting. My RE gave me the choice of taking misoprostol (which softens and dilates the cervix, causes uterine contractions, and induces labor), or having a D&C. I wanted the least invasive approach and I don't recall my RE explaining either of them much at that time, although my husband tells me he did. I had just found out I was going to miscarry and really couldn't process anything else. He gave me four vaginal suppositories, and said to take two and see if I started to have the miscarriage.

I went home, had a few glasses of wine with my best friend and husband, and just cried. When I decided it was time, I took two of the suppositories and went to sleep. My husband went out and bought heavy pads and an under-pad for the bed in case I bled through. About six hours later I began to miscarry. My RE had warned me about the pain and prescribed me Tylenol with codeine. I didn't think I'd need it but ended up taking half a tablet when the uterine contractions became very painful. I bled heavy amounts with large clots that morning and was sweating and in pain for about two hours straight, then on and off for a few more hours. My RE said the pain and bleeding should start to slow down after I saw the sac pass. I never saw it that day. I waited one more day, then called my RE. He advised me to take the other two tablets. I began having the painful cramps again a few hours later but they were not as bad as the first time. Finally, the sac passed. It looked large, kind of clear, and hard. After that I had painless heavy bleeding for about four days, then lighter bleeding and spotting for another two weeks.

If I were to do this over again I might opt for a D&C because of the physical and emotional pain. Having to see and feel everything pass was difficult. It's an experience that definitely changed me, and brought my husband and me closer together because we had to lean on each other for support to get through that time. It made me appreciate every step of my next pregnancy and the miracle it really is. (*Becky got pregnant with a baby boy on her very next injectable cycle.*)

Nico (D&C, 10 weeks): We found out about Schweffels' passing just before 10 weeks. Once we had some time to process, my ob-gyn talked to us about the different options for getting the remains out. I had a really hard time deciding; I had read about a few blog friends' natural miscarriages and I was somewhat intimidated by that prospect. I also had no idea when a natural miscarriage might occur and didn't want to be taken by surprise. But at the same time, the idea of a surgical removal just seemed so sterile—no mess, no pain, not seeing the baby—hard to get any closure. I called a few friends who I knew had also lost babies to find out about their experiences, and ended up opting for the surgical route. I was right; it was very surreal to go into the hospital pregnant and leave with nothing, and to feel nothing physically. Was it the best choice for me? To

> this day I'm not sure... but it did remove the pregnancy. After the D&C I actually felt more normal than I wanted to; I would have preferred some pain and cramping to help me process the end of the pregnancy. I bled for about the first week, similar to a period, spotted for another week, and that was it. (*Nico tried naturally for a year after her miscarriage with no success. She moved on to IVF and conceived her third son.*)

Conceiving Again

At some point after your miscarriage you will be ready to think about trying to get pregnant again. That can vary from almost immediately to after a few weeks or months of grieving. There is no "right" time—you will know if you are ready or not. As far as physical readiness, you may ovulate again or be given the go-ahead to start another treatment cycle once your beta drops to near zero. After your miscarriage is complete it typically takes around two weeks for your beta to become negative. However, be aware that the decrease in hCG can take longer—up to about six weeks—and it is not uncommon for the last 100 units or so to take a few weeks.

If you had used medications to get pregnant, some doctors will allow you to start another cycle once your beta drops to zero; others might make you wait a bit longer, and perhaps induce a bleed with Provera or birth control pills first. However, even if you needed medications to get pregnant, a chemical or early loss can sometimes be enough to reset hormones and lead to natural ovulation.

Natural cycles after miscarriage

Pregnancy type	Number resuming cycles	Percentage	Percent ovulating naturally post-miscarriage (by time)			
			2 weeks	1 month	2 months	3 months
Natural	39/40	98%	22%	67%	92%	97%*
Oral meds	8/15	53%	0%	25%	100%	NA
Injectables	1/6	17%	In the one case it took 107 days to ovulation, but betas were positive for 42 days after the D&C.			
IVF	4/15	21%	Ovulation occurred 42, 90, 90 and 100 days post-miscarriage.			

NOTE: Data from miscarriages were not reported proportional to the number of miscarriages from each pregnancy type.

* 35/36 survey respondents who provided data had ovulated by 90 days post miscarriage; the remaining person ovulated 109 days after.

The table shows information on how many of our survey respondents ovulated naturally post-miscarriage, as well as how long it took to ovulate after the miscarriage was complete. It is possible that more of those who used treatments would have cycled naturally post-miscarriage, but they started another round of treatment before that happened. Again, there is no right or wrong here—whatever plan you feel most comfortable with for trying again is the best plan for you.

The next table shows the route each of our survey respondents ended up using to get pregnant, depending on whether they ovulated naturally post-miscarriage or not.

Route taken to next pregnancy after miscarriage

Method by which next pregnancy was achieved	At least one natural ovulation after miscarriage (42 people)		No natural ovulation after miscarriage (29 people)	
	Number of respondents	Number of cycles to next pregnancy	Number of respondents	Number of cycles to next pregnancy
Natural	33	Median of 2 cycles. All but two respondents were pregnant by the 6th cycle post-miscarriage (with the remaining two pregnant at 7 and 15 cycles)	NA	NA
Oral meds	5	1, 2, 4, 4, and 9 cycles	5	3, 3, 3, 5 and 5 cycles
Injectables	3	1, 3, and 5 cycles	5	1, 1, 2, 3, and 5 cycles
IVF	1	One respondent was cycling naturally but did not get pregnant after 12 cycles, so moved to IVF and got pregnant on her first cycle.	19	Median of 1; those who took more than 3 cycles tried oral meds or injections before IVF, and took 4, 5, 7, and 8 cycles.

When Can I Try Again?

Many doctors, midwives, and other healthcare professionals will suggest waiting anywhere from one to three cycles after a miscarriage to start trying again. We were unable to find research supporting this waiting period.

What we did find were a number of studies in which an interpregnancy interval (IPI; the time between pregnancies) of less than six months was associated with a lower subsequent miscarriage rate:

- The live birth rate in a pregnancy occurring after miscarriage was examined among 30,937 Scottish women. Live birth rates were highest when the IPI was less than six months (85%)[19]. No adverse effects on the infants conceived after a less than six month IPI were found.
- Remarkably similar results were found in a study in rural Bangladesh that examined the outcome of a second pregnancy after a loss in 9,214 women. Live birth rates were higher in pregnancies occurring up to 3 months after a loss (87.7%), similar in the 3 to 6-month timeframe (84.4%), and at 6 to 12 months (84.0%)[20]. Somewhat higher rates of preterm labor and infant mortality were seen in this study with short IPI, but the authors postulate this is due to poor maternal nutrition in a developing country and not the IPI per se.
- Three additional studies with smaller numbers (64 pregnancies[21], 91 pregnancies[22], and 1,530 pregnancies[23]) found no increase in adverse outcomes with IPI less than three months.

So, in a nutshell, there is no reason to wait to try to conceive again once you are emotionally ready to do so. Among our survey respondents, 35% conceived on the very next cycle, 70% were pregnant within three cycles, and 90% within six cycles.

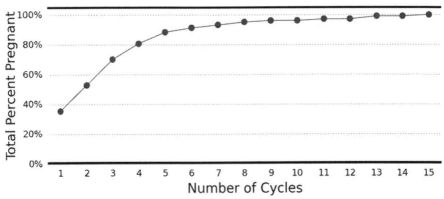

Number of cycles after a miscarriage to achieve another pregnancy (104 pregnancies).

Unfortunately, not all of these conceptions resulted in live births; 25% had another miscarriage (normal miscarriage rate). Repeat pregnancy loss, especially if you are trying to conceive your first, can make you wonder if you will ever get to hold your baby in your arms. Certainly among our group, continued attempts to get pregnant did result in at least one baby for every person. As far as whether there is anything you can do, the book *Coming to Term: Uncovering the Truth About Miscarriage*[24] provides an overview of recent research into recurrent pregnancy loss. Some have found it useful to read even after just one miscarriage.

Pregnancy After Miscarriage

> *Willow*: Thanks so much for the congratulations and welcomes! I am sure you all understand how nervous I am. When did you find the fear diminished? I'm hoping that seeing a heartbeat will help me relax, but I probably won't feel completely confident until the first trimester is over. I even feel nervous posting that I'm pregnant again, that I might jinx myself. I am trying to relax and not obsess, but it is hard! I hope I will have a good beta on Thursday, but until then I am going to enjoy being pregnant!

Many are aware there is a chance they may miscarry, so they understandably worry a bit about whether their betas are rising appropriately, or whether they will see the heartbeat when it's ultrasound time. But as each of these milestones passes it becomes easier to embrace the pregnancy. However, when you've had a miscarriage (or many), there may no longer be any excitement around these milestones, but rather a feeling of anxiety. It can be hard to enjoy a pregnancy after miscarriage, especially if you're always waiting for the other shoe to drop and crush your hopes yet again. All we can offer is the same advice we gave before—try not to wonder and worry too much about what will happen in the future because it is beyond your control. Let yourself be happy that today and in this moment, you are pregnant. Practice turning negative thoughts into positive ones when they arise. If you find yourself remembering the ultrasound where you found out the baby's heart had stopped, and worrying about the same outcome, stop yourself. Chances are good that the outcome this time will be different. It is impossible for a past miscarriage not to steal some joy out of a subsequent pregnancy, but do your best not to let your loss cloud your new pregnancy. If your angel baby could talk to you, he or she would tell you to never forget them, but also to cherish every moment in anticipation of their new baby brother or sister.

> *Stefanie*: I guess what I would like someone to know is that there is nothing shameful, embarrassing, or hopeless about miscarriages. Even

> with genetic issues (Factor V Leiden thrombophilia and a balanced translocation) causing an 80% miscarriage risk, I never gave up. I think people just need to know there is hope after a pregnancy loss. Most of the time a miscarriage is not the end of the story; you will have your miracle baby someday, and cherish your child that much more.

Parting Thoughts

There are no two ways about it; losing a baby is an experience we wouldn't wish on anyone, especially after working long and hard to become pregnant in the first place. But miscarriage is unfortunately a normal occurrence, experienced by over a third of our survey respondents. It is hard for us not to blame ourselves; in some ways the guilt we lay on ourselves may be easier than the idea that the miscarriage was random chance. If we did something, we can make changes to avoid another loss. As we discussed, however, almost all miscarriages are beyond our control. We just have to be brave and try again when we are ready. And hope. There is always hope.

> *Clover*: I went through a short period of bitterness. Not because of my miscarriage but because of the lack of support I received during that time. I remember there being a full moon; my husband and I were walking down the road with our two pups. I started sharing with him that a few "friends" didn't even call or reach out to me knowing that I had just found out my baby no longer had a heartbeat and I was waiting for my miscarriage to happen. I could feel my blood boil as I rattled on about "what I would have done for them" if the tables were reversed. Right at that moment it clicked. I thought, "We HAers and/or those experiencing miscarriages have become compassionate, empathetic souls because of what we have lost and endured." I share this with deep conviction and say with all sincerity that I am thankful for my sufferings (though regret the hardship my choices have caused others, like my husband). If it were not for those chapters in my life, I would not care with the depth I do, reach out to others struggling, and weep with those who are hurting. We HAers have true compassion and a strength that only comes through conquering adversity.
>
> While none of what I just shared will take away the pain of losing a baby, my hope is that it allows you to recognize that all is not lost with loss.

In remembrance of all our angel babies.

27
Postpartum, Cycling, and Conceiving Again

ONCE YOU'RE DONE with the pregnancy part of your journey and are holding an amazing little miracle in your arms, there will probably be a few questions that arise over time. At first your concerns involve deciphering the little creature that you are suddenly in charge of with no owner's manual. This often includes figuring out breastfeeding and sometimes apprehensions about your milk supply, or deciding on what formula to use if you cannot or choose not to breastfeed. A little part of you might also be wondering about losing the pregnancy weight—despite all you've done to try not to focus on the perceived negatives about your body, it is normal to want to "get your body back." As you get close to weaning (or if you did not breastfeed), a burning question is, "Will I start cycling?" or "When will I cycle again?" We wanted a crystal ball to know when we would get pregnant; now we're desperate to know when we will see some more of the crimson lady. And that leads right back to trying to get pregnant again, as many of us want another child, or more. The best way to answer these questions is with data, which our survey respondents were happy to provide.

The first issue, the question of milk supply, varies among HAers just as it does in everyone else. There is nothing inherent to HA that affects breast milk production. Some struggle to produce enough from the beginning; others have an oversupply and deal with big spots of milk on their shirts when they forget to wear breast pads. There are a number of factors that can have an effect on milk supply, including:

- Hydration: fill up a big water bottle to drink while your baby is breastfeeding.
- Supply-increasing medications: there are some supplements such as mother's milk tea and fenugreek, among others, that can theoretically help with milk supply. You can search online or get a lactation consultant's help with choosing those that might be right for you. Outside the US, domperidone is available by prescription and is excellent at increasing supply.
- Supply-increasing foods: some swear by lactation cookies, oatmeal, and/or beer (in moderation) to help increase their milk output.
- Supply-reducing medications: those that dry up mucous membranes (e.g., cold medicines) can also decrease milk supply, so it is best to avoid them.
- Nutrition: many find a correlation between sufficient energy intake (which can come from both consumed food as well as fat stores from pregnancy) and higher supply.

No matter what, it can be a challenge to learn how to breastfeed. Get help early on even if you don't think you need it because you can often learn helpful tips and tricks. There are excellent resources available to support you if you choose the breastfeeding route to nourish your baby. Most hospitals have lactation consultants (LCs); many health insurance plans cover home visits from LCs; some pediatricians have LCs associated with their offices; there is La Leche League where other mothers offer support and advice; and there are books you can get from the library, or online resources you can read such as kellymom.com. Remember: it sometimes takes meeting a few people to find one who clicks with you, so don't be afraid to shop around.

If you are unable to breastfeed or choose not to, it is natural to feel like a failure as a mother. But you are not. You are doing the best you can for your child, yourself, and your family. Breastfeeding can be wonderful, but there are many reasons that it might not work for you and your baby—allergies, physical issues, low supply, etc. Steph tried breastfeeding, but her son's dairy intolerance made for a miserable baby and a mom with postpartum depression. After a switch to formula, everyone was happier and healthier.

Cecily: The "Breast is Best" campaign does not acknowledge those who want to breastfeed (BF) but can't for physical or other reasons. I have

> inverted nipples, and even with a nipple shield wasn't able to BF my daughter after the first two weeks because she wasn't gaining weight appropriately. I pumped until she was a month old, but ended up going to formula since pumping was too overwhelming. I decided that a happy mom = a happy baby. But man, the guilt associated with stopping BFing was tough… "Breast is Best" makes you feel like you are ruining your child's life by not BFing. It's good to remember that our parents' entire generation wasn't breastfed and turned out OK! I finally felt much better about my decision to bottle feed after talking to my 90-year-old grandma, who also had inverted nipples and didn't BF her five children, all of whom have turned out to be fantastic, smart, healthy people. There's a lot more to successful parenting than breastfeeding, and I urge you not to feel badly if you aren't able to BF for long, or at all!

This leads us to the next common topic: losing the weight gained during pregnancy. This is a touchy one. In a perfect world, we probably wouldn't give our postpartum weight a second thought because it would be of no consequence. The importance would be placed on ensuring our health instead. But we live in a world so focused on physical appearance that it is really hard not to want to get back "in shape." Hopefully you can do both—think a little bit about getting back to where you were pre-pregnancy, but remain cognizant of your ongoing health, and prioritize that over how much weight you want to lose and how fast. A healthy postpartum weight might be a bit higher than where you were pre-pregnancy if you were still slim and hadn't gotten your cycles back naturally. Or it could be a little bit less if you gained beyond a previous high weight and resumed natural periods. Even if your pre-pregnancy BMI was on the higher side, we recommend not dropping more than 5 to 10 pounds below where you were pre-pregnancy, especially if you hope to conceive again. Keep in mind that as we continue to discuss this issue, we are generalizing. Every person is different. The key is to know yourself and your body, and maintain a weight that is healthy for you, even if it is not necessarily the number you want it to be. As you recovered from HA, you probably put in an effort to avoid letting your weight define you; after your baby is born is a wonderful time to continue that practice. If you must weigh yourself, we suggest no more than once a week; daily weighing makes it easy to fall back into old mindsets.

> *Kristen*: I just wanted to comment on the issue of "losing" your body or figure after pregnancy. For me, having had body image issues my whole

> life, I expected to have some difficulty with my postpartum figure. You know, it's one thing to be pregnant and carrying extra weight but much different after the baby is here and you still look pregnant and things aren't quite like they were before. But the experience of childbirth has given me a newfound appreciation for my body and what it has done to bring a healthy baby into this world. I think part of it is because I did it without pain meds—giving me a huge feeling of accomplishment and appreciation for the design of a woman's body. Having felt every bit of the process was truly amazing. So, when I look in the mirror and see some flab, I don't even think about it. All I see is a body that accomplished an incredibly wonderful thing: growing and giving birth to a beautiful baby girl. I hope that childbirth gives all of you the same positive boost in self-image.
>
> *Kasey:* A part of me wants to whip back into shape, but, like a lot of us, I want to have baby #2 naturally and I now know the best way to achieve that goal is to keep some of the flab around!

If you did not gain much while pregnant, you are probably going to struggle to keep weight on if you are breastfeeding. We hope that low weight gain is not something you aspire to if you're reading this chapter prior to or during pregnancy, because it really is not healthy for you, and can potentially have negative consequences for your baby as well as mentioned in chapter 25. These include low birth weight; premature birth[1]; and being afflicted with the "thrifty phenotype" that is associated with an increase in type 2 diabetes[2], cardiovascular disease, and obesity[3] over time.

If you're coming home from the hospital at your pre-pregnancy weight, that actually means you lost weight while pregnant because you still have increased blood volume and breast tissue that you will lose over the next few weeks to months, bringing you to a lower weight than when you started. And breastfeeding requires about 500 to 600 calories a day, so you will probably feel voraciously hungry. Feed that beast! You have no extra fat stores to fall back on, so you need to eat like it's your job. Well, your second job, after taking care of your little one. It's easy to let taking care of yourself slide, because you're definitely not top priority anymore. But it is important for you to stay healthy too—if you get significantly below your pre-pregnancy weight you will likely start experiencing HA symptoms all over again. Do you really want to have to go through the process of recovery another time?

If you are struggling to eat enough post-pregnancy, ask your partner to help you make time to nourish yourself, not only your baby. Keep calorie-dense snacks like nuts, whole milk yogurt, or energy bars within reach when you're nursing. As you sit down to feed your baby, grab a glass of water and a snack for yourself, and eat while your baby does. Some say they do all this and still lose weight; if that's the case for you, liquid calories are an easy way to make up the difference. Instead of drinking water while you nurse, have a glass of juice. Add a smoothie to your breakfast. Brainstorm with your partner or a friend to find some other ways to add more calories to keep your weight stable.

If you gained more than the minimum recommended amount while pregnant, you might find you continue to eat about the same amount post-pregnancy as you did while pregnant. You may also find yourself hungrier from time to time—or always. Almost all our survey respondents were back to pre-pregnancy weight somewhere between six weeks to a year after their baby was born. After the pregnancy weight is lost, if you're still breastfeeding, you may find yourself in the same situation as above: losing additional weight if you're not conscious about making sure to consume enough food. Your body may find its natural set point or, if you're not careful, fall below that. Keep in mind if you let your weight drop too low, even at many months postpartum, you run the risk of experiencing HA again, which we have seen. It can help to have a minimum weight in mind, below which you will not let yourself go, to keep HA at bay. And this minimum should be reasonable; dropping to a BMI of 18 or 19 is not going to do you any favors. It is true that weight is not the be-all and end-all, but if you are losing to a point far below where you were pre-pregnancy, that indicates you're back in an energy deficit... and now you know what that does.

> *Nico*: It was very important to me not to have to deal with HA, and all the stress and self-doubt it caused, a second time. While trying to conceive, I had gotten to an all-time high weight, a few pounds over what I consider my set point. After my first son was born, I lost the pregnancy weight slowly but steadily, and then a bit more. I wasn't restricting. I was eating normally—I ate when I was hungry and until I was full. I resumed exercising about five weeks post C-section; I started with some biking, then added back ice hockey a few times a week and some weight lifting. But I made sure that I ate more on the days I exercised. About six to seven months postpartum I hit my self-imposed minimum weight—a BMI of 21.5. That was around where I'd been before I went on my ridiculous weight-loss plan. It was quite a bit higher than my HA weight, so I figured

> it was a healthy place for my body. At that point, I made a conscious effort to eat some extra snacks each day. I'd bake a few loaves of banana bread and have a slice when I nursed mid-morning and mid-afternoon. Or eat some of the cookies my mom kept bringing over. Turned out I was right, this was a healthy place for my body—I ovulated and got my first period about 10 months postpartum, while still nursing my son morning and night.

On the other hand, there are some who find that they hold onto about five to ten pounds of weight above pre-pregnancy while breastfeeding. This can be hard emotionally, especially if you are around others who keep talking about how "the weight just fell off." Please remind yourself that every body is different. There are varied journeys to pregnancy, diverse pregnancy experiences, and a wide range of postpartum paths. If you find yourself struggling with not losing weight, or not losing as quickly as you had hoped, this can be a good time to go back to your affirmations, or maybe create some new ones that help you remember what amazing miracles your body has performed. In the end, it is not going to matter if it takes you a day or a year or more to lose your pregnancy weight, or even if you never do—those extra pounds may be exactly what you need to stay healthy. You will be the center of your child's universe for a long time to come, and what matters to them is that you love them and spend time with them. Nothing else.

> **Sheeza**: When you look at your post-baby body and resent it, think of all the work it has done to grow the healthy baby/babies that you now hold in your arms. Ask yourself, "Would I rather have my old body or my baby?" We spend nine months gaining the weight; I think it is unfair to hope for it to go away by two to three months after birth. Isn't the rule of thumb nine months on, nine months off? And for those of us who want another, from personal experience, keep the last five pounds on; it will help you to get pregnant that much faster. We suffered enough the first time and deserve a natural, stress-free conception the second time.

Regaining Cycles

Once you're postpartum, you may be wondering if and when your cycle will return, especially if you were not cycling naturally before pregnancy. You will be happy to know that overall, *83% of HAers resumed normal cycles between pregnancies, and 94% after their final child was born and weaned.* Of those who used fertility treatments for their first pregnancy, 90% eventually resumed cycling.

Out of the HAers who resumed cycling, 21% did so while nursing or pumping (14% of those who used fertility treatments; 24% of those who got pregnant naturally), with the remainder ovulating for the first time a median of two months after weaning. This timeframe was the same in those who had cycled naturally before pregnancy and those who used treatments to get pregnant.

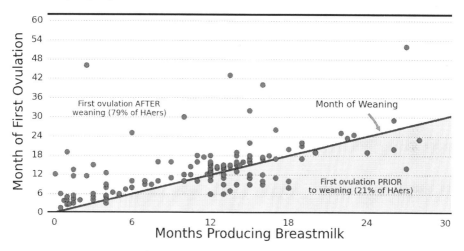

Cycle resumption and breast milk production. When each of our survey respondents (150 participants) resumed cycles in relation to when breast milk production stopped (black line) is shown. The points below the line indicate those for whom menstrual cycles began prior to weaning, points above the line are those for whom cycles started after breast milk production ceased.

Emilie: Twelve months postpartum, two weeks officially post-weaning, AND I GOT MY PERIOD!!!!!!!!! I was hopeful, but in the back of my mind never thought it would happen for me. So thrilled that my body is in a healthier state!

Steph: I stopped breastfeeding five weeks after my son was born. I was eager to get my period back. When I didn't see it within the first four weeks after weaning, I got nervous. (I encourage you, however, to be patient. I know now that four weeks was not a long time.) I called Dr. Hall and we scheduled an appointment for a month later. I walked into her office for my visit with a smile on my face, announcing, "I just started my period for the first time in over 10 years!"

There are two theories as to why breastfeeding prevents ovulation. The first is based on the hormone prolactin, which increases sharply when an infant suckles, and prevents the hypothalamus from sending GnRH pulses. The lack of GnRH means low FSH and LH, hence no cycles. Infant suckling decreases over time as formula and/or solids are added to supplement the breast milk, which reduces the amount of prolactin, eventually to a level where it is no longer inhibiting the GnRH. The second idea is based on energy availability. In this theory, ovulation is inhibited by lack of excess energy while nursing, through essentially the same mechanism as HA. The hypothalamus senses low insulin and other hormones indicating an energy deficit and shuts down GnRH signaling. This second theory better explains the wide range of time to resumption of menses, even when nursing intensity (and therefore the amount of prolactin produced) is fairly similar[4]. Researchers conducting a study on this topic collected information from well-nourished women in Formosa, where extended breastfeeding is common. Periods resumed at an average of 10 months postpartum, following one to three months of small weight gains as well as an increase in insulin, both indicative of an energy surplus[5]. It was theorized that the higher levels of insulin and energy surplus activated the hypothalamus to restart cycles.

In those of us who have recovered from HA, our hypothalamus has a bit of practice in shutting down GnRH production, and we tend not to resume cycling until an average of two months after weaning. However, that does vary based on the amount of time for which breast milk is produced.

Length of breast milk production compared to cycle resumption

Months for which breast milk was produced	Number of respondents	Percent regaining cycles while nursing	Median time to ovulation after weaning (in months)	Length of time after weaning for 75% to start cycling (months)
Less than 3*	35	0%	3	5.5
3 – 6	19	13%	2	4
6 – 9	12	0%	2.5	4
9 – 12	37	24%	1.5	3.5
12 – 18	64	37%	1	2
More than 18	20	57%	1 month before weaning	2.5

* This category includes those who did not breastfeed at all.

We also noted that while some were below pre-pregnancy weight (by an average of 0.5 BMI units), 85% of those whose cycles resumed gained from their lowest postpartum weight before cycles returned. This gain ranged from a couple of pounds to much more, depending on how low postpartum weight dropped. For some, weight gain occurred and cycles resumed while still nursing; for others, it was after breast milk production stopped. There were a few who took more than a year after weaning to regain cycles (we offer some suggestions below if this is your situation). In some cases, the return of cycles after this length of time was associated with a forced break from exercise due to injury; in others, stress was managed through therapy and medications.

There wasn't a correlation between exercise and cycle resumption—probably because most recovered HAers have learned to properly fuel their exercise, in which case it would not affect the return of cycles. However, there were some who did have to reduce or stop exercising in order to encourage the resumption of cycles. If you subscribe to the theory that it is energy balance that makes a difference, this makes sense—under-fueled exercise resulting in an energy deficit could very well be a culprit for absent cycles. Remember that our hunger signals do not adequately compensate for the energy expended in planned exercise, so you need to be conscious about eating at least one calorie for every one burned if you do continue to exercise. If you are waiting with bated breath for your cycle to start up again, you might consider cutting down on exercise for a month or two in order to get your cycles back. Also, note that in the study we discussed above, it took a few months of positive energy balance for luteal phases to adequately restore and to occur within a normal timeframe[6], which is also common after resumption of cycles in HAers. Getting cycles to normalize can be sped up by cutting exercise, and for some of us, any exercise can cause short luteal phases and other irregularities.

> *Nico*: Remember how I told you I got my very first natural period after HA while we were on vacation? Well, after my first was born and my cycles resumed, my luteal phase was super-short and I was ovulating late in each cycle. The first time I ovulated in a normal timeframe (CD 16), my exercise schedule had been seriously limited by snow-caused gym and hockey cancellations. That was the cycle my second was conceived.

Given all of this, we recommend the following as you try to recover your cycles after your baby is born:

- Ensure that you are in a positive energy balance.
  - The calories you expend on producing breast milk will naturally decrease as your child gets older, as solids are added, and especially if you supplement with formula.
- You may need to cut down or stop exercise both to decrease the stress level your body senses and to help attain an energy surplus.
- Gaining a few pounds from your lowest postpartum weight will help your body sense the extra energy, and you may need more than just a few pounds depending on how low your postpartum BMI gets.
- Patience! We recognize that this is hard to practice, especially if you are hoping to try to conceive again soon, but just as when you experienced HA the first time around, stress can absolutely play a part in suppressing your hypothalamus. Trust your body; it *does* know what to do.
- If your body is not following your timeline, you can speed up regaining your cycles by creating more of an energy surplus through any combination of the options below:
  - Weaning.
  - Eating more, especially foods that will increase insulin and leptin production.
  - Cutting down or stopping planned exercise.
- If you are a year or more post-weaning and cycles still haven't returned, the next section will offer some additional options to try.

> **Amanda D:** The twins will be TWO in two weeks, and I haven't gotten my period yet. I stopped pumping when they turned one, and weaned at 14.5 months. I went on one really low estrogen BCP for two months, then went off for a few months, and nothing. I called my ob-gyn and she put me on another pill, from which I spotted in October, then got a light period in November. I then went off again to see if this jump-started anything. Still nothing. My BMI is good and while I am working out, I am only running maybe once a week since it is too cold and I don't like the treadmill.
>
> **Seven months later:** *DRUMROLL, PLEASE* I got my period this morning! A whopping 31 months postpartum and 17 months after weaning! I guess this is the silver lining in being rendered immobile for a month. (*Amanda had been on bedrest for a month due to osteomyelitis. She continued cycling naturally, but didn't have 28-day cycles until she gained another 5 lb.*)

Options for Regaining Cycles

We mentioned earlier that 94% of our survey respondents regained cycles after they were finished having children, and this includes most who needed injectables or IVF in order to conceive. But that leaves 6% who have not resumed cycling. For some, the reason is persistence of the HA mindset and behaviors. Others are at a healthy weight and eat and exercise for health, not to control their weight, but their cycles haven't returned. Most of these people eventually go on birth control or hormone replacement therapy because, as we've discussed, artificial hormones are likely better than none at all. However, if you fall in this category, there are some options to consider if you are no longer in a chronic energy deficit and would like to try to regain your cycles. We discussed this topic in chapter 17, but will cover the salient details again here.

A simple option is to try a course of Provera. This does *not* work to restore cycles during initial HA recovery. However, postpartum, once there is no longer any milk production and assuming a fertile BMI and moderate exercise, there have been instances where normal cycles have resumed after a single course of Provera. Our theory is that the increase and subsequent decrease in blood levels of Provera mimic the progesterone rise and fall in the latter part of a normal menstrual cycle. This small change, *in a person who is at a positive energetic balance*, may be sufficient to then lead to the downstream hormonal changes necessary to start follicular recruitment and a new cycle.

Another area to explore is that of mental health. Cognitive behavioral therapy (CBT) in women with HA led to recovery of cycles in seven out of eight participants, compared with two of eight not receiving therapy[7]. This suggests that CBT is worth considering if your cycle is still missing despite being at a fertile BMI, limiting high-intensity exercise, and working on stress reduction on your own. Another idea to try is that of hypnosis. When a single session of hypnosis (described in detail in the journal article[8]) was performed, 9 of 12 women with HA menstruated within three months after the session. Supplementing with over-the-counter acetyl-l-carnitine (ALC) restarted menstrual cycles in 40% to 60% of women with HA in three studies[9] (http://noperiod.info/ALC). This compound has been shown to affect serotonin, dopamine, and beta-endorphins, reducing the impact of those molecules on the hypothalamus[10]. One final suggestion if you are plagued by stress and anxiety is to try anti-anxiety medications along with therapy. Controlling stress in this manner has helped a few people to achieve ongoing menstrual cycles.

Another avenue to explore if you and your doctor are open to the idea is the oral fertility medications: Clomid, Femara, or tamoxifen. The Clomid Extended Protocol[11] (EP), as we have mentioned before, led to recovery of ongoing menstrual cycles in all eight study participants, and has done so for a number of Board/support group members and clients since. Based on the similar ways in which the three oral medications work, we would suspect that the same result could arise from a few courses of Femara or tamoxifen.

Finally, there are a couple of medications that target other pathways. The first is naltrexone, which blocks the opioid receptor in the brain. There were a number of studies performed in women with HA in the early 1990s, leading to ovulation in approximately 75% of participants who took this medication[12]. As naltrexone targets an entirely different pathway from the oral fertility medications, it might be worth exploring if other attempts have been fruitless. The second drug with some potential is leptin. This was FDA approved in 2014 for treatment of a rare condition called "lipodystrophy" and requires an extensive application process to receive medication[13]. If one were theoretically able to acquire leptin, two small studies found that ovulation occurred in about 40% of women receiving treatment within eight months[14].

The likelihood of any of these treatments working is reduced in someone who is experiencing an ongoing energy deficit, overexercising, or underweight. There are no shortcuts. *We strongly suggest use of these methods only if you have put in solid physical and mental efforts toward recovery.*

Conceiving Again

One bonus of cycles resuming after pregnancy is that, even if you had to use fertility treatments the first time around, many are able to conceive naturally for subsequent pregnancies (if so desired).

Method of conception for first and subsequent pregnancies

Conception Method	First Pregnancy	Subsequent Pregnancy
Number of pregnancies	327	162
Natural	31%	62%
Oral Meds	26%	15%
Injectables[†]	27%	13%
IVF	16%	9%[‡]

[†] Pregnancies achieved using Clomid or Femara with injectables have been included in the injectables category.
[‡] Includes both fresh IVF and transfers of frozen embryos from earlier cycles.

You can see that there was much less medical intervention necessary than in initial pregnancies. In addition, the figure below shows how long it took to get pregnant when trying to conceive siblings. A number of pregnancies were unplanned (20%); that is, respondents were not specifically trying to conceive, but were also not using any form of birth control. Another 30% were conceived on the first cycle of attempted conception. Overall, 79% were pregnant within the first three cycles, and 94% within the first six*.

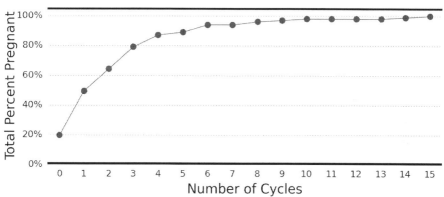

Number of ovulations to achieve conception, after first baby was born (101 pregnancies). Note that "0" indicates an unplanned (but not unwanted!) pregnancy.

Parting Thoughts

When we have HA and are working toward recovery, we all wonder if we will still be dealing with it after we have our first baby. Whether you do or not depends on how much you've been able to change your ways. If you

---

* A quarter of these pregnancies ended in miscarriage, similar to the rate of pregnancy loss when trying to conceive initially.

are continuing to operate at an energy deficit—through either undereating or overexercising—it is likely that yes, you will have to make additional changes if you do want to resume your cycles postpartum. You can always go back and re-read part 2 as many times as you need. If you got to the point prior to your pregnancy where you were eating enough and not overexercising, chances are excellent that even if you didn't resume cycles before pregnancy, you will afterward. Again, patience and time are key ingredients; if you are in a rush to conceive a sibling for your child, you might not be interested in waiting a few months to resume natural cycles. A small percentage (6%) of our survey respondents have not regained cycles yet, although this will hopefully change with time. However, if you're willing to give your body a few months, you will likely be pleasantly surprised.

> **Leslie:** I have completely stopped running and have just accepted the fact that I will need to carry these additional pounds until I conceive again. It is too much of a slippery slope right now, especially when I throw in the breastfeeding. I need to look at myself as a fertile momma and not the mom of a one-year-old who just can't shed the baby weight. As always, eating is no problem. I love food! That's part of what got me into this HA predicament. I love food so much I had to count every morsel that went into my mouth in order to lose weight, which led to binges, which led to lots of running. So I'm trying to just enjoy my little one and working on a sibling. That means I am not exercising (other than walking) and eat whatever I want. (*Leslie got her period six days later, and conceived the following cycle.*)

28
Long-term Health

WE'VE REFERRED TO fully recovering from HA many times, but before we go further we want to be absolutely clear as to what we mean by "a full recovery"—this includes both physical and mental components. Physically, the restoration of menstrual periods and other bonuses that come with providing your body sufficient energy. On the mental side, a shift in your view of what is important such that you no longer hinge your self-worth and identity on diet, size, or exercise prowess.

What does the life of someone who has fully recovered look like? Perhaps something like this . . . few rules about eating other than 1) not skipping meals, 2) eating when hungry, and 3) never training on empty. There is no "allowing" treats, because nothing is off limits. If there's a desire for something sweet or fatty or salty, they eat it, and then go on with the rest of the day. When at a restaurant, no attention is paid to the low-calorie options, but rather to the section with favorite entrées. Perhaps starting with the bread basket, sharing an appetizer or two with a dining companion, and looking forward to dessert at the end of the meal. Enjoyable exercise has been reintroduced, but the difference now is that when the session is over and stomach grumbling ensues, it's snack or meal time. Even if it is not "time" to eat. Food is viewed as fuel for activities, and exercise as fun and healthy, not to lose weight or burn off calories anymore. That is not to say there aren't situations in which the old mindset tries to creep back in. But our recovered HAer is aware of these negative thoughts, and is able to recognize them as unhealthy and ignore them, or call on the coping tools developed during HA recovery to deal with them without sliding back into old ways. Or even if there is a small slip up from time to time, like choosing exercise instead of a meal with friends, realization comes quickly, and more deliberate choices are made to support overall health. If our recovered HAer feels too challenged in making those choices, they seek help before backsliding too far down the slippery slope of HA. This is (one version of) recovery.

If you are not fully recovered yet, press on, keeping one foot in the door. It is never, ever too late. If you've been trying to recover but haven't been able to get all the way there, spend some time thinking about what's holding you back. You may be able to identify some of your barriers as you read this chapter; if not, speaking to a professional can often help.

> *Lisa*: What's "recovered"? For many of us it's a newfound appreciation for health and friends as well as enjoying the byproducts of weight gain: regular cycles, stronger bones, more energy, balanced hormones... along with freedom from food restrictions and rigid time schedules; the list goes on and on.
>
> Despite those commonalities, recovery does vary for each person with regard to food choices and amounts. I think that the difference between a non-recovered HA mindset and full recovery boils down to the anxiety caused by the thought of eating certain items. For example, the idea of eating bread with my meal as described above no longer causes me anxiety; I simply don't enjoy it much and therefore don't eat it. Put a chocolate dessert in front of me and that's a different story.
>
> *Steph*: Its 2 p.m. on Saturday afternoon. Aaron is driving through McDonald's for some coffee. All of a sudden I think, oooh, ice cream, and before I know it I am finishing off a delicious cup of soft vanilla. I didn't run long today. It doesn't matter. I will have pizza for dinner and probably M&M's for dessert, but this cup of soft serve does not give me a second thought. What does is the adorable little boy sleeping in the back seat, the growing baby in my belly, my husband driving us, and my sweet black lab resting quietly. This is my recovery and I am grateful.

Healthy Exercise Habits

In our description above, we said that someone who is recovered exercises for fun and health, not to burn calories. But that's a bit vague, don't you think? Would you rather have hard-and-fast guidelines? Well, in truth, there aren't any, beyond continuing to fully fuel whatever exercise you choose to do. For many of us, our exercise time is way more constrained by the rest of our lives than it used to be—work, possibly caring for and spending time with children, and household chores all make exercising as much as we used to nearly impossible. We squeeze in half an hour of exercise here, twenty minutes there, because we know that it is healthy to get our blood pumping and muscles working. Of course there are those that make exercise more of a priority; quite a few recovered HAers have run marathons and we even have a triathlete or two—all of whom continue to menstruate regularly. And you know why, don't you? They are adequately fueling.

> *Jennifer*: I'm still running, but at a nice, healthy weight and cycling regularly on my own! Plus, I'm way faster than I was when I was at my lower weight so it just goes to show you that some extra pounds won't hurt you. I'm done with having kids, but it's awesome to know that I'm on the right track (post-HA) with calories and body fat to be able to run and train as much as I do and still get my period each month. I was a 3:38 marathoner prior to trying to conceive. I gained weight, had two babies, and now I'm at a healthy weight, cycling regularly, and ran a 3:03 marathon this spring. You CAN train hard, still get your period, and be healthy!

Healthy Eating Habits

Just as with healthy exercise habits for the long term, there aren't fixed rules for eating habits either. We have recovered HAers who follow a low sugar meal plan to help keep (accurately diagnosed) PCOS at bay, there are vegetarians, and of course we each have our individual likes and dislikes. Again, the key is that we are eating enough. Our meals generally cover our caloric needs, and if we feel hungry beyond that, we eat more. Once you're cycling regularly, there is no longer a need to force yourself to eat extra calories, as you might have during recovery. You follow your hunger and fullness cues—eat normal meals (plus snacks, especially if you're breastfeeding, engaging in lots of high-intensity exercise, or pregnant again) of whatever strikes your fancy, and that's that.

You will have some foods that you like and want to eat because they are tasty and nutritious, and some that you really enjoy and eat regardless of the calories and ingredients (mmm... cheesecake). You will probably have some foods that you don't enjoy and don't eat for that reason. If you find that there are still foods you pass up because they make you somewhat anxious, you can carry on avoiding them, or work on taking away the power they have over you. Think about why the particular food makes you anxious. What is the worst that can happen if you consume it?

Postpartum Weight Loss

Many struggle with body image after having a baby. We are exposed to pictures of celebrities who have recently had babies and have to same figure as they did beforehand within just a few weeks of birth. This is not realistic!!! Many of these celebrities have personal trainers, chefs, and nannies; their body is their livelihood and therefore they often go to extremes to look like they were never pregnant. Most people will lose some weight at the time of delivery: baby, placenta, amniotic fluid. You might find that you actually retain some extra water in the week or so after delivery, this is normal and the swelling will subside within 1-2 weeks after delivery. Patterns of weight loss and body changes vary a lot from this point, with some continuing to lose weight at a somewhat steady rate, and others plateauing until 3, 6, 9 months or more postpartum. Some hold onto some pregnancy weight until they stop breastfeeding.

It can be challenging to come to terms with a body that looks and feels different from what it was prior to HA recovery, or prior to pregnancy, and it is quite easy to feel like it is important to lose some of this "excess" weight. We encourage you to work on accepting your body, appreciating it for everything it has done for you, like growing a whole other human being (or more!), and not on getting back into restriction and extreme habits to meet some societal ideal. If let your body reach its natural set point, by simply eating by following your bodies natural cues, you will find it takes very little work to maintain, other than perhaps some work on your mental acceptance of the changes.

On the other hand, you may find that you lose weight easily after having your baby. In this case, have a minimum size in mind, typically at least the low end of the "fertile zone," that you will not let yourself drop below, in order not to have to go through HA recovery all over again.

Recovering From HA After Baby

There are some folks who got pregnant without recovering fully. This is often through use of injectables or IVF, sometimes commenced prior to ever learning about the HA Recovery Plan, other times in concert with recovery. In any case, those who did not recover prior to pregnancy often want to do so before trying to conceive again. If this description fits you, you might want to go back and re-read part 2. Keep in mind that the first six months after your baby is born are challenging regardless of your circumstances; this might not be the best time to tackle recovery. It is probably best to wait until your baby is at least six months old so that you are not dealing with lack of sleep and the stress of figuring out your newborn at the same time as potentially struggling with a changing body image and altered exercise habits. But, as you start to think about weaning (if you were breastfeeding) and regaining cycles, going back to fully implement the Recovery Plan and experiencing all the benefits will serve you well, and give you an excellent chance of a natural second pregnancy.

The Slippery Slope Back to HA

While we've shared with you many quotes through the course of this book from people describing how much better they feel after recovery, there are still triggers that can spark unhealthy thoughts in each and every one of us even after we have resumed cycles and recovered mentally. Triggers that bring back the want—the need—to find control by reverting to old behaviors that feel safe and comfortable, even as we rationally know how unhealthy those behaviors are. We can never become complacent about our recovery. For some, these thoughts are fleeting and far between, while for others, they're a daily conflict. True recovery comes when you recognize the negative impulses, put them away, and continue to nourish yourself appropriately regardless of what your demons are telling you to do.

> *Elissa*: I think no matter how far we have come, we will always need little reminders to check ourselves. I truly feel in a completely different place than I was in HA land, and back to my usual self. However, I worry that I could slowly slip into overexercising and underfueling again if I become overly stressed. During my HA recovery, I adopted a habit of doing the opposite any time I had even the slightest negative thought about myself, felt the urge to overexercise, or thought about choosing the "healthiest" item and skipping the "unhealthy" one. Instead, I would think something positive about myself, have an extra dessert, skip my daily walk/workout or cut it short, etc. That approach helped me banish those negative thoughts and took away their power. Having a daughter now is a *huge* motivator for me to never pass these HA tendencies onto her, especially when she will already face a body-centric media and society.

Rachel: I absolutely still struggle and it's good to get a reminder that I need to pay attention to what I'm doing with my body. I do believe that HA recovery is like recovery from alcoholism—a lifelong journey, always with you, always requiring mindfulness.

Sarah W: I'm going to say this... I like being thin. I like how I feel thin. I was big for so many years and so miserable. Problem was when I got to my smallest (still technically a healthy BMI), I got negative attention again. I thought I couldn't win. And you know, I'm a very healthy 22-something BMI now and this should be me winning—I've been maintaining for months while eating well, indulging regularly and exercising healthfully—but no. I'm still plagued by wanting to be thinner. I'm not trying too hard obviously since I haven't lost weight in months. I know rationally I look good and am at a great physical place. The brain just has some catching up to do. There was a period in my mid to late twenties I weighed more than I do now and exercised similarly with zero issues. None. I was happy. I want that back, but since I've been off the deep end my head won't come to shore, sadly.

Phoebe: I struggle Every. Single. Day. My daughter is three, we're trying to conceive, and I cried on Saturday when I had to buy bigger pants. Ugh. I descended right back into my eating disorder and HA after she was born. I think it's the stress and having no control or time for yourself. Treatment is great, but it doesn't make everything go away all at once and it certainly doesn't make you not struggle. I will instinctively restrict if I don't consciously eat and it's such a constant still. I'm not saying I'm not better, I very much am, but I'm not perfect and I struggle. Remember that to be a mom you have to be a person first and you have to take care of yourself. My therapist always says that your "ED voice" goes away last. It's a matter of putting YOU first.

Natalie: I think it's nearly impossible to avoid the old thought patterns from time to time... even if we didn't have a history of HA, we are bombarded with terrible messages about how to look. I have overcome a lot of my issues and feel really good about where I'm at... but it's definitely a conscious effort to stay on that path and there are days where it's easier than others.

Liz S: I still struggle too. After I had my first I was better with eating, but I was working out as much as I could. I had less time to work out so I was not doing as much. I think most of us still struggle to find that healthy balance and to really accept who we are and know our self-worth is not based on a number or size.

Laurie: I'm not as hard on myself if I miss a workout or eat something high-calorie. I just always think about it and am aware in the back of my mind all the time, especially now that I'm not pregnant anymore. But we are all strong, overcoming, sensuous, so much more... and have to remember that.

Stacey H: I still struggle and actually made my husband promise me yesterday that he'd step in if I get any thinner. I haven't weighed myself since about 12 weeks postpartum but given how my clothes fit now I'm quite a bit below my pre-pregnancy weight (although still well above HA weight). I have to admit, I like it and don't do a lot of exercise but have started avoiding the heavier foods I used to eat... for example, I didn't replace the peanut butter when I finished it because I thought I went through it too quickly... stupid and I'm working on it. I think I may need to go and talk to a therapist as well.

Identifying, Preventing, and Coping With Triggers

It is valuable to recognize the causes of your self-doubt and negative thoughts so you can avoid them, or at least learn to respond differently. One way to think of your triggers might be to compare them to an ocean rip current. When a swimmer gets caught in one unawares, they are quickly swept out to sea with no control. Yet when prepared, they know to stay calm and not waste energy swimming against the current. Instead, they swim parallel to the shoreline, then slowly angle toward the beach—or waves their arms and yells for help until safely out of the strong current pull. For those who have recovered from HA (or are working on recovery), being confronted by triggers can result in old HA behaviors. But when prepared with a plan on how to respond, we can dodge the unhealthy reactions. Just like rip currents, triggers can be imperceptible, but when we learn to identify warning signs in advance, we can strategize how to cope. Whether it's setting boundaries with those who bring about negative thoughts, stepping out of the room to make a phone call to a friend, taking a deep breath and recalling affirmations, or seeking a counselor, having a plan in place to deal with triggers when confronted with them can make a productive difference.

Various circumstances, such as those listed below, can increase vulnerability to old ways and thought patterns:

- You feel your family is complete and therefore a working reproductive system is less critical.
- Stressors crop up in your life that you used to handle by food control or exercise.
- Time is at a premium and eating falls down your priority list.
- Specific people (often family) make comments, not understanding the potential effects of their remarks.
- Being around others who suffer from disordered body image, eating, or exercise habits.
- Returning to daily or weekly weighing.
- Feeling self-conscious about your postpartum body.
- Experiencing postpartum anxiety or depression.

Recognizing the situations that pertain to you can help you reflect on proactive steps you can take to prevent any relapsing.

Maintaining recovery after children. If you hope to have more children, the promise of another pregnancy soon to come makes maintaining recovery easier. With no additional children planned, remind yourself of all the other positive changes you have experienced. In fact, write down five reasons for remaining recovered right now.

Managing stress. If you are used to handling stress by controlling your food and exercise, it can be easy to fall back into those ways. Work on recognizing the issues and situations causing you to feel pressure, and use the tools suggested in earlier chapters to resolve the emotions.

> *Celena*: Stress is a trigger for me. I find when I am experiencing a stressful time, I have a tendency to increase my exercise. I am aware of it and try to eat more during these times. If I slip here or there, I have a pact with myself to stay above a certain BMI. I probably feel best even higher than that though.

Not finding or making time to eat. When you have small children, they come before you. Often they are so needy that you just don't manage to feed yourself while you're feeding them and changing diapers and doing the umpteen other things small children require. Or, if you're in the middle of a big project at work, it can be hard to take a break to feed yourself. If you find this is true for you (and perhaps find your HA self taking pleasure in the missed mealtimes), you have to be extra vigilant about adding extra calories when you *can* find the time to eat, such as after work or when the kids are in bed. Don't forget to make yourself some easy on-the-go, energy-dense snacks so that even if you can't eat a full meal, you aren't running on empty for hours.

> *Lindsey*: I am totally still struggling. While I'm not completely losing on purpose, I have a hard time finding time to eat during the day, and have started running again (because I love it, not to lose weight).

Family. Family can be particularly challenging. Years of ingrained patterns and responses are incredibly difficult to break. This in particular might be an area in which talking to a therapist or impartial outsider could be useful in order to find ways to defuse thorny situations.

> *Leah*: For me it's not so much a "what" as a "who." My husband's younger sister is freakin' thin, doesn't eat much, and runs marathons. She's also materialistic and shallow and I have a totally superficial relationship with her now. She's my trigger.

"Gym friends." If you feel jealous or wistful about your old body or training habits when you're around certain people, especially if comments about your new habits are made, you could consider avoiding those settings (e.g., the gym) or people. Other options include repeating your affirmations, and reminding yourself how healthy your lifestyle is, even if it doesn't conform to the ideal of "perfection."

> *Nicole*: Ugh, it's so hard for me now because I am a fitness instructor. I started teaching Zumba, which I love, but watching all of the super fit people walking around the gym obsessing about exercise is so hard for me to deal with.

Returning to the scale. Going back to frequent weight check-ins and letting your mood be affected by whether the number is up or down is another common sentiment. Most of us come from years of controlling our weight, and believing the societal decrees that "thin is good" and "thinner is better." If you did not get rid of your scale when you were recovering, or brought it back, consider reinstating your limits on weighing (i.e., no more than once a week), or tossing the scale altogether. You may even find that you enjoy the added freedom when you fuel yourself based on listening to your body instead of the scale.

> *Dawn*: I'm not restricting, doing moderate exercise three times a week and feel like I'm at a happy place ... but I still weigh myself and get upset

> if I see the number getting higher (though for the most part, it seems to have stabilized)—I get that panicky feeling and urge to restrict.

Body hatred or dysmorphia. If you find yourself feeling negative about your body, you can return to some of the ideas we discussed in chapter 11. When these thoughts arise, try to remember how incredible and miraculous your body is. It was able to reverse course, restore periods, bones, improve heart health, libido, GI distress, the list goes on and on. Maybe it was able to get pregnant, carry a child, and give birth to that child. It did this because you treated it well. Your body is an amazing gift. Turn those thoughts around and think of all that your recovered body has done and can do!

> *Nadia*: I don't have an outer trigger. My trigger is being over a certain weight. I was a bigger kid who was teased and bullied non-stop—including by my own family members. No one ever noticed me or listened to me. Then I lost weight and started getting attention. For me, being thinner means people like me and I won't have to face judgment. I am not OK with being heavier than that weight I've got stuck in my head.

> *Clover*: I was recently at the beach and a really attractive woman with a nice figure asked me how she could get rid of her "muffin top" so her stomach would look "flat" like mine. I cringed inside when she asked and replied by asking if she had children. She said she did, and I responded, "Consider your 'extra fluff and skin' a beauty mark of fertility and my flat stomach a mark of no babies." She smiled, recognizing the truth of that statement. Ladies, enjoy your baby-making body and whatever comes with it. There is absolutely nothing wrong with wanting to look hot, but please consider the truth that functional postpartum bodies are beautiful.

No matter how far you have come in your recovery, it is common to experience times of self-doubt. Just because you have some of these thoughts doesn't mean you are heading back to HA land; you now know how to stop those negative thoughts in their tracks. Even recovered HAers experience similar moments of past thoughts and behaviors from time to time. Here's a quick checklist of what DBT would call red flags (situations that put you on alert of impending slips). If you find that more than one applies to you, you may be falling back into HA ways and want to evaluate your choices:
- spending more than a few minutes a day thinking about negative aspects of your body
- eating on a time schedule
- consuming the same "safe" foods

- becoming irritated when you don't get your workout in
- frequent (daily or more often) weighing
- counting calories
- trying to "lean out"

If you recognize one of these red flags, what can you do? We suggest paying extra close attention to the situations you are in when these behaviors present themselves. Take some time to analyze your emotions. Can you identify what is precipitating the red flag reaction? Consider everything we have discussed so far in this chapter, or other potential triggers unique to you. After you discover what is causing your feelings, you can make plans to change either the situation or your response. If you need help, check in with your partner, a friend, or your therapist. Catch yourself early before you end up with HA again.

> **Sarah**: Work helps. Distraction is one way of coping with anxiety. Your brain is occupied with other things, unlike when you are at home with an infant or toddler and you have less "complex" things to worry about. You're also around adults and have more adult conversations. Honestly, I am just so busy with work and the kids that I don't have time to think or even really care about my appearance. Work is also a way to explore other parts of you. It's another identity to fill, rather than the HA/skinny/healthy one. Telling yourself a big mental STOP is helpful whenever you find yourself thinking numbers. Or even just asking yourself why you care so much. If you catch yourself calculating how many calories you've eaten or wanting a run, start asking yourself what is really going on… what are you really feeling? Are you trying to distract yourself from an uncomfortable issue or cope with pain or stress? There are a lot of body image books that can help. If you haven't, get rid of fitness magazines or women's magazines in general. Don't follow fitness blogs, etc. None of that stuff is healthy.

Bones and Other Systems

We have already discussed the evidence that weight gain and restoration of periods can have a significant positive effect on bone density, even in those in their late 30s and early 40s (well, at least it did for Amy S. and Clover, which means that it probably can for you too). There is much evidence that shows amenorrhea is detrimental to bone health and suggests that your heart and brain can suffer too. We hope the desire to keep yourself healthy through old age is enough of an incentive to prevent you from returning to your old ways. Many of us have said, "Well, I can always lose the weight after I have my babies," but have come to see over time that this is not a healthy mentality. We need our bones, heart, and brains to be in tip-top shape so we can continue to look after our babies for a long time to come—as well as to continue enjoying ourselves well into old age, rather than being prematurely relegated to a wheelchair, hospital, or assisted living. There are so many reasons to stick with recovery once you've gotten there.

> **Beth**: I have to keep reminding myself that it is not just my reproductive system or the other noticeable things like my hair, skin, and nails that have been harmed, but also the less obvious, more important areas like my heart, brain, bones, etc. When I read Gwyneth Olwyn's blog post[1] "Insidious Activity", which describes the damage to the heart that can result from restrictive behaviors—physical damage to muscles, electrolyte imbalances, and de-myelination of nerves—I remember thinking, "Wow, this is a lot more serious than I imagined." I thought that my recently low resting heart rate in the 40s (when most of my athletic life it had been in the 60s) was a sign of extreme fitness, when in fact, in the presence of restrictive behaviors, it could actually have been a sign of bradycardia. I was also experiencing tachycardia (sensation of my heart speeding up and beating hard for a couple seconds even when I was just lying in bed, often combined with the feeling of it skipping a beat) these past few months and realized that the last time this happened was when I was slimming down before my wedding a few years ago. I would also feel very dizzy many times when I stood up after sitting, even if I had just eaten and could rule out low blood sugar. Apparently this is a circulatory issue called "orthostatic hypotension" and can also be dangerous. I am thrilled to report that in the past month since I have been eating more and avoiding the gym, all of these issues have gone away. My resting heart rate is back up in the 60s!

Parting Thoughts

The main reason we wrote this book was to help others work through their eating and exercise issues, and come to realize that in the long term, life can be so much more than just focusing on being thin (for us) and fit. We hope that you are able to arrive at a similar place as many of those who have walked this route before you—one of eating freely, exercising for the enjoyment and health benefits, and having lots of time for the other important parts of your life, such as family, friends, and hobbies that make you smile.

> *Nico*: It has been almost nine years now since I overcame HA. I eat freely when I'm hungry, and sometimes when I'm not but there's a tasty option available. If I'm writing late at night and feel peckish I have a handful of nuts or a bowl of cereal or ice cream. When I'm eating, I stop when I'm full, unless dessert calls, in which case my second stomach takes over (witnessed by both Steph and Lisa). I enjoy my exercise. My motivation is no longer to burn calories; it's for the health of moving my body and pure enjoyment of my sport. Between raising my three boys and writing this book, I'm lucky to squeeze in ice hockey three times a week. I know that what I'm doing is healthy because I get my period every month. Despite nine years of recovery, though, there are times when my thoughts drift back to losing weight, often triggered by comparisons with others, the blatant posting of calories, or when I'm feeling sad about something. At those times, dropping a few pounds to "feel better about myself" seems attractive for a few minutes, but then I remind myself of all the good that is in my life, that I could probably use the "extra" calories, or that losing weight is not going to have any effect on the root of my unhappy feelings, and I get over it. My life is so much more now.

> *Steph*: About twice a year, I share my story of recovery with those fighting eating disorders in the hopes of inspiring them to never give up and to realize there is more out there. I want to leave you all with a similar message. Beyond our struggles with eating and exercise, there is a life worth living out there waiting for you. It took me years to get there. It was not easy and it was not fun, but it was 100% worth it. Each of us deserves that life. Never give up. Push through. Know that there is a light at the end of the tunnel and that we are always here for you.

> *Lisa*: I do believe for most it's a lifelong struggle. Even those of us who completely recovered at times sense the monkey on our backs, which seemingly comes out of nowhere. I personally equate the disordered eating and exercise journey to birthing pains, with varying intensities and frequencies. During really hard times is when we need to remind ourselves that these feelings will pass. It's all so temporary! Keep working on this and facing it head on … building healthier new coping skills to deal with life. This is the freedom we have all worked so hard for and earned.

Part 5:
Stories of Hope

Steph: During my first week of eating disorder treatment, I attended an event called "Hope and Inspiration." A monthly occurrence, this forum features a speaker who has recovered from an eating disorder. I felt privileged to listen, and I knew that one day I would be up there telling my story. Not just because it was important for me to regain my health, but because I wanted to help others and give back as well. Being able to hear a recovered person's story along with their struggles and successes aids in healing and gives the motivation to persevere, fight, and win. The speech helped me immensely at the time. And since *my* recovery, I have now spoken at Hope and Inspiration on many occasions.

The evidence of the continued success of the Recovery Plan in helping people regain their periods and health, and get pregnant if so desired, is contained in tens of thousands of posts on the Board. It takes weeks to read though the entire thread, if not longer. But the motivation gained from seeing the transformation of each person over time is priceless. In fact, it is often reading the story of someone "just like me" that finally convinces new members that their story can and will have the same happy ending. We've excerpted a number of stories in this section, and will include more on our blog at www.noperiodnowwhat.com.

29
The Road to Recovery

OVER SIX HUNDRED have posted on the Board sharing their battles with HA. Before actively participating, many found it helpful to read through earlier posts, gaining confidence from reading about others in a similar situation whose story culminated in recovery (and pregnancy). While each person's experience is specific to her, categories emerged that are more relatable depending on the HA factors in play. For example, your HA may be caused by overexercise or you may have both HA and PCOS. Therefore, we categorized the narratives we collected here to make it easy to find those that most resonate with you. Please keep in mind many of these stories were written in a time when we were still focused on body size, and didn't have an understanding of Health At Every Size, or how body size has been stigmatized.

1) HA caused by overexercise, undereating, or both—with some stress mixed in too
2) "normal weight" HAers; those diagnosed with HA at a starting BMI over 21
3) formerly larger HAers; lost significant weight and gained HA in the process
4) HA and mis-diagnosed with PCOS
5) HA and true PCOS
6) HAer with bone density issues
7) medical issues resulting in underfueling and therefore HA

Category 1: HA Caused by Overexercise, Undereating, and/or Stress

By far the most common form of HA involves both underfueling and overexercising, often along with stress from various sources. We share full accounts of Shirley, Erica, Helen, Katherine, and Casie, with short recaps from Emilie and Dawn. The accounts include steps that were taken to reach recovery as well as how pregnancies were achieved: some natural, some Clomid or Femara, along with injectables and IVF. We are confident that by reading through these journeys you will be equipped with more motivation through first hand insights as to the process of recovery and self-acceptance, and the journey to getting pregnant.

Shirley—Exercise and Undereating (recovery focus, natural cycles, then pregnancy with oral meds)

July 21, 2010—When I was 20, I was inspired to live a healthy lifestyle. I started going to the gym daily, eating healthier, etc. I unintentionally took it *too* far and didn't get my period for four months.

My doctor then prescribed Birth Control Pills, which I've been on for five years. A Band-Aid solution, but I didn't know much back then. Anyway, over the past five years, I recognized it wasn't healthy to restrict food and overexercise, but I continued to try and live a very active, healthy lifestyle.

I'm now 25, and ready to start trying for a baby...however, even though I went off BCP this past April, I still have not had a period. It's been three months.

I'm 5'7" and a BMI of 18, but keep in mind that I am VERY small-boned, so I am not as "skinny" as I sound. I definitely have love handles.

I visited the doctor last week; she agrees I'm lean, but doesn't think I'm *so* lean that it would impede ovulation. Perhaps it is the low-calorie diet (which I can agree with—1300 calories a day probably is low)... so she suggested to perhaps try to reduce exercise and increase calories to about 2000 a day. She said to check back with her in two months. So here I am, *very* motivated to ovulate and therefore eating a TON. For the past week, I have been eating probably close to 2500 (or even 3000) calories of healthy foods a day. It's kind of fun.

Lots of nuts, fruits, cheese, etc. And I want to shock my body a bit so I am not exercising at all. Just a few walks here and there. I want my period back as soon as possible!

August 7, 2010—I'm currently on week three of my "weight gain bonanza"—unlimited calories and no exercise. I'm waiting very patiently for my period to show up...

All my clothes are getting so tight, I feel bigger—and I'm worried that I'll just end up bigger *and* infertile.

August 23, 2010—A quick "what would you do" question: I've been off BCP for five months now, and no period. But thanks to the awesome advice on this Board, I'm six weeks into lifestyle changes, and have gained a bunch. Love handles abound because I have a very small frame, but I'm willing to do *anything* to get my period back. Anyway, I am definitely a "fertile" weight now, and walking briskly for 30 minutes just two to three times per week.

I'm hoping to go the natural route—waiting and waiting for my cycle to come back. I'm only 25, so time is on my side, but you know how once baby fever strikes, you want one ASAP! And of course, I'm worried that even if I wait six months, my period still might never show up. Arghh.

So, how many months do you think is reasonable to wait for my cycles to return naturally before jumping into treatment... Three months? Six?

> **Katherine N**: There are definitely differing opinions on this, but I would say to wait three to four months *after* reaching a healthy state. Right now your BMI is in the normal range, but with HA sometimes we have to get a bit higher to start cycling again. You have come really far in six weeks, awesome job! So maybe you try to gain to a BMI of 21 or 22, and once you are at that point, wait four months? That is what I would do; some people are willing to wait longer.

August 25, 2010—I'm just patiently waiting... I do notice I'm getting increasingly moist down there (sorry, TMI), and my beloved long-lost boobs are filling out my bras quite nicely.

September 19 2010—am making a list of **Reasons to Stay Positive** because I always feel better reading other posts like this.
- Out of all the causes of infertility, HA really is the "best" one to have. It's reversible; our parts are in working order but just on hiatus right now, which is *definitely* a reason to be grateful. I HAVE OVARIES! I HAVE EGGS! I HAVE A UTERUS! Score!
- It's a life lesson: Because I am so motivated to get pregnant, I am motivated to gain weight. And through this, I've learned that *life is too short* to restrict calories. Life is too short to cut giant bagels and alfredo

pasta from my life ... And after I eventually have a baby and try to lose the post-pregnancy weight, I will *not* go back to my old habits. This experience has taught me all about BALANCE ... and that truly, nobody cares about extra wobbly bits on me!

- In fact, this is a genuine wake-up call that it really *is* healthier to have wobbly bits. The media and health/fitness industry have skewed us into thinking you need a flat stomach to be "healthy."
- My definition of fitness is much more sustainable and fun—instead of working off as many calories as I can on a boring machine, fitness now consists of trying different classes: yoga, Pilates, dancing, etc. Who cares if I'm burning fewer calories per hour? Fitness is now something I can truly enjoy for the next 50 years, instead of being a chore.
- Realizing that everyone has a struggle. Whether it's infertility, financial, other health problems, relationship woes ... we don't get to pick our tough spots, but we sure are in control of how we respond.

October 2, 2010—I'm 2.5 months into lifestyle changes, a "healthy" BMI of 21, and my estrogen has gone up since two months ago. I tried the progesterone challenge but it's been six days since the last pill and nothing yet, so ... bleh.

October 14, 2010—I used to think it would *suck* to gain, say, 5 or 10 pounds ... so much that I would choose Diet Coke or aspartame-filled yogurt instead of natural, etc.

But now ... man oh man. It has been a blessing in disguise to go through this and gain some weight. I forgot how tasty lasagna is, how much more free time I have without the gym, and how fun it can be to eat a cookie or two without secretly counting how many calories need to be worked off later!

And actually, my former "potbelly" that always bugged me (when I was at my lightest!) now looks in proportion with the rest of my body—it doesn't make me look like a skinny pregnant woman anymore, which suggests that my body really was not balanced before.

October 18, 2010—So I called the ob-gyn to ask about getting an appointment. Apparently there are 70 new referrals ahead of me ... so I won't get in until February or March. *&&^^!! Can you imagine if I need a referral to the RE after that?

I am really, really, really hoping my cycles return before then. March would be a whole year after ditching BCP. Seeing as how I've already gained

25 pounds and stopped all cardio, I don't know what else to do. *has a pity party*

November 1, 2010—I am excited because I manage to score an ob-gyn appointment for December 16th. I am looking forward to her officially diagnosing me with HA... fortunately I figured that out myself months ago!

I'll beg and plead for a referral to an RE, since I bet the wait list is at least a year long (no joke). According to the receptionist, this ob-gyn does not do injectables, but she does do Clomid. If I still don't have my cycles by mid-January (six months after lifestyle changes), I decided I will go ahead and start the Clomid extended protocol.

In other news, for the first time in my life, I've been feeling sore nipples for about three days now. Some of you girls say that often happens after ovulation... but the thing is, I've had no egg white mucus? Maybe I did ovulate anyway? I guess we'll have to wait and see, I'm not getting my hopes up though.

November 13, 2010—I THINK MY PERIOD IS FINALLY BACK!! I have a light brownish stain on my panties (sorry for TMI, but it is from my girl-hole, because I rubbed a bit of tissue up there to make sure). I guess I'll know more in a few hours, but is that kind of what a light period (or "spotting") can look like? It's not all that reddish colored, though.

If it IS my period, that's *awesome* because roughly two weeks ago, I was suspicious that I was perhaps ovulating. And if I actually did ovulate when I felt those symptoms, it was a decent luteal phase too!

November 30, 2010—I'm chugging along. Feeling out-of-shape and so fatigued lately. I wonder if I've taken the whole "eat whatever" and no exercise thing too far. I tend to be an all-or-nothing kind of gal.

I'm 5'7" and roughly a size 8-10 now, which I have *never* been before in my life. I'm feeling rather helpless. I'm very small-boned, so this is bigger than I need to be. I know I should just let it be *for now*, as I don't want to scare my cycles away again as I got my first natural period in 5.5 years last month. I try and tell myself that I can lose a bit of this excess weight after having my baby, but still, it's hard to feel all my new rolls but not be pregnant to make it worthwhile. *sigh*

December 29, 2010—My biggest challenge these days is keeping busy. I find myself twiddling my thumbs in the evenings after work, not sure of what to do.

The weeks just crawl by ... I would really like to press "fast forward" on my life for about four weeks (or until my next ovulation). I'm sure many of you can relate to this "empty" feeling.

December 30, 2010—Dear Reproductive System,

It's me, Shirley. I really *really* want to make a baby. But I am not sure what's happening: I am spotting right now. What is it? Ovulation? A mini-period?

I confess, I secretly got excited and took a home pregnancy test with the two drops of pee that I could muster, which obviously came out negative.

Please don't forget about me. All I really want is to ovulate on my own, preferably every month. I think I'd be a good mom someday.

Sincerely,

A very confused Shirley

January 2, 2011—The Bright Side of HA Recovery:

- Boobs! Bazookas, or whatever you call 'em. Need I say more?
- Half my clothes don't fit anymore ... which means MORE ROOM IN MY CLOSET!
- And related to that ... an excuse to buy more clothes!
- Va va voom—forgot how it feels to be turned on!
- Ice cream! Chocolate bars! Muffins too!
- Less time at the gym equals more time with friends, family, and hobbies.
- The feeling of pride with every little thing my body does right, like cervical mucus (CM). I mean, who else would be proud of seeing CM?!

January 10, 2011—CD 57 and feeling so darn frustrated. ARGHHHHH :'(I'm getting so many mixed signals—it's good because it keeps me hopeful, but it also sucks because there are so many false alarms. On Saturday I had EWCM (I *think*, anyways), and dark OPKs (70% as dark). Sunday there was nothing—not much CM, and only faint OPKs. Today (Monday) my OPKs were 90% dark (internet cheapie and a Clearblue Ovulation test to confirm), but yet not much CM at all! On the other hand, no sore nipples, which is (retrospectively) what happened when I ovulated for the first time two months ago. I dunno, is it common to have different symptoms for each ovulation? *sigh*

We've been having sex every day (and will do it *at least* every second day) to cover our bases, but I am so sick of the rollercoaster of emotions. I've heard from others on the Board that it's normal to have several "false alarms" ... but sheesh, it's been almost TWO MONTHS of false alarms!

goes off and sulks

January 13, 2011—I had two *very* positive OPKs the last two days, and this morning my temperature was up. My nipples are a bit sensitive too, but maybe it's because I keep checking and rubbing them! Ha ha. Eeek! My first two week wait!

January 24, 2011—Today is 12 DPO. I was spotting yesterday and today too, I'm assuming it's the start of my period but I still have a wee bit of hope—it ain't over till the real flow arrives, right? Even though I told myself I wouldn't test today, I did, and got a Big Fat Negative of course. :(

March 24, 2011—Ugh. My temperature dropped way down today, 14dpo, and dear old Aunt Flo showed up in the afternoon. Boo. Back to "square one" (or Day 1, ha ha). I feel kind of cynical because both last cycle and this cycle, we had sex at all the right times. Waiting six weeks to ovulate each cycle is getting old.

I have my first appointment with the fertility clinic at the end of April—maybe they will let me try Clomid. I feel like I gave my body a real chance (no exercise, +25 pounds, and waiting for 8.5 long months…) I tried to stay positive throughout this entire journey, but now I'm tired of feeling so helpless. I'm ready for a little nudge from Clomid.

May 14, 2011—Now that I am on the "other side" (as in my cycles have returned), I am truly a thousand times happier than I was when I was restricting calories even though I'm still not pregnant. Food is enjoyment, and this basic enjoyment is an important part of living a happy life.

This is truly a lesson that our bodies do indeed need those calories—a lesson I was too scared to believe earlier. I worried that my metabolism was busted and that I needed to stay at 1100 cal/day forever… but our bodies bounce back! Believe me, *your body will speed up to accommodate the extra food intake!* And it will eventually find a happy, healthy weight to sit at.

May 16, 2011—I was frustrated and disappointed that it was CD 45 and no signs of an upcoming ovulation (last cycle's was CD 45), so I started taking Clomid *without* a bleed. For my own calculations, it was a "pretend" CD 5 through 9 dose…and now I here I am on "CD 14", about to ovulate in the next day or two! Woo-hoo!!

May 27, 2011—I am 11 DPO. I wasn't planning on testing until 12 DPO, but this morning I couldn't take my temperature because my cat knocked my thermometer off the bed stand and I couldn't find it. So I decided that to replace that very important morning ritual, I would pee on a pregnancy test… (and see a negative, and then move on)… but…

TWO LINES.

Then I used the Clearblue that I was saving for the weekend and got a +. Oh… my… gosh…

I am in utter shock. I really can't believe this at all! When I imagined what a positive test would feel like, I thought I would be dancing with joy, but I'm just completely SHOCKED!

After Shirley's daughter was born, she nursed for 16 months, ovulated four months prior to weaning, and got pregnant again on her first cycle trying to conceive. Shirley is still nursing her son (20 months), and her cycles resumed when he was eight months old.

Erica—Exercise, Undereating, and Stress (recovery focus, natural pregnancy)

April 29, 2012—I'm new to the forum, looking for some insight and advice. I went off the pill in February of 2011 and have not had a period on my own since. I was recently diagnosed with HA during my first visit with an RE. I'm trying Clomid to see if I can ovulate and get pregnant.

I'd never heard of HA until I was diagnosed and from what I've read so far, it seems it's often caused by being under-weight, overexcising, and stress. I love to eat—and I do—however, for the most part I am very healthy (lots of fruits, veggies, nuts, and whole grains) and I do track my calories. My average intake is around 1500 a day, maybe 500 more on weekends when I "let go." I work out four to five times a week for about an hour. It's mainly boot camp type classes, a spin class or two, 45 minutes on the elliptical, or an occasional outdoor run. My BMI is on the low end (19.5) but still in the "ideal" zone. My doctor thought that even if I gained five pounds, it wouldn't help me cycle and didn't seem too concerned.

In addition, I've been on medication for anxiety since middle school so stress is a constant factor in my life. I'm sure this is not helping matters.

I want advice. Do I need to completely stop exercising!? Working out is still healthy and helps relieve stress so I don't want to give it up completely.

May 1, 2012—I'm trying to wrap my head around HA. Like I mentioned in my first post, I never had an eating disorder, although I admit that for about the past three years, exercise and calorie awareness (definitely not normal) has been a constant in my mind. I always worry about how much

I eat and what I'm eating. If I'm out, I allow myself to eat because I love food (no self-control) and just count that day as a wash. I try not to have many of those. If I do eat more, I hope that working out will somehow even out the calorie intake. My gym advised me scientifically, 1500 calories a day would maintain my weight, which I thought was fine. Clearly not.

From what I've read on this board I could probably stand to eat some more, especially because of my exercise. If I ate more but still worked out, maybe skipped spinning, could this help? I just don't see how gaining fat and becoming out of shape is healthier. Maybe I'm taking it too literally.

I am thin but have always been. I am not emaciated looking in any way, I have some curves, good muscle tone. It is really scaring me that I might have to completely quit working out and gain weight to *maybe* get pregnant and if not, just be out of shape? I'm sorry if this sounds so shallow, I'm just trying to understand how to fix this so I can regain my cycles and get pregnant!

> **Laura**: Erica, I like you, was never diagnosed with an eating disorder, but I did not eat enough fat and ran and exercised too much! I was too thin and had barely any body fat. It has been hard for me to stop exercising, but not as hard as I had imagined. I used to be such a health *freak*. But now it is so nice just to relax and eat whatever the heck I want, and not worry about "when will I exercise today?" I want a baby so badly right now that I will do whatever it takes to help me to get pregnant. I know it's hard, but if all of us ladies can do it, you can too!

May 17, 2012—Update: I'm starting round two of 50 mg Clomid. I found out that from here on out, I have to pay $500 a visit for basic blood work and a two-minute ultrasound. It doesn't look like we're going to be able to keep this up, which is sad. The total is $1500 for one cycle's worth of monitoring!

I'm feeling defeated. I'm afraid I have a long road ahead of me, and I'm frustrated. I don't want to have to worry about this. I wish I could just throw my hands up, eat some more calories, and get my period back in a few months, but it's a lot easier said than done.

May 18, 2012—I've been laying low the past four weeks. I've been doing a couple days of 30 min elliptical routines and some yoga, mostly just walking. Is that too much? I *really* miss all my friends in my boot camp classes. It takes everything not to join them when I'm at the gym. I sit there like a sad puppy on the treadmill watching them. LOL. It's driving me nuts. I also feel like all my clothes are tight already (perhaps a bit more in my head than reality but we'll see).

I went on vacation for a few days last week and weighed myself the morning I got back and my BMI was up to 20.6. Granted that was probably a lot of water weight since we ate like absolute crap. But I think I could easily put on some pounds, I just want to see something positive come out of it.

I talked to my RE and we can reduce the cost to about $500 for the entire cycle (three weeks or so) by eliminating some ultrasounds. I may give it one more go then wait for a while and see what we can do on our own.

May 19, 2012—This past week, I've allowed myself to order a grilled cheese and fries (normally only allowed on weekends) and I had cookies and cream ice cream, wine, and cheesy pasta (non-whole grain). I was very anxious at first but you're all right, it is *so* freeing not to obsess about my food! I'm sure there may be a few setbacks but it's a step in the right direction. As I was writing this, I was debating whether or not to go to the gym this morning but you all helped pull me back. I'm going to put in my yoga video, do some housework instead and be OK with it. Wish me luck!

June 27, 2012—On the issue of pants being snug, I've finally gotten to the point where I pull them up and if they're too tight, I immediately throw them in the "giveaway" pile so I'm not tempted to try them on again and feel like crap. Buy some new ones! I like to buy a little big too because it makes me feel better than wearing tight clothes all the time.

September 8, 2012—Just wanted to give you an update that we're taking a break from meds until January so I've been taking a mental break from the board and thinking about things. Side note: it's actually been quite refreshing. Knowing that I might not be able to get pregnant for the next few months has made me focus on other things. Anyway. I started temping for the first time after my last period from Femara and I ovulated *on my own*, on CD 16. Today, I'm 11 DPO and my period arrived lightly this morning. I'm *so* thrilled to have a natural ovulation, despite not being pregnant.

I asked my doctor if any meds were still in my system and she said, "Absolutely not, it's all you!" It gives me huge peace of mind that I'm able to do things on my own again. I hope you all find some comfort in this and know that with weight gain (I gained about 15 lb, into the "fertile" zone), decreasing workouts, and eating more fats, you can achieve a natural cycle again.

January 19, 2013—OK ladies, I'm cautiously optimistic but I took a pregnancy test today (11 DPO) and it was positive! I almost fainted!

I emailed my RE since I had no idea where to go from here since I'm not being monitored by her. She wants me to come in for blood work so we'll see what happens. Fingers crossed!

January 31, 2013—I wanted to update you and tell you that I unfortunately miscarried. It's an awful feeling, very defeating after all the work I've put into this, but I want a healthy baby and if this wasn't one, then I understand. It doesn't make it much easier but it's a bit comforting. I'm feeling OK, I miscarried naturally and the doctor said everything looks clear on the ultrasound so I should just be able to continue doing what I'm doing and the bleeding should stop in a few days. I know some of you have gone through this and it is reassuring to hear that many of you got pregnant again with successful births. I hope that I can get here again too.

Erica got pregnant again two months after her miscarriage and now has a healthy baby boy. She weaned at 2.5 weeks postpartum and her cycles returned 1.5 months later. Erica conceived again 18 months later on her first cycle trying.

Helen—Exercise and Undereating (recovery focus)

October 25, 2012—I'm new to the Board but have suffered with HA for 10 years. Here in the UK they simply say I have "unexplained infertility" but I know it is a result of HA. I'll be honest I'm my own worst enemy with exercise and food but this Board is giving me hope I can change!

My stats: I'm 5 feet exactly, BMI around 19. Because my BMI is "in the healthy range" I've always resisted weight gain but reading your stories it sounds like I might be wrong! I have reduced exercise to half an hour gym sessions three days a week and a two-hour bike ride on the weekend which is a huge scale back from the 60 miles a week I was running. Recently I had a stress fracture of the hip and I am worried now about my bone density. My HA began when my first marriage broke up—all at once I started running, came off birth control and lost 7 lb to my current weight. I am 32.

October 25, 2012—I am interested to find out if weight gain is the key to recovery? I've been told so many times it's unlikely to help. I'm sure going to give it a try though! It seems stress is also a huge factor in body responses—I am sure it was divorce that triggered mine. Problem is, now it's stuck on off. No health care professional has been able to help me; I've been trying to reverse my HA for 10 years now. I'll pretty much try anything for fear of osteoporosis.

October 27, 2012—Increasing calories is not proving as difficult as I imagined mostly due to a suppressed love for food!! Exercising is a different story, I love to cycle, run, and swim, so am missing it massively. I know the end result far outweighs anything but without your support I'd weaken I know it! I can't believe after 10 years I am finally going to do this!

October 29, 2012—It hurts me to think of all I missed out on the first time I was pregnant and the subsequent damage I've done. I conceived my daughter on Clomid with a BMI around 20, but was so scared to gain through my pregnancy I swam a mile every day to the day I gave birth. My little girl was fine but six days after she was born I had no energy or milk to feed! I was so proud upon leaving the hospital that I was already back to my pre-pregnancy weight, having gained nothing at all. My daughter is two now and I have spent many a day baking with her and refusing to eat the cookies etc. What a waste of a beautiful gift. As I write the tears roll down my face realizing what I do on a daily basis to further compound my HA and potentially deprive her of a brother or sister. I am so determined to get better and finally have the life I want. I do not want to be the one who spends the entire day stressing on when I can fit a workout in, or not have a beer for fear of the calories!

Today I feel terrible, bloated, and really low. The demons are there but we must use the support to get better. I ask myself, do I want to be the person everyone looks at and says "what a wonderful fun loving woman who enjoys life as a mommy" or the one they describe as "sick and skinny looking who's no fun with no energy"? Three years ago I refused to gain and pushed my RE for medications. I refused see the simplest solution. Don't do it. Don't waste any more of your life.

November 17, 2012—I had my first session with my alternative therapist today. We spent 90 minutes discussing a lot! The therapy element really helped as it's the first time I've put everything together that's going on in my life and looked at the whole picture. She believes most of my fertility problems stem from nourishment issues (no revelation there!). She helped me look in depth at the real problem areas for me like planning meal times rather than eating whilst driving or working etc. She was not concerned at all about weight when she saw I was gaining but did raise concerns that I was still not nourishing myself with protein and fat (I exist on bagels, cereal, coffee and OK I'll admit it, a gin and tonic most nights!) I know my calories are high enough as I'm gaining but I'm still a long way from being healthy and nourished. My "homework" this month is to add protein to *every* breakfast: eggs, fish or cheese. A typical morning meal right now is tons of sugary cereal, extra dried fruit, and no milk! We also worked on other stress areas in my life and finished with half an hour of reflexology and acupuncture, which was wonderful.

Totally unrelated my nipples are tender today... maybe my body is responding to the gain? My CM is still quite plentiful too. Here's hoping hey!

November 18, 2012—Who sent the exercise sabotager (is that a word?) out after me?? I decided as it was such a beautiful day and I've gained 10 lb, to treat myself to a leisurely cycle with a friend. Just 30 seconds into the ride, I lost the back wheel and hit the deck, hard, head first. Twenty minutes later I ran over something and my tire was punctured. Just after I fixed that, punctured again and had to be rescued by car! OK I get the message, NO EXERCISE!

November 21, 2012—All my symptoms (cramping, CM) disappeared so I'm not sure what's happening. An ultrasound showed a very thin lining three weeks ago so can't imagine too much. I guess it's carry on eating and falling off my bike (hahahaha!). I just got cinnamon rolls out of the oven for breakfast tomorrow... oops, one didn't survive to breakfast!

November 25, 2012—Today I got my period!! It was totally unexpected—no symptoms, it was just there. My husband thought I'd completely lost it when I ran into our kitchen shouting and yelling but given the last time I had a period without the aid of medication or BCP was 1996 I was pretty darn excited! He just rang now as he's gone back to work to tell me how proud he is of the changes I've made to allow this to happen. I know the road to conception might still be a long one but I can truly say that without the support of this Board I would NEVER have done this by myself. So thank you, sincerely!

November 26, 2012—When I found the Board in September I decided that enough was enough: I wanted to live again but more importantly I wanted to start trying for another baby. From then on I've gone all in. Exercise has decreased from upwards of four hours per week (which is actually still low for me, I was doing around two hours daily from 2005-2008) to a bit when I feel like it—because I want to, *not* because I have a requirement or have indulged. I also started to regard food as it should be, necessary and a pleasure. For as long as I can remember it has only been a reward or to be avoided. I've upped my weight 10% in 12 weeks so pretty full on giving it my all—eating a lot more healthy fat and generally more calories. I'm far from a perfect example; most evenings are a series of snacks with no meal in sight but I do try to eat a big cooked lunch and have generally just relaxed about everything, tried to forget numbers both in a calorie sense and time spent exercising. I also haven't fixated on where I want to gain or not gain, I have just let go. I'll be honest the softening of the belly and expanding of the thighs has been a killer but each night I've gone to bed having not restricted or exercised through compulsion I've smiled and realized, "OK I'm not skinny anymore—I'm normal in many ways and that's something to embrace!" then I get up and try to do it again. To those of you not giving recovery your all, I've been doing that since 2008 and got *nowhere*. It wasn't until I dived in head first and stacked the weight on quickly that things really changed for the better. Maybe I just kicked the heck out of my system finally!?

January 17, 2013—On other matters I have ditched the scale; weighing myself makes me feel worse than I should about my body. Looking in the mirror I am beginning to accept things but then I see the numbers and freak out. So there you go—now I don't know my weight or BMI and don't want to! I have been unable to do any exercise for a week due to various circumstances and this has freaked me out a little. I got marginally panicky about it yesterday, so I know the demons are there... that said, I did just slap them back with a Cadbury Fudge chocolate bar!

February 9, 2013—I'm on CD 2 of my fourth natural cycle since joining the Board in October. I'm not pregnant but heck it looks like I might actually have beaten this damn HA. This cycle was 36 days so coming down in length too (42 and 40 previously) although my LP was still only eight days so progress is still needed. I may say I have beaten HA although I have certainly not beaten all that resulted in it—but you know what? I actually believe now I can and I wanted to share this with those who believe this is only about getting pregnant. When I joined I thought, OK, I'll do what I need to have another baby and then great off we pop to the track to run the "baby fat" off—WRONG, BAD! Answer these questions honestly: do you want to be liberated of the feeling of compulsion to exercise? Do you want to wake up full of life ready to embrace the simple pleasures in each day? Holding on to destructive tendencies (as I have done for too long) will never allow you to recover. If deep down you think "Once I have this baby I'll go back to my old ways" you will be back here again and again; that I know firsthand. I feel like the luckiest person alive—I have a beautiful daughter—and yet here I am unable to give her a sibling (which she asks for weekly as all her friends have brothers and sisters). I have told them in person but a few people on this board gave me some really smart advice that has finally given me my life back: some days I'm low, some days I battle but I don't give up! I stay off the treadmill and still eat and yes, I'm gaining, yes I'm softening—but I also smile more, I have more energy, and I *love* having time to do fun stuff like cake baking and nature walks or building snowmen! Before when life was consumed by fitting in workouts I never did these things and that is a real shame!

April 30, 2013—Officially I am now only a cheerleader; we are taking a break from trying to conceive until Christmas as I will be starting nursing school in September.

August 21, 2013—For everyone struggling it gets easier I promise! I made changes in October of last year, by December I was cycling naturally having gained 14 lb and cut all exercise. Since May I have added in small amounts of regular exercise. My weight gain stopped but I have never tried to drop any of the gained weight as I know by eating and fueling I can be active and healthy and hopefully again soon conceive naturally. The recovery is hard but it is so worth it! Living a balanced life where food is a pleasure and small amounts of exercise promote wellbeing is a liberating feeling and one you will all get to as well as getting pregnant along the way!

I have to stress though you *must* in the initial stages be committed to change. Gaining can be emotionally draining but I am firm believer that all my problems stemmed from lack of fuel! Stopping ALL exercise and eating is the only long term solution. Currently we are not trying to conceive for family reasons but I am confident all the changes will make the whole process a whole lot easier in 2014.

Helen conceived just a few months later on her 14th natural cycle. After her baby was born she nursed for 12 months. Three months later, she's hoping to start cycling soon!

Katherine—Overexercise and Undereating (recovery and pregnancy focus, oral meds)

April 12, 2011—I'm new to HA and wanted to introduce myself. What a wonderful, supportive community you have here! I am a pediatrician and a runner. I had normal periods as a teenager that became irregular when

I was a scholarship athlete in college. I've been on BCP from the end of college until six months ago when my husband and I decided we wanted to start a family. I'm 5'7", BMI around 21, and 8.3% body fat according to the recent analysis by the nutritionist. The same nutritionist measured my resting metabolic rate based on exhaled CO_2 and apparently I require 1941 calories per day *without* any exercise.

I haven't had a period since going off the pill. My common sense suggested that I had HA (the first three months off the pill I was running five to six miles every morning, biking about 12 miles at lunch every day, and doing P90X with my husband in the evening six days a week). I am not a restrictive eater, but I tend to have a very healthy diet and don't consume enough calories during the day to make up for all of my activity (then tend to be starving in the evening so I'd eat a big bowl of ice cream every night). So, my eating is kind of disordered since I have a relative calorie deprivation during the day and lots of calories in the evening. And I have a huge problem if I am not allowed to exercise. Seriously, running to me is like a cigarette to a smoker or a shot of vodka to an alcoholic. I do not know how to enjoy my day if I can't exercise. I feel sad and anxious if I can't run, whereas I feel like a totally normal, happy, well-adjusted person if I'm allowed to get my fix.

I had convinced myself that I had PCOS, which is why I was refusing to give up my running for the past six months (feared I would gain lots of weight, become hairy, and have acne). However, failing the Provera challenge solidified the HA diagnosis for my ob-gyn.

I think it is time I face the truth about the cause of my amenorrhea and start some lifestyle changes. Today I walked instead of my morning run and I cried the whole way. This makes me seem like a total psycho to normal people, but I would imagine many of you can understand. So, I'm starting the road to recovery.

May 2, 2011—Do any of you ever feel like this is AA for running addicts where we come for support and encouragement as we try to break an addiction that is interfering with our life goals? In AA tradition, I should say, "Hello, my name is Katherine, and I am a running addict. It has been one day since my last run." I must admit that I really fell off the wagon this weekend and went for a nine mile run. I had been very disappointed this week feeling like I wasn't making any progress, and I just cracked today. I ran far and fast, and it felt terrific. But I know it was a set-back from my goals and it will make it even harder to work on running less again this week. Cursed running-induced opiates. I swear I crave them like a smoker craves a pack of cigarettes after a Trans-Atlantic flight.

May 3, 2011—I have some great news to share this morning—my first ever positive OPK! It was so exciting to see the smiley face! It is a good thing I was using them this week because otherwise we were planning on abstaining today and tomorrow because my husband's semen analysis is scheduled on Thursday. Also I have an appointment with my doctor today where I was about to cave in to my desire to hurry things along and try Provera again in preparation for Clomid. But it certainly looks like we should try to give this a shot on our own this month.

May 3, 2011—Thanks for all the congratulations on my (hopefully impending) natural ovulation! It has really helped me to be reading this board for the past six weeks (that is the only time I have been *really* consistent about my lifestyle changes). For the six months preceding that, I would cut back on exercise for a week or two, then freak out and exercise a bunch again, etc., never making any progress until six weeks ago when I finally saw the hard facts (low estrogen, body fat <10%, and no withdrawal bleed after Provera). It took all of that data for me to really admit it was my exercise and inadequate caloric intake causing this problem. Knowing that you are all going through the same thing really helped me stay consistent with reduced exercise and increased fat and calories.

I know this may be only the beginning of a long path to pregnancy, but I'm certain that eating more and exercising less are going to be key to my recovery. For those interested in what changes I had to make to get my first natural ovulation, my BMI increased by 1.5, exercise went from three times a day run, bike, strength train, to a two mile walk/jog and 30-minute slow beach cruiser ride with at least one day completely off per week, and for my diet I added nuts, peanut butter, eggs, and more ice cream. I may have to cut back more on the exercise to successfully get pregnant, but I think the ovulation is a good sign that I'm making progress.

I do think we are all on the right track with the lifestyle change even though it is so hard to get used to. Thanks for all the support!

May 9, 2011—Today was a really bad day for me. I had blood drawn to confirm that last week's positive OPK actually translated to ovulation, but the progesterone level showed that I did not in fact ovulate. It was *so* incredibly disappointing; it was all I could do not to cry until I got home from work. I guess I will start Provera today and see if I have a withdrawal bleed. I haven't before, so I may not again, but either way, I'll start Clomid five days after finishing the Provera. Ugh. This is so discouraging.

May 16, 2011—My withdrawal bleeding started today! Exactly 72 hours after the last Provera pill. I am on track for Clomid on Wednesday—yay!!

May 18, 2011—I forgot to mention a funny story from today. I was riding my bike at lunch. Got a flat tire. Stopped, changed the tire. Two miles later, another flat. Now I was running on a gravelly road in my socks (since my bike shoes have clips on the bottom), carrying my road bike, in the rain, trying to make it back to clinic in time for afternoon patients. All this time I have my thumb out trying to hitch a ride back. Finally, a nice man stopped and drove me back to work. Now I have blood blisters on the bottoms of my feet from running in the gravel.

Does anyone else think fate is conspiring to try to get me to stop exercising? Two flat tires in one day, now blood blisters on the bottom of my feet makes it very difficult to run and bike. I will try to sit still tomorrow!

May 27, 2011—The second line on my OPK was a bit darker today, my boobs are getting much bigger, and my ovaries kind of feel like they might explode. So I think Clomid is doing something. Whether or not it is doing the right thing remains to be seen, but I'm feeling good about it!

May 29, 2011—Can someone tell me some success stories of girls on this Board who ovulated late with Clomid and ended up pregnant? I'm getting nervous that today is CD14 (the seventh day after my last Clomid pill) and I haven't seen an LH surge. I'm getting a faint second line on the OPK still and I've been doing it twice a day for the past four days). I am terrified that it isn't going to work and I had been so optimistic for the past three weeks. My biggest fear this cycle is not ovulating even with the help of Clomid. Ugh.

June 1, 2011—I'm still waiting to ovulate. I think I may not have cut back enough on exercise for the Clomid to work even though my weight and body fat are fine now. We'll keep "trying" daily through the weekend but I'm just not sure it is going to work.

June 9, 2011—Effffffffffffffffffff. Progesterone 1.41. I didn't ovulate.

I really think you all are right that I need to stop exercising. Even though I have cut down my overall exercise substantially, I still have been jogging a slow two miles four to six days a week and biking at lunch several days.

What this seems to have accomplished is make me miserable but still not convince my body that it is safe to make a baby.

I think I need to NOT run. *At all*. I remember a month ago when Nikki said she was going to go cold turkey and I thought she was so brave and I hoped it wouldn't come to that for me. You know how you always hope if you just cut down a little bit more that it will do the trick? I thought adding Clomid would get me over the edge since I had cut down so much I hardly felt like I was exercising, but it seems my body is refusing to ovulate until I stop running.

I read one of the studies posted way back on this board about LH pulsatility in recreational runners[1] (who were only running 18 miles a week) and even the ones who were menstruating were only ovulating 46% of the time. So I really think the running must mess with LH pulsatility enough that I can't get a decent LH surge. Both times that I've gotten a positive OPK have been after two consecutive days of no running (this is rare for me), so it must be related.

I think I am going to try to not run at all for one solid month and see what happens. No new meds, just no running. Will you guys try to keep me sane during this?

June 18, 2011—To those that have asked about how I'm doing with the exercise ban, it is going really well. There are days where I am angry that other people can work out and still have babies, then there are days where I look in the mirror and see my curves and think I look quite fertile now, this must be what nature intended. My husband has taken to calling me "curvalicious," which is pretty funny. He digs the new shape, and tells me a thousand times a day how great I look, which really helps. He is such a trooper for putting up with my insanity. The stir-craziness sometimes gets bad, but most days I'm handling it pretty well. Getting rid of caffeine really made a big difference; I didn't feel so much of the constant urge to "get going."

June 27, 2011—My RE appointment was beyond disastrous. To start with, the RE refuses to see patients on the initial visit. So I was meeting with a nurse practitioner who would leave the room to talk to the RE and then come back to me. The highlights of this visit:

1) "You should try one more month of Clomid at 150mg and if that doesn't work, then do injectables."
2) "I'm not sure if your diagnosis is PCOS or HA, it doesn't really matter, the treatment is the same."

3) "You are lucky you are meeting with me (the nurse practitioner) and not one of the first year residents. You know it is almost July, right?" (When all the new residents start.)

4) "We don't do ultrasound monitoring with Clomid, either you'll ovulate or you won't. If you don't, then move on to injectables."

5) After me asking a few questions about different possibilities like Clomid with an hCG trigger, she says "If you think you can manage yourself better than the doctor, then go ahead."

6) "The most important thing is we repeat your FSH on day 3 since you might have premature ovarian failure and not respond to treatment at all." For the record, I've had my FSH checked three times and it was always between 5.8 and 6.3, so clearly I do not have premature ovarian failure.

After all of this, they conceded to do an ultrasound today, which showed multifollicular ovaries and no dominant follicle. Boo.

The "plan" they left me with is to wait two weeks and take a pregnancy test. If it is negative (i.e., I do not experience an immaculate conception from my non-existent dominant follicle), then they will have me take Provera. On the seventh day of withdrawal bleeding from Provera, they want me to have an HSG. After the HSG and repeating a bunch of labs I've already had drawn, then the doctor will actually meet with me to "discuss what to do next."

Since I am in the military my only alternative to this doctor is to go out in town and pay entirely out of pocket. I have been crying for the past two hours and I can't believe I have to see patients in 15 minutes.

June 28, 2011—Thank you girls all for the support. It really means so much to me. I know you all understand, and that really helps. I'm feeling much better today. I think I'm going to give Clomid another try. If I ovulate, I'll do the HSG after I get my period then follow up with the RE. If I don't ovulate with the Clomid again, I'll take Provera, get the HSG and follow up with the RE.

I'm hoping the doctor herself won't be as terrible as the NP I met with. I don't think they'll push me into injectables before I'm ready, but it does sound like I'll have to choose to continue Clomid without monitoring or go onto injectables. I imagine I'll give Clomid a few more rounds with my lifestyle changes, then if it doesn't work, it will be OK to move onto injectables. I guess I had just expected with some tweaking (trigger shot or estrogen/progesterone supplements, etc) that I'd eventually get pregnant with some sort of Clomid regimen, so I hadn't really faced the idea of injectables.

Being a pediatrician, I've worked in the NICU and many times triplets and higher order multiples do not do well so it is not something I am willing to risk. That means if I end up doing injectables, I'll either be more likely to have to cancel cycles if I overstim or face the possibility of selective reduction, which I know would not be easy. This is what scares me about doing injectables.

So, now to decide whether to try Clomid 50 mg again as I'm not exercising and at my body's "happy weight" or 100 mg. Pregnancy rates are higher with 50 mg than 100 mg since there are fewer anti-estrogenic side effects, but if I don't ovulate, then obviously my pregnancy rate would be zero.

July 8, 2011—It is official. My hypothalamus has finally returned from its long vacation! It took many positive OPKs for me to believe this is not a false alarm, but they kept getting darker throughout the afternoon and now the control line is a faint glimmer compared to the test line. So, I'm no longer worried about getting my hopes up. This is totally different from my other mini-LH surges in the past; I'm actually going to ovulate this time. Hooray! (Today is CD15, six days after my last Clomid pill.)

July 19, 2011—OMG. I peed on a stick when I got home from work (11 DPO). There was a *very faint* second line. I thought I must be hallucinating. I took a second test, same brand, *very faint* second line. Third test, different brand, no second line.

I read the test within five minutes (the line appeared at about the three-minute mark). So it shouldn't be an evaporation line, right?

I'm so excited but also afraid it isn't real at the same time. The second line is so faint I'm too embarrassed to ask my husband to look at it and give a second opinion because I'm afraid he'd say, "What second line?"

Why don't any of you live in my town so you can come over and look at my pee stick and tell me if it is for real?! Please, oh please, let it get darker tomorrow!

July 20, 2011—It's the real deal. Big Fat Positive!!! The line is darker than yesterday and my temps started climbing again today at 12dpo, so I'm sure I'm pregnant! Thank you so much for all the congratulations—I never could have done this without you all!

Katherine regained cycles at 21 months postpartum, while continuing to nurse her daughter. She conceived her second child, a boy, one month later on her first cycle trying.

Casie—Exercise, Undereating, and Stress (recovery focus, IVF for male factor that failed, natural cycle)

March 28, 2012—I have never posted on a forum before, but it seems that there is a lot of info and experience to gain from others. I am very interested in timeline to recovery. I know that everyone is different and BMI is just a number, but how long from achieving a good BMI have others experienced a spontaneous cycle? As for my story... I use exercise to reduce stress since my job is very high stress with demanding hours. I was on BCP for more than 10 years, and stopped in the spring but no period. I have now cut my exercise like crazy and am eating more, mostly carbs because those are my favorite. I added fats too, except for the week when I was on Provera where I could barely tolerate food (counterproductive much?). My BMI is already up to around 22ish.

April 5, 2012—I am very encouraged to give the lifestyle changes a fair try. In fact, I haven't exercised more than walking for two weeks. Plus, with all the fat and carbs I've added I am sure I will hit a good weight in no time. I actually went on a scale for the first time in months, and my suspicion was confirmed that I have gained 10 to 15 pounds since January (BMI 21.9). As I didn't truly cut the exercise to this extent until now, I hope this will pay off sooner rather than later. A friend recently scared me with her IVF stories and having to take off work for a month. It definitely made me reach for extra sweet potato fries when out for dinner with my colleagues last night.

April 26, 2012—I have definitely put on the pounds. I don't own a scale so hop on occasionally at the hospital at work. I have gained around 20 lb in just over a month, which puts my BMI at about 22.8. I know that's good, but now I want to stay put. I don't really count calories but my guess would be that I have been eating way over 3500. Plus, I think I had mostly an exercise problem—so maintaining will be a new challenge I guess. Sadly, I don't look curvy, I pack it on like a football player in my arms and torso and face... Hence the tears.

May 4, 2012—No real news on my front. Now CD 30 after Provera. No + OPK, no period, and definitely no fitting into my clothes. I went and bought a new wardrobe for work. I'm still having CM but there's no pattern to that either. It was the most last week while I was out of town. Then drier and sticky, now more clear?? It's so hard to tell. Either way I will get labs done on Monday to check my TSH (as it's been crazy high in the past), and will check estradiol and progesterone then too...

May 25, 2012—I have been at a BMI of 22-22.6 (depending on how tall I stand up) for almost two months. No period yet. As of my last blood work, I'm still stuck in the follicular phase with low E_2. I have been titrating up my thyroid meds since I was under treated in February and was quite hypothyroid (high TSH). Since it's not recommended to even "try" to conceive until my TSH is under 3, I am waiting another week and half to see if that's at target. I will recheck the other hormones then too.

June 18, 2012—I am a bit overwhelmed with the weight gain. After I stopped the exercise, I gained 25 lb in about three months! It was intentional, but it still hard. (It raised my BMI 2ish points, getting close to 23). The worst part I guess, is that nothing has happened yet. No period.

Actually the worst part is that my husband was tested and his numbers are suboptimal as well. I am really hoping to hear if anyone has had experience with this, as far as I understand this likely destines us for IVF only?

June 21, 2012—My mom told me that it's time to stop gaining; shouldn't this be enough? I tried to explain rationally that who knows what enough weight gain is and what is too much exercise. But then I get frustrated and just stop talking about it.

September 16, 2012—Eating is great as always–I never had trouble with that (likely why I gained weight so quickly). Now that my BMI has settled into the 22.5-23 range, I have gone back to some healthier eating... I stopped the extra unnecessary foods like cookies etc., unless I want them. A big change for me was cutting the low-fat yogurt (which was a staple) and replacing it with copious amounts of almond butter and other fats with every meal. Really though, trying to eat like a normal person. The exercise I still desperately miss. Since I have to wait for two months until IVF (due to sperm issues) I have now added back some light elliptical (my equivalent to "walking") and mostly on the weekend but I never sweat and don't even get close to the hour plus mark as before. I look forward to exercising again in the future. The stress part... well eight weeks and counting until my life gets less stressful. I just need to start enjoying my new curves, since that stress is unnecessary and I need to completely get over it... as you all know, there are good days and bad days.

October 21, 2012—The last time I was on here, I was taking estrogen pills to see if my lining would respond. A test run to give the RE some prediction of future response I guess. My lining perked up to about 6 mm in two weeks. Now I'm on progesterone (with the estrogen too). Ugh. I've taken it for two nights and already broken out. But not as much cramping as last time.

Ten nights to go then it will be CD 1 and IVF starts. I'm quite nervous. But I have been amazed at the number of colleagues and mentors who have told me they are or have gone through this so I have a support system in place (other than this one of course).

We are thinking of this round as a trial run to see how I react. After the orientation a while back, my husband couldn't believe how many stages there were for failure. It's amazing that this ever works!! But at a BMI of almost 23 I am doing everything I can to give it the best chance.

November 12, 2012—I started my IVF stimulation just about a week ago, it's now day nine. Things are going OK I think. My scan showed steady growth. Today my E_2 jumped up from 492 to 1700 pmol/L (Canadian units) so I am continuing as is with my next appointment on Wednesday. Perhaps then we can talk about retrieving. "Lots of moving parts" as my hubby says. We're taking it one day at a time. It helps that I am really good at following directions. The monitoring is interesting. It's a first come, first serve clinic—super annoying. But obviously I am the first or second one there each time, I am sure you all would be too.

November 19, 2012—I had my egg retrieval this morning. It was OK—a lot of prep time for a short procedure, like most things. They "snowed" me with the drugs so I actually slept through most of it, in fact missed the watching the first ovary on the screen (this was not intentional apparently, as they were anxiously arousing me in the middle). Then I was nauseated for a bit after. I had lots of eggs retrieved. My E_2 level on Sat was only 8764 pmol (2387 in the USA units) so I think that calculates to about 10 mature eggs. If there are that many, I will be very pleased. Cautiously optimistic I guess. I will know more on Wednesday afternoon when I get "the call."

Otherwise, I had to be weighed at the hospital today (to dose the drugs) and I am much closer to a BMI of 23 than a 22 ... so hopefully this will help the cause. Oh, and if it makes it that far, this clinic doesn't do betas until 17 days past "ovulation." This is to be sure that the 5000 IU trigger from Saturday is out of my system.

November 21, 2012—Firstly, I'm still feeling quite ill. My nausea has gotten worse and I am crazy bloated and tender. My afternoon call let me know that I have a good selection of fertilized embryos (13 were mature, and a good chunk fertilized) so it will be a day 5 transfer. I now have to mentally will them to live until then.

November 23, 2012—Ugh, I'm still feeling under the weather and looking four months pregnant with extremely stretched ovaries. I am hoping it will be worth it. There has been no actual vomiting (although I have spent quite some time on my bathroom floor contemplating if it will just happen). But I think things are getting better, slowly. I feel like such a wuss. No updates from the lab so I will take that as a good thing.

November 24, 2012—I'll cut to the transfer, which was fine. The fellow first showed me my large ovaries and pockets of fluid in my abdomen, lucky me… although he said this is pretty typical and as long as I have good urine output (and I do), I am doing fine—but it may take *weeks* to get better. Ugh. I really liked the doctor today, she was funny. Oh and we transferred one embryo. We won't know if there were any good enough to freeze until Monday, their freezing criteria are quite specific. They called my lining a "nice home." Hopefully that will be true. And then the doctor told my husband that she thinks that diamonds really help implantation. Told you she was funny.

November 26, 2012—I tested out the trigger—today was way harder to make out the purple haze on the cheapie test. So I am feeling confident that it will be totally gone by the time I test. Then it hit me that it will be really hard if I feel so awful for this week and the embryo still doesn't take. I know that many way more perfect cycles don't work, but I would *really* like to be on the good side of the coin flip this time.

That being said, I have no idea when to test. I am scared to. I am scared to talk about it. And have always been told by my grandmother to not even say congratulations to someone who is pregnant until the baby is out, so I know that a positive beta (if that) is a huge way away from a baby. Although it would be a really nice (and crucial) start. I'm starting to feel a bit better, although the fluid in my belly has overstayed its welcome.

December 3, 2012—Spotting this morning and a negative pregnancy test confirmed that I am out this round. Big shame. Now there is the all-important blood confirmation tomorrow, and then a month off, apparently to let my ovaries fully shrink. And I had to remind them that they have to bring a period on rather than just wait for the next cycle.

So hopefully, if things thaw properly, we will do a FET in January. I have heard horror stories from ladies I met at cycle monitoring of like 10 frozen embryos all dying during the thaw... urg! Not the best way to start the week.

December 6, 2012—I am hanging in there, no crying today. So I guess that's good. My plan from here is no meds until my appointment in January. Then I'll do an ultrasound and if my lining is thin then start building. If a lining is present, I'll take Provera to shed it and go from there for the FET. So I will have this month for my ovaries to "settle down" and I guess concentrate on non-fertility parts of my life.

January 4, 2013—I had my scan yesterday. My lining was 7 mm, but the even bigger shocker was my progesterone of 45 (= 14 in USA units). The RE told the nurse that I won't believe this. So my "non-medicated rest month" led to an ovulation and now I wait for CD 1 to present itself within the next two weeks. Before you all get excited, we still have the male factor so I'm probably not pregnant. Still this is wonderful news. Another case to show that weight gain, self-care and laying off the running works! So keep it up all of you!!

What do I think led to my recovery? Weight gain and stopping running completely. There is no other way. I limited my exercise to walking, yoga/Pilates, light elliptical or recreational rollerblading.

I consumed copious amounts of nut butter (more than four tablespoons... possibly a lot more) almost daily. Nonfat dairy was removed from my diet. My weight gain was quick (20 lb in two to three months).

I think we are lucky to have one of the only conditions that is treatable with chocolate. 'Recovery' is our choice. In terms of infertility, although there may be guilt stemming from the "self-induced" component, remember that this is the most treatable infertility issue and generally has favorable outcomes.

Casie got pregnant on her frozen embryo transfer in the next cycle. After her daughter was born she breastfed for 13 months, but did not get her cycles back within the first four months of weaning, though blood work looked promising. Due to another medical indication, she was put on BCP that masked her body's progress for the next six months. When she wanted to conceive again, she started another round of IVF due to the male factor.

Emilie—Overexercise, Purging, and Stress (backstory, recovery focus, little bit about oral meds for pregnancy)

November 24, 2012—I was always a normal cycler in high school and college, despite running cross country, track, and cheering. At 5'2, my BMI was around 20. I went on BCP in 2005 before getting married in 2006. After getting married, I put on weight, up to a BMI of about 22. (This was due to working, less running, and eating what my skinny husband who never gains a pound liked!) I went on Weight Watchers in January of 2008 at a BMI of 22.7, the highest of my life. I joined the gym and started running a bit more. The weight came off quickly, but as I was always a perfectionist and goal setter, I thought I'd go a little more. I remember being so excited when I saw the scale back down to my college weight.

In the meantime, my husband and I went through some critical life events that included taking over a family business. It was super stressful, he wasn't home much, and I felt terribly neglected. I ate to comfort myself and put on a couple of pounds, but I figured I could get that back off by working out more. I upped my cardio and weight sessions from two to three times a week to every day. That got the weight off plus a few more pounds. One night while my husband was still at work, and having had an awful fight with him and a horrible day at work, I ordered a pizza and ate over half of it. Freaking out, I went to the bathroom and threw it up. Until this point, I had never had a bona fide eating disorder.

As my work stress continued, I went to church less, my relationship with God and my husband dwindled (I was so angry at both of them—that's another story in itself). I got wrapped up in my "gym" identity. People told me how fabulous I looked, how they wanted to look like me, etc. I did my first body show at a BMI of 19 and 12% body fat. I was going to the gym at 5 am for one-hour spin classes or running (I would find a way to run 35-40 miles a week one way or another); then during work or after I would run or do other cardio again, plus do circuit training. I kept this up for three years, dropping to about 7% body fat and a BMI of 18. I was consistently tired. I ached. I drank five cups of coffee a day and took caffeine pills before the workouts; I used glucosamine for my aching joints; took Tonalin CLA for body fat reduction; and only fueled my body with half a banana after my workouts (even after 8 mile runs!). I never had any time for friends or for my husband, and I would get frustrated when plans or meetings were made that messed up my workout schedule. I threw up in bathrooms in shopping malls, airports, and my workplace in sheer desperation when I ate half a bagel. Then, just in case I didn't get all of it, I'd go do another workout.

I went off BCP in October 2011 in hopes of re-establishing normal periods before we started trying to conceive in the summer of 2012. The funny thing is, I didn't think I'd have an issue since I still got a "normal" period on the BCP. I remember that October as such a low point... I was supposed to be honored with an award from my company one night, but during the afternoon I ate a few too many brownies and forced my bulimia so hard that I wound up in a carb hangover, with a bloody nose and a migraine. I remember feeling like such an imposter that evening, pretending to be so successful and having it all together when on the inside I was such a mess. Even when I was taking photos with the award I remember almost crying because I hurt so much on the inside. SUCH A FAKE! The entire time I'd been able to keep the bulimia my secret, but I finally told my husband so he would hold me accountable. I remember him crying and praying for me right there, telling me how thankful and hopeful he was that his "old Emilie" would come back.

At my ob-gyn appointment in January I remember being *so pissed* when she told me to gain 5 or 10 lb after I failed the Provera challenge. I hadn't thrown up in a few weeks, but I had been severely restricting and exercising *not* to gain. During my research over the next few months (in the meantime I was so exhausted I had to let up on my exercise and eat some more), I realized I likely had HA. I came across Nico's blog and the FoodNFitness Diary Blog, and made an appointment with an RE in May. By the time I went there I had gained a few pounds.

It wasn't an easy process to go all in. I would have days I would eat up, and the next *hate* myself for "giving up" what I had worked so hard for. I would be up two pounds, then down two in April/May/June. I think I had an anxiety attack on a work trip in New Jersey over a pair of pants that didn't button, but that was the day I decided how ridiculous I was. I had been eating more and hadn't been ballooning! So, I started eating but not so much that I might gorge myself and start bingeing again. I stopped my "kinda-intense" workouts and only walked or did super light weights, and honestly, many weeks I did not work out at all. In the meantime, my marriage flourished, my faith grew by leaps and bounds, and I reconnected with friends and family I had completely neglected. My life became rich again!

I started my first Femara treatment in August (2.5 mg with no response); Second round I did an extended protocol of Femara (5mg) followed by Clomid (50 mg) that did not result in pregnancy, which was killer... but something I needed to experience to ready myself for the positive I just got (Femara 5 mg extended protocol). It is still unreal! This cycle, I had not worked out in well over three weeks (aside from walking) and got my BMI up to the "fertile zone."

I wouldn't have made it without constant encouragement from so many ladies on this Board and I will encourage those now reading to stay in and fight the fight. Lay it down as soon as you can. Be uncomfortable, and get used to the worry—whether waiting for your period or ovulation, for the two-week-wait, positive pregnancy test, for next cycle, for the beta, for the heartbeat... and I don't think it gets any better once you actually have a child!! I know it's not easy, but the great things in life never are. You wouldn't be here in the first place if you weren't driven, intelligent, successful, and caring, because that's what we continue to drive toward—perfection! Just remember it's time to drive toward a different goal, and while it seems *so backward* some days... when you see those two lines, or THAT BABY, who's really gonna care if you weigh a couple more pounds or have some cellulite on your tushy? You will be a mother and maybe a grandmother one day, surrounded by family who loves you. I can't think of a blessing any greater than that.

Emilie nursed her baby for 12 months and regained cycles one month after weaning. Her second child was conceived naturally the first cycle she tried.

Dawn—Stress, Exercise, Undereating (recovery focus, little bit about pregnancy – oral meds and injects)

November 24, 2012—Prior to medical school I'd always been "slim" and relatively healthy. I gained and lost a few pounds here and there, but never overdid the food restrictions or exercise. I didn't weigh myself often but I estimate my normal healthy weight to be a BMI around 20. Cut to end of med school and internship year. I started doing "power yoga" and running more, lost a few pounds and liked the way I looked. As stress increased during internship (I was also planning my wedding this year) I started feeling like I was losing control. I was constantly terrified I would screw up and hurt someone at work. I had awful periods of anxiety; on one intensive care rotation, I found it difficult to eat as my stomach was always in knots. I was still exercising like mad and began religiously counting calories and writing down daily tallies. I ate "a lot" and regularly but it was all low calorie foods (soups, salads, etc.). Needless to say, my weight plummeted. Was everyone around me concerned? Oh yeah. My mother was beside herself with worry. Was I concerned? Nope. I thought I was super healthy, with a tiny figure I thought everyone envied. I don't know exactly, but I think that at my lowest, my BMI was around 17. On my wedding day, I looked sickly and my hair looked thin. All this time, I was on hormonal BC (Nuvaring) having normal monthly withdrawal bleeds. I thought absolutely nothing of it.

Once I started working during my residency, my lifestyle changed a bit. I finally started heeding others' words and thought, OK I could stand to gain a few pounds. I gained maybe five pounds over the course of a year, but was obsessed with keeping my weight low, and would not let myself go over a BMI of 18. I exercised five to six days a week: running, spinning, and power yoga. I still wrote down everything I ate and restricted when I thought I had indulged too much. I ate Arctic Zero instead of ice cream—anyone familiar with that crap? I did this for about four years. I never truly felt I had an eating disorder, but I'll admit here for the first time, I did purge once or twice after eating too much. I felt horrible after and vowed not to cross that line. But I see now how dangerously close I was.

Cut to August 2011, my husband finally convinced me it was time to start thinking about kids. I was hesitant since I worried constantly about how my body would change. I went off the Nuvaring and of course, no period...one month, three months, six months...nothing. I finally went to see an ob-gyn who patted me on the back and said, "Don't worry, you just need some more time, go home and call me when you're pregnant." After I failed a withdrawal bleed to progesterone, I said, "No more waiting!" and went to see an RE in January of 2012. The thought of HA was in the back of my mind, but I was in complete denial at this point...I mean, I was not a marathon runner, Olympic athlete or anorexic, right? I was just a normal skinny girl, obsessed with fitting into her size 2 jeans. Well, I finally had to face facts when all else was ruled out and tests came back consistent with HA. I was initially offered treatment, but I wasn't desperate for a baby just yet and I feared the "infertility" world. I decided to commit to six months of cutting back on exercise and doing herbs and acupuncture. Well, I half-heartedly cut back on exercise, from six days to three or four. I loosened up my diet a teeny bit and gained four pounds (that's being generous). After five months of consistent acupuncture and bottles of Chinese herbs, I did another round of progesterone—still no response. I should mention I found the Board back in Feb of 2012 when I was first facing the HA diagnosis, but like others have said, I absolutely resisted the weight gain mantra. I thought, "Nope, not me... I don't need to do anything drastic, just tweak my lifestyle a little bit." Ha ha ha.

So come June 2012, after one year of "trying to conceive" and no progress, I went crawling back to the RE with my tail between my legs, asking for Clomid. My nurse congratulated me on gaining a few pounds, but I should specifically point out, *no-one* in the medical field told me to gain *any* weight. They offered me drugs and said gaining weight couldn't hurt, but they never said I *had* to do it. So I didn't. I did my first round of Clomid 50mg and didn't respond. The RE gave me his "last ditch" dosage of 100mg for 10 days and finally, I had a late response. I triggered one follicle, and had a ton of "symptoms" in my luteal phase; I was really convinced I was pregnant. I still remember taking that first test and not believing that it was negative. I was crushed. Having the idea of being pregnant being taken away hurt a million times worse than I expected. Not to mention, after months of being patient, I was now desperate to be pregnant (my younger sister-in-law was pregnant with her second and it killed me). I didn't care what happened to my body anymore, or what it was going to take, enough was enough. I started reading though the Board again, and it finally clicked. If I was really going to get pregnant, I had to commit to this weight gain thing, there was no avoiding it anymore. I started posting and *eating*! Those first few weeks, I was a garbage disposal. I think all the restricting reversed itself for a bit and I just ate to my heart's content. I ate the junk in the break room I would never touch before, I ate when I wasn't even hungry. And I started to see the changes in my body... I was starting to look like the "old me" again—not rock hard and lean, but soft and slim. I gained 10 lb and I hated it. I thought *everyone* would notice. I was especially ashamed of people finding out my situation, that I finally had to admit that all those people who told me I was too skinny were right. As if my friends and family would say "Haha, we told you so... now you're just ordinary." It took a long time to get over these feelings: weeks, months. Maybe I still haven't let go of my skinny self completely, but I can say with certainty that I'm surprised at how good I feel now. I threw away my old clothes and have no interest in trying to be a size 2 again.

Through these months, the Board was critical in helping me manage my feelings. Because I'm almost 33 and wanted to be pregnant, like, yesterday, I continued with treatment and thus never attempted to cycle naturally. I was responding to treatment nicely at this higher weight and I continued to feed my body and almost completely eliminated exercise (gasp!!) except for walking and some light elliptical and yoga once in a while. After three heartbreaking rounds where I didn't get pregnant and a few weeks of being sidelined with cysts, I got pregnant on my first round of Menopur and IUI. Would this have worked back in January when I was a BMI of 18? Maybe, but I doubt it. And I'm actually *glad* I had to go through this; I'm not so scared of how my body will change during my pregnancy. I won't hesitate to nourish it and rest when I need to. I also feel better: my joints hurt less, my hair is thicker, and my overactive bladder (which was always a bother when I was underweight) has greatly improved. Why? Who knows, I just think my body is happier. And big surprise, I'm eating as much as I want and my body size is just stable! All that panic and self-control was completely unnecessary. Things are still very early for me, but I'm so grateful for the wonderful women who were good examples to me and pray that I continue on to have a happy and healthy baby.

After her baby was born, Dawn breastfed for 13 months, with cycles resuming three months after she stopped. She never went back to undereating and over-exercising.

Category 2: Normal Weight HAer

Many people think losing monthly periods only happens to the "skinny." However, it is completely possible for someone of "normal" weight to stop having cycles; as we've described, weight is just one of many factors (including undereating, overexercising, stress, and genetics) that go into causing HA. Someone who is "normal" weight or above can feel even more lonely and misunderstood because many people won't see the need to change habits in order to recover, and comments from others can be free-flowing and often unhelpful. However, our survey respondents who fell into this category had essentially the same rate of recovery as the "skinny" HAers. Here we share Anna's story.

Anna—Exercise, Undereating, Stress (pregnancy focus, injectables and IVF)

February 8, 2014—My story is a little different from most. I exercised a lot and didn't eat enough to match my calorie output, but I was never underweight, so my HA was overlooked and I made excuses for it for a *long* time. My lowest BMI was only around 21, which isn't quite a "fertile" BMI (that's probably more around 22), but it's still not what most would expect to be low enough to lose your period.

I've always been an active person. But in my early twenties, life took a bit of spin and in my effort to try and take back control and be healthy, I started exercising an hour a day, mostly jogging and the gym. After a year of my new routine, I noticed my cycles were getting longer and my period lasting for fewer days. I didn't think much of it until my period completely stopped. I hadn't lost a heap of weight according to the scale, but my family and friends noticed that I was shrinking. I saw my doctor after two missed periods and had blood work and an internal ultrasound.

Looking at those results now, they screamed HA, but instead I was diagnosed with PCOS. I wasn't entirely convinced this diagnosis was accurate, after all my androgens were fine and I didn't have insulin resistance or other symptoms of PCOS. I convinced my doctor to refer me to an endocrinologist, who also said PCOS. This was based on missing periods and the immature follicles seen in my ovaries. He put me on a low dose estrogen pill. I was told to come back when I wanted to get pregnant if I couldn't conceive naturally. In the meantime, I was working in a diabetes clinic and I asked the endocrinologist there about my results. He didn't think I had PCOS, but he didn't quite know what was going on with my hormones either. I decided to see a different private endocrinologist who took me through extensive testing and said that I had "a signaling defect" where my hypothalamus wasn't signaling to my ovaries to allow my body to cycle. She also said to take the pill and come back when I wanted to get pregnant. She was closest to nailing my diagnosis but her advice in the meanwhile wasn't very helpful. I told her about my exercise and she felt it wasn't excessive and I was technically a healthy weight, so she wasn't sure what to recommend.

About six years passed, and life got really crazy. I maintained my exercise routine—after all, no one told me stop and I liked how strong and toned I felt. But I was working more than full time (across multiple sites and at two private practices on weekends and evenings) and I took on a teaching gig where I taught one subject per semester. I mainly did it because I felt I could and the money was good. I married my boyfriend of nearly 10 years and I felt in control of my life. As far as eating was concerned, I don't think I ever *meant* to restrict; I was the person to go back for more cake at a party, but because I worked so much, all my meals were planned and prepared ahead of time. As I was being "healthy," I ate whole grain, low fat, and mountains of vegetables. Once I ran out of food that was it for the day, as that's what I had decided was a reasonable amount.

After being married for three years and working long tedious hours, we decided we wanted to start a family. I stopped the pill hoping to get my period back, but secretly knowing there was a chance I wouldn't. When I didn't get a period after 40 days off the pill, I made an appointment with the endocrinologist, as I knew there would be a wait. By the time I saw a doctor, I had been off the pill for three months with no period. My estrogen, LH, and FSH were all pointing to HA (I knew this from Nico's blog and this Board that I stumbled on during one of my zillions of Google searches). I halved my exercise load—at my peak, I was doing 90 minutes a day, five days a week, which consisted of 40 km jogging each week, 2.5 km of swimming, and 40 minutes of strength training twice a week. The doctor thought my exercise level was fine, again he told me that I had PCOS and he asked me what I wanted to do. I told him I wanted to get pregnant, so he said let's start with ovulation induction (which is the injections) to grow a follicle. He skipped Clomid/Femara as he felt that they wouldn't work for me (which is probably not true, as I now know lots of lovely ladies with similar blood work to me that the oral meds did work for). Anyway, four months after stopping the pill, I did my first injections cycle. It was long and annoying. They started me at 12.5IU FSH, and would only increase by very small amounts. I was having internal ultrasounds every second or third day and nothing happened for a long time. After more than 40 days of injections, my follicles took off. In three days I had four follicles that all looked like they would mature. The clinic was not about to risk quads so the cycle was canceled. They induced a bleed with Provera and then I started again.

This time, I knew I had to make lifestyle changes if I wanted the meds to work. I started reducing my work commitments, which naturally meant I started to eat more and I gained about five pounds, but my second round of treatment ended the same way—after 40+ days, there were 10 follicles that took off. I begged the doctor to switch me to IVF and harvest the mature eggs, but she wouldn't hear of it. She told me that our next attempt would be IVF and we would get results. The IVF fortunately went much faster. I only needed 14 days of injections, then had about six mature eggs retrieved, five of which fertilized. I had a 3-day embryo transferred and at 12 DPO I got a positive pregnancy test (who's having his morning nap right now as I type).

From the time I went off the pill to the time I got pregnant was around nine months. I know this is a faster than others have experienced, but I really went all in. I completely stopped exercising by the time I got to my second attempt at ovulation, and I was eating freely; not just the amount I had planned to eat for the day. For me, I think it was about letting go of controlling my food intake and feeling that "need" to exercise most days. I started to just see how I felt on the day and exercised if I could be bothered, which is my overall style now.

I'll be honest, I think the years of energy deficiency messed my metabolism up a lot, and I gained weight quite quickly when I wasn't controlling or monitoring food and exercise. I peaked at a BMI of 23.8, and it took time for my body to sort itself out.

Unfortunately, I never regained my cycles before conceiving my son. This worried me a little as I wondered what would happen when I stopped breastfeeding. When my son turned one, he was only nursing once or twice a day, and I started to get antsy about my body's ability to conceive. I could feel that something different was happening, but I wasn't sure. I was back to jogging every day I could when my son was about six weeks old, but, being a stay at home mum with food at arm's reach, I never quite returned to my pre pregnancy weight. When my son was about 13 months old, I noticed a faint line on the OPKs. It darkened a little, but never gave me a true positive. The day after it was at its darkest, I felt like my ovaries were about to explode. I told my husband that evening that I thought I had ovulated, and asked if he was ready to give another kid a crack. Well, it turns out that I did ovulate, and not only that, at 11 DPO I found out I was pregnant again—all natural! So I got pregnant breastfeeding without ever having a period.

Be kind to yourselves ladies—and trust me, you really need to eat freely and exercise gently if you want things to happen. And they will happen! But they do take time. And, I have to say, nobody is going to notice if you gain weight, or become less toned, and if they do, they are losers and you need to block them from your thoughts as they will get in your way of you achieving what you want! Good luck lovely ladies!!! XOXOXOX

Here are a few other posts from Anna that you might find worth reading:

February 19, 2011—My doctor seems to think I'm not thin enough to have HA but due to low estrogen has diagnosed me with having mild HA on a background of PCOS (due to lots of follicles in my left and right ovaries). From what I've read HA is not always a result of low body fat or weight, more about adequate energy and carbohydrate availability so I'm not too sure about some of his ideas. In the last month, I have increased my carbohydrate intake (and my weight, which I am not liking at all!). When I told the doctor I had increased my weight, he said, "Oh no, don't do that!" His advice was to "exercise less and eat less." Hmmm, not to sure exactly how to do that! I don't think I eat heaps now.

February 24, 2011—I saw an exercise physiologist today. She started by asking me what my goal was, and my response was "I want to get my eggs cracking but remain in good shape." We had an interesting conversation, which really helped me to realize that regardless of what we eat and whether our exercise looks fine on paper, if we are having hormonal imbalances, something is not right and needs to change. I have realized that I have been rationalizing my excessive exercise routine for too long. Yes, I have a "healthy" BMI and body fat percentage, but my body is telling me there isn't enough energy to make getting pregnant viable. She also asked me why I jog so much... after all, who in their right mind would get up at 5:15 a.m. before work and work out for 90 minutes?? This is when I had to get real. I think I'm still trying to figure out how this obsession with exercise happened without me even realizing it.

June 6, 2011—According to my scale, at my lowest, my body fat was 22%, now it's up to 30%! Weird, because since gaining around 4 kg, I have definitely noticed that I am nowhere near as cold as I used to be! So, I guess, even though my body fat was probably not typically considered low before, perhaps my body is just happier fatter.

Anna regained her cycles eight months after her second was born, while still breastfeeding. She has had regular cycles since and is still breastfeeding her 19-month-old daughter.

Category 3: Formerly in Larger Bodies

About 18% of folks with HA were at one point in much larger bodies then lost a significant amount of weight and acquired HA during the process. These large changes in weight can't play a part in your thinking around recovery—the same basic principles apply. It is important to be adequately fueling, not overexercising, and reducing stress. We will follow Lisa Marie's journey, and read Laurie's HA recovery summary.

Lisa Marie—Weight Loss, Exercise, Undereating, and Stress (pregnancy focus, oral meds and injectables)

March 24, 2012—I've been reading the posts on this Board for a while now and it's a relief to find some others who understand what I'm going through. Not that I would wish this frustration on anyone, but I need to vent sometimes and I'm a pretty private person. I'm sure my husband is sick of my whining (though he doesn't show it and is very supportive)!

Anyway, I have not been officially diagnosed with HA but I think that's what I have although I don't fit the "typical" profile. I'm a "healthy weight" for my height (BMI around 22). I've never been underweight but I used to be much larger. I was on Paxil for 12 years, from age 16 to age 28. During that time I gained a lot of weight—gradually at first, but it seemed to accelerate during those last few years. At my highest, my BMI was about 32. Back in 2007 I decided enough was enough, and I turned my life around. I quit smoking, I got off Paxil. (Side note: quitting smoking was easier!) I started to lose the weight I'd gained all those years without even trying. In May of 2008 my BMI was about 25 and I started dieting and exercising to "lose the last 20" or so pounds. I accomplished that in about four months. I took up running. I was on the pill at the time, and my cycles were getting weird (breakthrough bleeding, two week long periods, etc.) I tried different pills but I was sick of the various side effects so I decided no more. I got to my goal weight in Sept 2008 but I kept running and eating healthier. I didn't get a period after going off the pill, and this went on for about a year and a half. My doctor prescribed Provera but it didn't work. In August of 2009 my fiancé and I relocated from upstate NY to FL so I didn't see a doctor for a few months. The stress of moving probably wasn't good for me either, looking back. The new ob-gyn in Florida took my history, did blood work, etc. She couldn't figure out why I wasn't getting a period either, so I went back on BCP for a while (starting in April 2010, I think), because at the time I didn't want to get pregnant. My husband and I got married (finally! we'd been together almost nine years) in August 2011. I went off the pill in October, knowing it would probably take a while for my cycle to come back. I suspected that the problem before was the weight loss (almost a third of my body weight) combined with running (20 to 25 miles per week). I thought for sure I'd get my period by now though, since I've been at the same weight for over three years.

A few weeks ago I went back to the ob-gyn and she prescribed progesterone, 50 mg for 12 days. I didn't get a withdrawal bleed. Now I'm on estrogen patches combined with progesterone after a couple weeks, to induce a cycle. I started cutting down on my running, but I think I'm going to just stop completely for the time being. Which *stinks* because I love running. It's my antidepressant. The last time I really ran was last Sunday. Today I did a little... I took my dog for a walk but he started running and it just looked like so much fun! So I ran for a few minutes but then I stopped and just walked again. I'm feeling OK with less exercise, mostly. I'm trying to tell myself that it's only temporary. After I have babies I can run again! I'm now 33 years old—I don't think it's wise to wait any longer to try to have a baby, especially when we want at least two, but I wish my body would cooperate! The last time I had a real period without pills, I was much larger and a smoker. What. The. Heck!

March 25, 2012—Thank you for the warm welcome everyone! Laura, I know exactly what you mean being nervous about ballooning up to the weight you were at. I always thought that if I stopped running I'd gain a ton of weight. Oddly enough, since I've been running less these past few weeks I actually lost a few pounds! Weird because at the beginning of this year I had resolved to lose five pounds so I started running more, but my weight wouldn't budge. But no more... walking it is for now. It's convenient that it's starting to get hot again here in Florida, almost too hot to run outside unless you go out really early. In the summer I have to do most of my running on the treadmill, and I *loathe* the treadmill.

I'm pretty sure I'm getting enough calories now, especially without running. I never felt like I was depriving myself, but maybe I was when I was running a lot. I have a major sweet tooth, and I would make room for sweets almost every day, but that is the key I guess—I'd exercise more to compensate for that piece of cake, or I'd eat less other food that day. Not very healthy after all. Well, I'm hoping that not running and eating when I feel like it will do the trick. I complained to my husband, "I don't want to gain weight! I'll have to buy new pants!" and he pointed out that if I get pregnant, I will gain weight and need new pants anyway. He definitely has a point there. I just hate the thought of not being able to run, getting bigger, and having to wait months and months while it seems like every other woman I know of child bearing age is getting pregnant no problem. But I'm determined to do it, and I know from losing weight that I can set goals and achieve them. So I'm going to do it right!

April 7, 2012—I don't know what to do. I don't see how I would possibly need to gain more weight. My BMI is 22.3 but my body fat is around 26% (probably, I didn't actually have it measured but I calculated it). I did exercise a lot, but I don't feel like I restricted calories. I've never had an eating disorder. I just don't understand what's wrong with me.

Here I am 33 years old and everyone else my age or even younger is having their second or third kid. I wish I hadn't waited so long. We were waiting for things to fall in place like my husband's career and buying a house. We're still not quite there but I don't want to wait any longer. Ultimately I blame this all on Paxil... if I'd never been on it I wouldn't have gained and lost all that weight.

April 8, 2012—I am hoping that ovulation is just around the corner! I randomly had some EWCM today, out of nowhere. Here I thought maybe I was going to get my period finally, then today EWCM? I don't know what to make of it. My body's all confused. My husband and I took advantage of it today but I'm not getting my hopes up just yet. I entered it into my chart on Fertility Friend and it took away my "ovulation" from two weeks ago. *sad face* I'm now on CD 173 and it needs to end!

April 12, 2012—I'm wondering if there is anyone else out there like me—started in a larger body then lost a lot and acquired HA. I want to know if you've successfully recovered from HA naturally and if so how long did it take? Before I gained all that weight and when I wasn't on the pill I had really normal, regular cycles. I've been about this weight for over three years now. And, this was about how much I weighed before I went on Paxil. Will cutting out exercise and eating more fat help me? I don't know, I'm just having one of those days where I miss being able to run (it's been a month now), I feel blah, and what if I never ever get my menstrual cycle back?

> **Willow:** My story has some similarities to yours. I was a normal weight (low end of normal BMI) for all my life. When I was in my 20's I went on an antidepressant and in the 10 years that I took it I gained a bunch of weight. When I came off the antidepressant, I developed some stomach/digestive issues and ended up losing a lot and this weight loss is what caused my HA. I have regained my cycles naturally. I am not yet cycling regularly, but I am cycling! I gained 10 lb to get my first period. I am still working on gaining more, to hopefully get more consistent cycles. My weight loss was not exercise-related, so I can't advise on that aspect, but many of the women here who have regained their cycles have done so by cutting way back on exercise. I just wanted to let you know that you are not the only one!

April 20, 2012—I'm getting a little frustrated but I know I need to not stress out about this so much, as stress certainly isn't going to help, and may be why I *still* haven't gotten my cycle back. I guess I need to give it more time.

It's been about five weeks since I quit running. I walk (with the occasional jog to keep up with my dog) three times a week for about 30 minutes each time. I feel like I eat tons. About once a week I have EWCM, but then it goes away and I don't ovulate.

Sometimes I worry that I'll never get my period back, no matter how much weight I gain or how little I exercise. I know my history is different from most of yours, as I was larger in the past and it might take longer for my cycle to come back, but good lord it's been almost four years since I lost that weight. This is getting ridiculous.

April 28, 2012—Since I've stopped running and eating whatever, I haven't actually put on any weight (maybe a pound)... but my pants are tight and I feel flabby. I guess I need to go shopping for some new pants in the next size up, maybe some scrubs for work so I'm more comfortable. When I get pregnant I will need them anyway right??

May 2, 2012—Not much to report here. I was feeling a little down today, looking at my body and how it's changed in the past six or seven weeks since I quit running and worrying about how many calories I was eating. I swear I have rolls on my stomach now that weren't there before, and my boobs are huge (they have always been on the bigger side; I'm a C cup and I really don't want them to be any bigger!) I feel like I'm two months pregnant but I *still* haven't ovulated. But I'm not giving in to the temptation to run 10 miles and eat salad for dinner! I did yoga today and it was quite enjoyable!

May 16, 2012—I had my appointment with the RE today and I wanted to share my experience with you all. After a long wait in the waiting room the nurse called me in. She took my blood pressure and it was 139/70 something. It is never that high! I was really keyed up and nervous.

We went into the doctor's office space and discussed my recent blood work. He mentioned that the LH/FSH ratio is supposed to be close to 1:1. Mine was like 1:3 and he said that indicates "hypothalamic suppression," which can be caused by stress, weight loss, or heavy exercise. It felt nice to finally have a doctor agree with what I've been suspecting all along! Then I had an ultrasound. So cool to finally get a look inside and see what's going on, but now I'm even more confused! Here is the rundown:

1) My uterine lining was very thin, only 2mm. I didn't expect it to be really thick or anything, but I guess I'm not getting my period anytime soon.

2) He noticed a lot of fluid in the cul-de-sac, which is the space in the abdomen between the uterus and the colon. He said that is highly suggestive of endometriosis. If that is the case, that explains my general pelvic pain and bowel issues.

3) When he scanned my left ovary, it had a TON of small follicles, like 30-40. The whole time he was explaining things to me but I was still stuck on the endometriosis part so I think I missed some of it. But I guess that's way more follicles than I'm supposed to have, and now I'm wondering, doesn't that sound like PCOS? I do have some PCOS symptoms (acne and facial hair on my chin—UGH!) but when I had my testosterone tested it was normal.

So at the end, I'm thinking this looks pretty grim. I (possibly) have multiple causes of infertility. He didn't seem concerned at all, "No worries, we can get you pregnant!" I'm glad he has faith cause I'm not so sure anymore!

It's all good though, I'm just really glad I went to an RE because if I just stayed with my ob-gyn I don't think I would have had a good outcome. I feel like I'm finally going to get to the bottom of my issues. The next steps are: more blood work, semen analysis for my husband, and an HSG for me, which means I have to take a round of BCP's so I get a period. I have some pills left over from last summer so I'm starting them tonight. It's just weird that here I am, trying to get pregnant without success, I finally see an RE and now I'm going on BCP. I'm really, really glad we're doing all these diagnostic tests before starting any treatment. I have a feeling my insurance won't cover any of it, but it would be a pity to waste money on treatments without resolving *all* underlying issues first. At least I can get my blood work done for free at the lab I work in.

May 20, 2012—The more optimistic side of me was thinking today, maybe I'm going through this for a reason—to learn to be patient before I have kids, who will most certainly test my patience! I am really lacking in this department. When I was on Paxil for so long, it kind of numbed me and I didn't get worked up about anything. Then when I went off of it, I had to learn how to not flip out over the tiniest things (like getting caught in traffic). I've gotten a lot better, I think, but I've got to work on it still. If it's going to take me as long to get pregnant as I think it will, hopefully in that time I will learn to relax and be patient!

May 28, 2012—I was feeling so anxious and depressed this morning, and I couldn't snap myself out of it. Finally, I said **** it and I went for a run. I know, I know, I shouldn't have, but it was only about two miles in 20 minutes. I'm way slower than I used to be, and I was impressed that I could even do that much. I felt so much better afterwards. I think there are three things that contribute to HA: overexercise, undereating, and stress. Stress is something I have a difficult time dealing with without exercise. This morning I felt like I had to get that energy out somehow. I know it's bad, it's only going to hurt me in the long run and I have to find some other way to deal with stress. I'm hoping how I felt this morning was mostly due to the BCPs! I guess I thought that it would be better for my hypothalamus to stop all those feelings of anxiety, even if it took a little running. I know I can't do this all the time if my ultimate goal is to get pregnant. I need to figure out what else can I do to get rid of all of those anxious feelings!

May 29, 2012—Thanks to everyone for the advice and comments regarding exercise and stress reduction. I do know that overdoing the exercise will hurt me if I want to respond to the oral meds, so I'm not going to go crazy.

June 19, 2012—Today was my appointment with the RE to discuss the next steps. Much to my relief he wants to hold off on the laparoscopy (for those of you who missed it, when I went for my first appointment about a month ago, while doing the ultrasound he found "free fluid" in the cul-de-sac, the area behind uterus and in front of rectum, suggestive of endometriosis). Thankfully he realizes that my major issue is that I don't ovulate. He also said that many women get pregnant and have this fluid and it doesn't cause any issues, so that is good to know. Also, much to my relief, he wants to start out with less expensive meds, so after I get my period (more birth control pills OH JOY) I'll be starting Femara from CD 3 to 7. Then, around CD 11 I'll go in for a scan and see how things are progressing. That seems awfully early to me, I'm worried there won't be any action going on at that point, but I guess we'll see. If I get some mature follicles, I'll take a trigger shot (Ovidrel) to make me ovulate.

June 24, 2012—I think I'm finally coming to terms with the fact that yes, I've put on more weight, but it's OK because it will help me get pregnant that much faster. You know I honestly think seeing the before and after pictures of all you ladies really played a role in my realization. Such an awesome idea! I checked out pictures of me at BMI 32, 21ish, and 24.5 (because that's what I had) and I don't think I'm meant to be a BMI of 21. I was trying so hard for so long to stay there, and that's why I have HA (well, a major part of it, anyway!) I think 22.5-23 and up is where my body is happy.

June 30, 2012—I always thought that running helped with my stress but I now know that wasn't the case, it was making it worse! I'm so much more relaxed since I quit running (back in March). But I still don't have my cycles back. I'm not very patient and I feel like I'm getting older so I'm getting help from an RE. Anyway, so yes, stress is a big factor for me. What I find helps is keeping busy with things that I enjoy (cooking, baking, gardening, spending time with my husband and his family, and friends) that take my mind off having a baby. Because when I'm not immersing myself in something else, it's all I think about! Also, sometimes I think it just takes time at a higher weight to get cycles back. It doesn't happen right away for all of us unfortunately.

June 30, 2012—I took the last BCP last night and I predict that my period will show up Friday morning. Then I have to call my RE to see about what to do next, and get my prescription for Femara. As I said before, I really hope that my weight gain/increased body fat and limited exercise will help me respond. I went shopping yesterday and got some new clothes: some new shorts, a cute sundress, a couple of tops. As I looked at myself in the mirror, I definitely could see how much less muscular and flabby I am but I didn't let it get to me. I thought, I still look fine, and being buff and muscular isn't going to help me get pregnant! I can deal with this!

July 12, 2012—I took the last dose of Femara tonight. I can't believe I have an ultrasound in four days. I can't believe there will be anything going on because I feel *nothing*. And practically negative CM. It's just hard for me to believe that I'll have any follicles of decent size. I almost just want to get this over with so I can move on to whatever WILL make me ovulate. I don't know why I'm being so negative. I guess I'm thinking—the last time I ovulated (probably 2004) I was much larger than I am now. So I'm worried that I still have a long way to go to get to my body's set point for ovulation. I just have a feeling that my body is going to need a bigger jump start to ovulate. I'm hoping to be pleasantly surprised on Monday though.

July 20, 2012—My RE wants to cancel this cycle due to the poor response. Besides the poor growth and thin lining, my E_2 is dropping (and it was only 31 on Monday. The nurse who called didn't even tell me what it was, but it doesn't really matter if it went down.) I have an appointment to discuss other options in August. I didn't even get to talk to him today, so I didn't ask about piggybacking, but I will ask if that will be an option in future cycles at my next appointment. I would *definitely* prefer if I could somehow ovulate with oral drugs because of the cost. Anyway, I'm trying not to be too discouraged but sometimes I wonder WHY I didn't respond. I quit running months ago and my BMI was over 23 last time I checked. I know those aren't the only factors, but still. Frustrating! I just want to ovulate already!

July 26, 2012—Every time I think there's something happening, I start to get my hopes up but I know deep down that I'm not going to ovulate on my own any time soon. My hypothalamus is still asleep. Sometimes I wonder if something else is wrong with me, but what could it be? Is it just because I was larger before and now my brain still thinks I'm underweight (even though I never was, and now I'm at a "fertile" BMI)? I just want to ovulate and get pregnant!

August 10, 2012—I had my appointment with the RE today. He has recommended moving on to Menopur for the next cycle. I had a feeling that he would, and I had already made up my mind that I don't want to waste any more time with oral meds if he didn't think they would work. I had such a poor response to Femara that I don't think even a higher dose (or EP) would help. I'm impatient and I just want to ovulate already! It's going to be expensive but I'm prepared for it.

September 10, 2012—I'm feeling kinda depressed right now. I made the decision to cancel this cycle due to my husband having the flu. Last night I thought he was getting better, but then his temperature went up to 103 again in the middle of the night. I could hardly sleep. I kept thinking why am I doing this if I think it's going to be a failure? Plus, I was so worried about him, so I thought the stress of continuing this cycle on top of that was just too much when it probably won't work. Ugh. Now I guess we have to wait two months, boo. (I'm basing all of this on this article I found: History of febrile illness and variation in semen quality[2]).

Canceling this cycle felt like the right decision this morning, but why am I having second thoughts? It's too late now, I have no more Menopur for tonight. Why does it seem like every obstacle to getting pregnant, even ones that I never even thought of, is getting thrown at me?

December 2, 2012—I FINALLY went through my closet and pulled out all of the pants that don't fit anymore. I had thought about saving them in case I lose weight after having children, but I decided eff it, I'm not going to try to fit in a size 2 again. My body is definitely happier where it is now.

I'm giving the pants to Goodwill. Two more birth control pills until I can start my next cycle!!

December 10, 2012—I've been on this board for nine months and if there's one thing I've learned it is that everyone is different. I don't think there is a set weight or BMI that any one of us has a menstrual cycle at. Some people only have to gain a little bit of weight, and others more. Some ladies just need to stay at a higher weight for a longer period of time before their cycle comes back.

December 16, 2012—I went for my scan this morning and it was just as I expected; not much going on yet, but it's all good. I have many follicles but nothing over 10 mm. On my right there were 7 and 8 mm follicles, and on the left, a few 6's that the nurse measured. My lining is at 4.1mm, E_2 was 50. This is pretty much where I was last cycle at this time, before I over stimulated. So the plan now is to go up to 1.5 vials, and go back on Wednesday. At first she told me to come back Thursday but I convinced her to let me come Wednesday instead. I told her my whole sob story about over stimming (not sure if she had looked at my chart) and how I'd feel much better coming a day earlier. I feel good about this plan now and I hope only a couple of those follicles continue to grow. At least we know it won't be like last time, where I went up to two full vials for four days without a scan. That was a nightmare!

December 23, 2012—My E_2 was 297. I have to continue injections tonight and tomorrow, trigger Tuesday night and IUI on Thursday morning! Can't believe I'll *finally* be in the two week wait! Hopefully I can sleep better tonight because I'm exhausted. Now I'm not as worried and anxious, but excited, and as my husband pointed out, that might keep me up, too. When I texted him this morning with the news, he replied, "I told you not to worry so much!"

December 26, 2012—I triggered last night at about 8 PM. It felt so surreal to finally be able to use that Ovidrel syringe that had been in my fridge since my failed Femara cycle in July! I also asked the nurse today about progesterone and she said they would give me a prescription to start on Friday. I thought for sure they would give me a hassle, and I had a whole speech prepared if they were going to deny me the progesterone. But I didn't need it! Can't believe I'll be in the two week wait tomorrow! Sorry for the wordy post but I'm excited like a kid at Christmas, if you couldn't tell!!

January 7, 2013—Good morning ladies! So... I wasn't going to test today. I was going to wait until tomorrow (12 DPO) but I couldn't stop that evil little voice that said, "Do it do it do it... just an internet cheapie... come on!" I thought the test would probably be negative, so I wasn't going to get discouraged just yet. *But it wasn't negative*!!! I'm being cautiously optimistic, as it's still so early. I hope it sticks!

January 10, 2013—I got my beta back today (14 DPO)—203! I feel good about that number. Repeat on Saturday, along with a progesterone level, and ultrasound in about three weeks (not scheduled yet, they'll probably have me do that after my beta on Saturday, assuming it's doubling appropriately). This is almost starting to feel real.

And having a baby in my belly is totally worth feeling yucky the last several months. It's so worth putting on the weight and giving up running. A year ago, I never would have believed this, but I'm glad I woke up!

Lisa Marie nursed for 18 months after her daughter was born. She ovulated for the first time while still nursing (12 months postpartum) and got pregnant naturally with twins!

Laurie—Weight Loss, Exercise, Undereating (recovery focus, natural cycles and pregnancy)

September 22, 2013—I always had normal cycles my whole life up until HA, however my weight was all over the spectrum through different seasons of my life. I believe my "happy" weight is somewhere around a BMI of 24 to 25. I've never been thin but I was healthy and settled here for a long time. In my early 20's I went through a *lot* of traumatic events leading to some depression and weight gain, mainly after my father's passing. I found myself at a BMI of 33; still cycling but *so* unhappy. I was addicted to drugs, ate horribly, smoked, drank, blah blah blah, so I decided to embark on a "mission for me" a.k.a. getting healthy. I lost weight slowly by exercising moderately and eating well. But as soon as my weight began to plateau around a BMI of 26 I felt I needed to go to more drastic measures like doing cleanses, fasts, shakes, Weight Watchers etc. I decided to give up animal products and became a vegan. During this time, I also took up running—as I'd never run before I started slowly but then my mileage crept up with no moderation. I was barely eating, running six miles every morning before my two-hour kickboxing classes, then it was another nine miles before bikram yoga, then more kickboxing at night. Whenever I could fit in exercise I did. Plus, I'm a massage therapist and worked like a dog. I somehow survived on no protein and between 1200-1500 cals a day while doing all this. It became an obsession! I stopped cycling without noticing at around a BMI of 25 but didn't think much of it; I was actually kind of happy because no periods right?! *Wrong!* After almost a year of not cycling I was down to a BMI of 20.8 and yet still dissatisfied about my body.

With missing periods, I also began to wonder whether I would ever be able to have children. So I went and saw a doctor who gave me Provera, which did not work. I was convinced that if I went on hormone supplements I would gain weight again and I was *never* going back to the size I was before, so I refused anything of the sort. After another year and a half I met my current husband and we decided together that I needed to start eating meat again for protein and to get my periods back. However, though I began eating meat again I continued with even fewer calories because now I was gaining muscle mass. I dropped my calories to about 1000 a day while continuing to run, kickbox, and practice yoga. My HA seemed even worse. I lived in anxiety and always worried about my weight. While my fiancé was deployed in Afghanistan I dropped to a BMI of 19.8. I stayed there until married life settled in; then I got *really* worried about not having children. I found the Board and began doing the hard stuff. I gained a total of 45 lb. My cycles came back after about 35 lb—back at my happy weight, BMI 25. As my cycles regulated I continued to gain about 10 more pounds—eeek!—currently BMI is about 27. I never fully stopped exercising but I am *convinced* that my continued exercise is why it took so long to get my cycles back. When I stopped running my cycles finally came back. And now I am 10 DPO and just got a positive test! I can't believe it!!! I'm still in shock!!!

Laurie nursed her daughter for seven months and regained cycles six weeks later. She returned to her "happy weight" postpartum without "going on a diet." When she started trying to conceive again, she got pregnant on her third cycle.

Category 4: Misdiagnosed PCOS

It is remarkably common that people with HA are misdiagnosed as having PCOS because of the lack of periods and often multicystic ovaries. However, the lifestyle recommendations for the two conditions are very different, as we described in chapter 6. Jessica O's misdiagnosis caused her HA to worsen; Dana was not convinced by the PCOS diagnosis and proceeded to find another doctor.

Jessica O—Weight Loss, Exercise, Undereating (recovery focus)

October 4, 2010—Throughout my mid-twenties, my BMI was around 23 and my cycles were regular. I was on birth control for a little while, but when I went off, they went right back to 28 days. I ate a reasonably healthy, but unrestricted diet. I jogged very slowly (12 min miles) three to four times a week and walked and biked some for transportation.

Everything changed when I started dating my now-husband and hanging out with his group of friends. Their attitude towards exercise was a new experience for me. We were "training," always pushing to bike farther, run faster, bike a steeper gap. It felt good, and before long I was making changes to my diet as well; I wanted to look lean and cut like my new friends.

A few months after we got married we started trying to conceive. At this point, my cycles had started to get longer and occasionally would skip a month. My ob-gyn assured me this was normal and had nothing to do with my increased exercise, after all my BMI was a "healthy" 21.5 and I wasn't a "real athlete."

After a year of not getting pregnant, I went back to the ob-gyn for a full work up. Everything appeared healthy and normal but I had some cysts on my ovaries, so they diagnosed me with PCOS, put me on metformin, and sent me home. A few weeks later, right after Christmas, I got pregnant, but had a miscarriage in February.

After my loss, I got really serious about attacking my "PCOS." In addition to the metformin, I went on a low carb diet, got really strict about my exercise regime, and pushed myself to lose more weight. Surprise, surprise, my period never came. The longer I was unsuccessful, the more restrictive my diet became, and my BMI dropped to 19.5.

Then in July, I stumbled upon some stuff on HA and thought OMG, this sounds like me. Nothing I had read about PCOS (and I read a lot) had sounded right to me. Eventually, I found Nico's blog and the Board. I'm now up to a BMI of 22. My only exercise is walking and yoga. This month I had lots of CM for the first time in years, and Sunday, I got my period for the first time since last November!

Jessica conceived for the first time two months after writing this post, but unfortunately had three miscarriages before conceiving her son. She nursed for 14 months, with cycles returning two months after she stopped. Jessica's second child, a daughter, was conceived naturally after one more miscarriage. When not nursing or pregnant, she's had regular cycles and no sign of PCOS.

Dana—Weight Loss, Exercise, Undereating (diagnosis focus, natural pregnancy)

June 12, 2006—I'm 29 and my husband is 32. I went off BCP in July 2005 to try and get pregnant, but never got a period. I went to the first ob-gyn in October and he gave me Prometrium, which didn't bring on a period, so he did some blood work that came back normal. He then gave me Clomid, which also didn't work (surprise!). He wanted to just up the dose the next month, but I was pretty curious as to why I still hadn't gotten a period so I didn't take it. I had a sneaking suspicion it was HA, because I'd lost about 20 lb several years back when I started running and became a vegetarian (my low BMI was about 17.2; I've since gained up to 18.4, started eating meat, and exercising less). Although when I asked my ob-gyn if it was possible, he said "No, that only happens to really skinny people." So I went to a second ob-gyn, who did yet more blood work, which all came back low-normal, in addition to an ultrasound that showed multiple small follicular cysts on my ovaries. Based on the ultrasound she diagnosed me as having PCOS, despite the fact my LH: FSH ratio was < 1, let alone 3:1, I had normal testosterone, normal insulin and glucose, no hair problems, no fat problems, a family history of HA and *not* PCOS, and with overexercise and diet issues obvious. Anyhoozers, she wanted to give me Clomid *again* after I started hormone replacement. At this point I figured I'd bite the very expensive bullet and go to an RE, who said definitely HA. He said polycystic ovaries don't equal PCOS (you can have multiple "cysts" and not have PCOS and you can have PCOS and not have polycystic ovaries). I read that up to 50% of women with HA have PCO[3]; they can be caused due to chronic anovulation for any reason. So I just underwent my first cycle of Follistim+low-dose hCG injections, but the cycle was canceled when I over stimulated on account of the polycystic ovaries (I would have ovulated like 20 eggs!).

February 29, 2008—A quick recap of my story: I ended up doing two cycles of injectables, both of which produced too many follicles and were canceled. We were out of money at that point. In August 2006 I finally quit running and gained 15 lb—my period returned in just under six months (January 2007). I conceived on my natural third cycle but had a missed miscarriage (the baby had died but my body didn't recognize that fact) discovered at eight weeks (August 2007). I conceived again on my third cycle after the D&C, December of 2007.

Dana nursed her first son for 21 months, regaining cycles 1.5 months after weaning. Her second was conceived naturally after gaining a few pounds and cutting exercise again, after trying for 3 months. After this baby was born, she nursed for 16 months, again regaining cycles 1.5 months after weaning. Her third was a surprise, conceived on her 8th cycle. After her daughter, Dana's cycles returned one month prior to weaning, at 17 months postpartum. There has never been any indication of PCOS other than multifollicular ovaries.

Category 5: HA and PCOS

In some cases, people do in fact have both HA and PCOS, although PCOS symptoms are often minimized when HA is active. Here we follow the stories of Grace who had both HA and PCOS, and Shayla who had some high androgen levels suggestive of PCOS but whether the diagnosis was correct was never entirely clear.

Grace—PCOS, Weight Loss, and Exercise (combined recovery/pregnancy focus, injectables)

April 16, 2014—I have been reading this forum for the past six months or so and am now finally gaining the courage to post myself. Although I may never meet any of you ladies, you all have offered me support, encouragement, and wisdom these last several months.

To make a long story short, I have a history of irregular cycles starting from puberty. My period would often show up at the most inopportune times: on vacations, while I was in clinicals for nursing school in my white scrub pants, and, my favorite one, while I was on my weekend retreat with my husband and other couples at a remote Catholic retreat center. Lovely. Now I am wishing so hard for a period. How times have changed!

I was an avid runner and exerciser and most doctors didn't really care that I didn't get a period because I wasn't "trying to get pregnant." When I got married I started birth control so that I wouldn't get pregnant right away (ha ha). I had regular periods on the pill but eventually developed ischemic colitis from the hormones in the pill that resulted in a 10 lb weight loss. I had to stop the pill in November of 2012, so we decided it would be a good time to start trying to conceive but I still have not gotten a period on my own. Multiple rounds of testing with my RE resulted in a dual diagnosis of HA and PCOS. I have the clinical signs of PCOS, including awful dark hair on my face (hot, I know ... thank goodness for waxing), cystic ovaries, and 2:1 ratio of LH: FSH. I also have the HA piece due to the exercise and weight loss. Since the diagnosis was finalized in January, I have just been walking and doing yoga and have gained to a BMI of about 21.5ish.

In February, I got a bleed from 25 days of estrogen with 10 days of progesterone and did one round of Femara. It failed miserably as I could not even grow follies big enough to trigger. The growth stopped at 14 mm. My doctor prescribed Provera to see if I'm finally where I need to be to respond, and it is now 11 days past my last pill with no signs of a period. I am just frustrated at how long it seems to take to do *anything*! We started this journey almost a year and a half ago, and I only have one round of fertility treatment under my belt. I am a pediatric nurse, and it has been getting hard to hold all of those little newborns. I just can't wait for one of my own.

April 24, 2014—I had my appointment with my RE today. I was looking forward to seeing him because I figured he would let me start another round of Femara and go from there, however, I was wrong! I got weighed, which is never fun, and I am up to a BMI of 22. With the walking and yoga and increased BMI, I was happy with my progress and feeling like I was in good shape to really get things moving with oral medications. He was surprised, though, that I did not respond to Provera, especially given my progress. He did an ultrasound and found that my lining was super thin. He was also concerned that I may have endometriosis because of prior symptoms and continued stomach pain. To make a long story short, he told me he wants to look into the endometriosis before moving forward with treatments. I really do trust my doctor, but I am so, so disappointed about taking a step back. This process just gets longer and longer. I pretty much have cried on and off all day. I know that ultimately, all of this will help me get pregnant and maintain a pregnancy, but I'm just sad.

April 27, 2014—On a positive note, yesterday I did a two mile walk for an organization that fundraises for premature babies, miscarriages, birth defects, etc. with a bunch of people from work. Back when I was running miles and miles, I would never do walks like this because they would take all morning and they weren't worth the time or money because it was such a short distance and would interfere with my morning run. However, I had a blast even though it took us about 50 minutes to walk the distance with the big crowd. No matter what happens with this process, I have already gained so much from just learning that I don't have to be defined by how much exercise I can do. I used to feel like I couldn't start the day unless I got my run in, and I would get upset if it was interrupted or something would get in the way. It feels so freeing to not worry anymore. I know I will still enjoy exercise when I can do it again, but now it will be because I want to (and in moderation), not because I have to.

May 1, 2014—I had another RE appointment today. After seven days of estrogen my lining grew to 9.5 mm. We decided to go forward with the surgery for endometriosis after I bleed, which means another one to two months before we can start fertility medications again. I am bummed, but I know that I need to get these procedures out of the way first so that I can move forward. I don't know the last time I have ever had a lining this thick, so I'm kind of worried about what my period will be like! I was joking with my doctor today about how I've never been so excited to start bleeding. Funny how our priorities change, right?

May 10, 2014—Just took my last dose of Provera so we will see what happens this week. I am feeling really, really down about myself. I went to get a pedicure with one of my friends this morning and she took a picture with her phone and posted it to Facebook. I should not have looked at the picture. It was just a reminder of how different I look; in my opinion, a lot less pretty. All of the hormones have caused my PCOS symptoms to increase, like the dark facial hair and the acne, and add to that the weight gain, and I basically just want to crawl in a hole. These last couple days of Provera have made me feel extra bloaty, and I just want it all to go away. I know it is important to stay the course because I want a baby more than I want my fit body, but it is hard to just feel like you don't want anyone to see you.

May 19, 2014—I had my HSG today. I had heard that the procedure was "uncomfortable," however, I was crying the entire time. They were very nice to me and kept asking me if I wanted them to stop, but of course, I just wanted to get it all over with. I have never felt pain that like before. The right tube looked good but the left tube was blocked for some reason. He said that when they go in for surgery he will take a better look at it and try to either see what is causing the blockage, or fix the blockage if he can. I still pretty much just want to cry all day. I feel like every time I go to the RE there is something new. I am thankful that this surgery will give me more answers, but I am also getting a little nervous. Sorry to vent, I think I am just a little exhausted. Thanks again everyone for the support, advice, and encouragement

May 29, 2014—The surgery went well! The RE said he found endometriosis and removed as much of it as he could. Also, he got a good look at my uterus (he diagnosed it several months ago as a "congenital anomaly of the uterus"), but said he won't do anything about it unless I have multiple miscarriages. The HSG had showed that my left tube was blocked, and during the surgery, the RE said he could only see a "trickle" of flow through the tube but didn't want to do anything yet so as not to damage it. I have my follow-up appointment in two weeks where he will discuss everything in more detail. I am anxious to hear what he has to say!

June 26, 2014—I have been reading the posts about struggles with weight gain and not seeing results and just wondering if it is all worth it. It is. Trust everyone on here when they say that increased body fat and decreased exercise *will* make a difference. I went in for my four-week follow-up after surgery with the hopes that I would be able to start treatment again. Lo and behold, I somehow had a 5.8 mm lining which is more than I have ever had on my own. And this is without any drugs or help whatsoever! That is me and my extra fat churning out some estrogen. The doctor was so pleased, and when I told him about the weight I gained, he was very, very happy. I know some of your REs said that your weight was fine, activity level fine, etc., but mine clearly said that there is evidence that increased body fat increases fertility and the response to medications. I even have PCOS too and the RE was still happy with the BMI increase. My doctor graduated from Cambridge with all of his degrees, so I believe him and trust him! I have been at this since January and the weight gain is *worth it*!

July 20, 2014—It has been quite the month. So full of ups and downs and everything in between! Last time I updated you all, I had just started 7.5 mg of Femara for five days. Long story short, nothing really happened—my lining actually decreased and I had no follicle growth. This was quite disappointing because I responded better to the 2.5 mg Femara that I did back in March. So, we decided to move onto injections. I took 75IU of Bravelle for four days then went in for an ultrasound. And, holy crap, my ovaries *blew up*. I grew five mature follicles as well as tons more that were smaller. My RE said we should cancel the cycle due to the high risk of multiples and OHSS. I was devastated. I know that over stimulating like this is common with PCOS, but I was on such a low dose for such a short amount of time. So, we canceled the cycle—then I got my period eight days later! I went back in for a CD 3 scan and I have three cysts on my right ovary, so I have to wait one more week and get another ultrasound to see if they shrink before we start the next round.

The good news is that it appears that I respond to injections (understatement), so we will try again this month with 37.5IU of Follistim for four days. I know that it can take several months of trying to get the medications right, so I just need to be patient. It is just difficult sometimes because we haven't even been able to get to try an IUI yet. Someday though! Patience is a virtue, right?

August 3, 2014—I did the 37.5 IU Follistim for six days, then I was ready to trigger! I had a lead follicle at 18 mm and three smaller ones. My husband and I even left a concert early so that we could trigger exactly on time. People must have thought something was wrong considering we had to leave right as the main act came on, however, we have new priorities now. I triggered Wednesday night and then went in for my IUI Friday. Everything went really well. It was strange to return to work right afterwards and pretend that I didn't just get inseminated by my doctor... but when you think about everything, it is somewhat humorous. I started the progesterone gel last night and then I test Friday August 15th, which seems so far away! I want to thank all of you on this board for your prayers, support and words of wisdom. My husband and I prayed and prayed for just a chance, and we got it. I can't believe that I will be taking my first ever real pregnancy test in a couple weeks after almost two years of trying.

August 6, 2014—Regarding the question of whether PCOS symptoms will get worse through HA recovery, I have both PCOS and HA, but I have not "androgenized" as I've gained weight. I do have quite a bit of dark facial hair (had it since I was a teenager), but I get it waxed every three weeks. I used to obsess about how awful it was. But people close to me know I have excessive hair and constantly tell me that they don't notice it. We are our own worst critics, so we are more likely to notice anything peculiar about ourselves way more often than other people. If you do in fact have PCOS, it can be regulated by lifestyle changes, so all hope it not lost!

August 14, 2014—I GOT A POSITIVE!! I just cannot believe it. We are in absolutely shock. It took about four seconds for the pregnancy test to turn positive. I went and got a beta drawn, so I'm waiting on those results, then the doctor wants to see me tomorrow to do an early ultrasound. They don't expect to see much, but I think they want to make sure that everything is where it is supposed to be. I think with the PCOS, endometriosis, and bum tube, they want to be extra careful. But I don't care, I am relishing this moment!!

Grace had her baby boy at the end of April, 2015.

Shayla—Possible PCOS, Exercise, and Undereating (recovery and diagnosis focus, then pregnancy – oral meds)

November 8, 2011—I have a past of disordered eating and overexercising and was on the pill for about 10 years. I went off the pill in March 2011 in the hopes of getting pregnant. Summer came and still no period. I went to the doctor to have a work-up done and was diagnosed with hypothalamic amenorrhea in July 2011. Since then I've gained a couple more pounds to get to a BMI of 21, and have decreased my exercise but still have not gotten a period. I also failed the Provera challenge. Now I'm wondering where I go from here. Do I reduce my exercise more? Currently I'm exercising five days a week at an hour most, either cardio (elliptical, walking) or a mix of cardio and strength training. And should I be upping my fat intake? Gain more weight? It's hard to know what exactly to do and all of you are such inspiration and I would love to hear any of your suggestions and learn more from you all.

> **Michelle S:** You sound like me about a year ago. I was in the same place; failed the Provera challenge, then put on some weight while continuing to work out 5-6 days a week. Finally, this past June I cut out all cardio and have continued to eat more in an effort to get my period back. I've taken Clomid twice and it worked well both times though I haven't gotten pregnant yet. I think you have to pay attention to your body. My RE originally told me to run just four days a week but after reading over this board I decided to cut it out completely. Again, I still haven't ovulated on my own yet but I know I'm closer now than I was a year ago. If you don't cut exercise out completely, definitely reduce it. Maybe cap it at a half hour per workout. And make sure you're getting enough fat.
>
> **Stefanie:** You're still working out a lot. Consider cutting back to 30 minutes and see how your body reacts. Decreasing the cardio really helped my body.

November 10, 2011—I'm eating around 1800 calories and from what I'm hearing here that's most likely not enough, especially with the exercise I was doing. Granted, at the time I thought that was an improvement! I should most likely be aiming for 2,000 calories or more with healthy fats and only walking for exercise.

> *Ciara*: I would actually suggest around 3,000 calories if you are trying to gain quickly. That may sound crazy but that's what I am eating. My nutritionist always told me to try and aim for 1,000 calories by noon. When she first said that I thought she had lost her mind! But now, I totally see what she means. I hope I don't sound preachy at all, I just know that I bummed around for a while making little changes and it wasn't until I really let everything go and ate like a football player that things started to turn around!

Ha-ha eat like a football player, love that! That's the thing… these past five months I feel like I've just been making little changes here and there (although I thought they were pretty big at the time), but it's obviously not enough. You're right, 3,000 does sound like a lot but it's probably easy to do once you add in all those healthy fats—they add up quickly! I'm definitely going to reevaluate my diet, make some changes, and like you said, just let everything go! My husband won't mind me eating this way either.

November 14, 2011—Thank you so much for your support and advice. You've convinced me that cutting down to a half hour of elliptical or walking will help. And you're right about not doing it on the treadmill—once I get on that I want to up the incline and speed and that won't help my situation. Then if I find that little amount of exercise is still too much I may just have to cut all exercise out until I get a cycle. It will be hard but taking baby steps will help.

December 4, 2011—Seeing the positive happenings and successes here that are happening for the ladies on this Board is so motivational and inspiring. My husband and I just had a serious talk Friday night about how I need to make more changes since my not getting a period yet is concerning him. I need to once and for all get my BMI to 22, keep eating lots of healthy fats, and reduce my exercise to just walking—no more elliptical. There are some days I'm in denial about it all and want to get that intense cardio workout in, but then I come to the Board, see the progress you've all made and how much those lifestyle changes help, and it reminds me to stay on track and not revert back to old habits. Thank you all for reminding me of that. It's truly so helpful and I'm now more motivated than ever!

December 31, 2011—Yesterday I went to have blood work done to see if my levels have improved and I haven't gotten back my estradiol results yet, but my LH was 14.3 and FSH 5.8. In July when I was diagnosed with HA my estradiol was below 50, LH 2.5 and FSH 4.1. Since they've both increased is this a good sign? I'm assuming we don't know much until I know if my estradiol has increased. Your thoughts/advice would be much appreciated.

January 4, 2012—My ob-gyn just emailed me and said that despite my higher LH level, the blood work results are still indicative of HA and I've made no improvement. My heart sank when I read his email. I thought my numbers did show improvement so I'm not sure why he feels this way—perhaps because my estradiol is still low? All he could advise was to see an RE but my insurance doesn't cover it and paying out of pocket is just not feasible right now. In any event, I'll just keep trucking on with my lifestyle changes and pray that I either ovulate or get my period soon.

> *Nico*: I don't think anyone on this board has had an $E_2 > 50$ except when just about to ovulate or on treatment. The E_2 level also doesn't seem to matter as much with regard to recovery as LH; mine was actually lower when I was cycling than not (around 30). One thing that I actually find interesting is that your LH was almost double your FSH. That suggests one of two things to me: either that your body was trying to ovulate (and many of us have our body try a few times, about two weeks apart, before the real deal happens—if you've been tracking your CM you may notice patches of EW about two weeks apart); or you perhaps do have a mild form of PCOS that was masked by your HA exercising and eating habits. I don't think that is a big deal, except in that you may end up with longer cycles or not cycling because of PCOS. It is possible that metformin might be helpful, and Clomid or Femara should also take care of any cycling irregularities that may be due to the PCOS. I would suggest that you get another set of blood work done about a month after the last one, and see if your LH: FSH ratio is going up. If it is, and you're not showing signs of ovulating, I think at that point you should talk to your doc about the possibility of PCOS.

January 8, 2012—I'm very happy I made these lifestyle changes because even if I weren't trying to get pregnant, I would have wanted to heal from HA in and of itself. This whole experience has made me a healthier and happier person: I've really learned to be more balanced with my exercise and eating; to accept my body at its happy weight; and to just live life. I like to think everything happens for a reason and I've definitely learned a lot from this experience!

January 11, 2012—Well I got my results back and the PCOS diagnosis is inconclusive, but chances of trying to get pregnant naturally seem slim to me. The email from my doctor said:

"Your total testosterone level is 56 (slightly elevated), and the free testosterone level is 4.6 (normal). Free testosterone is the active component in your blood, so this is the more important value. Your LH value is elevated in relation to FSH. But lab values are not the only indicator for the diagnosis. With regards to the diagnosis of polycystic ovarian syndrome, it's inconclusive. We will discuss this more at your visit."

**Edited to Add: I just read up on some symptoms of PCOS and while I don't have all of them, I do have some like mild acne (face, chest, and back), blood sugar swings, high cholesterol, and no period. So I may have a mild form of PCOS.

> *Jil*: Whether or not you have a combined PCOS/HA problem it doesn't change the fact that you need to keep doing what you're doing! I don't think acne necessarily means you have PCOS even though it's part of the diagnosis. For me, I had perfect skin until I was 18 and lost a ton of weight/began exercising like crazy. In my opinion my hormones were totally shifted from my low weight/body fat etc., not because of PCOS. Keep your chin up!

January 27, 2012—From July to December, I had a couple of setbacks: adding in a bit too much exercise, being in denial about it all, and taking my stress out by exercising. This month I gave myself a reality check and realized that I absolutely need to lay off the exercise if I want to do this naturally. Now I'm just walking, 45 minutes four times a week. Had I not had those silly setbacks and swallowed my pride I'd probably have my cycles back by now, so my advice to you is to really start NOW at gaining weight and lowering the exercise—you can do it!!

February 8, 2012—I met with my endocrinologist (who I started seeing because of the possible PCOS) this morning and it went really well. She's confident that I should have my cycles back in a few months if I just maintain my weight and reduced exercising. She reminded me that although I've been on this journey since I was diagnosed in July, I have only maintained this weight since the beginning of January (along with my reduced exercising) so she feels I need to give it time. And like you all said, she also thought I'd respond really well to Clomid if I chose to go that route. However, she still wants to do further blood work to either rule in or rule out PCOS since my testosterone was high. Results are best when you've fasted so I'll go in to the lab this Saturday and results should come in about a week.

February 15, 2012—I met with the endocrinologist, and based on my latest blood work she says I probably do have PCOS. With that, I'm starting to get irritable and anxious about my period coming naturally and with turning 30 coming up in May, I really want to get the ball rolling, so I think I want to give Clomid a shot.

March 5, 2012—I finally have the green light to start Clomid—yay! I got the prescription yesterday so that I was ready when she gave me the go ahead. I'll start Provera tomorrow morning for 12 days and hopefully I'll get a bleed. If not, I'll contact my doctor for an estrogen/progesterone pill to induce a bleed and will start Clomid after that. She firmly believes I have PCOS and that I'll have great success on Clomid…we'll see.

March 18, 2012—I wanted to let you all know that my period is here!! The Provera worked and I am over the moon, so thrilled. It started this morning as brown spotting and now I've got full blown cramps and blood. My last Provera pill was yesterday so I'm happy that my period came right away (I think that's a really great sign) and things are working. Now I start Clomid on CD 5. I am so excited!

March 19, 2012—To those that are struggling to gain and waiting to get a period— I've been in your shoes and please don't lose hope. If there's any advice I can give, it would be to give it TIME. It's been a year since I went off the pill, nine months since I was diagnosed with HA, and three months of consistently being at a BMI of 22. I've been (mostly) patient throughout all this and I truly think that helps. You need to give your body time to be at that healthy weight so it can trust you again and knows you'll stay there and not get overly thin again. I know how hard it is. I shed many many tears wondering what was wrong with my body and having bad body image days, but remember, it WILL work and your body will respond, with time. I know, easier said than done, but if I can do it given the damage I had done to my body, I know you can too. Yeah, I have my moments where I'm feeling a bit jiggly in spots, but it is so very worth it to know that those jiggly bits are what's helping me produce estrogen and I responded to Provera. I also want to say how much of an advocate you have to be for yourself in all this. My ob-gyn was sure I wouldn't respond to the Provera since I failed it last year, but I pushed him to have me try it again and it worked! You really need to stand up for yourself and do what you feel is right. Give your body healthy fats, keep exercise intensity and duration low, get to a fertile BMI, and give it time.

May 17, 2012—I'm ashamed to admit that though I've maintained a BMI of 22, during my last cycle I added in a bit more intensity and duration of my workouts than I should have. I feel like such a sham doing that but it's the truth—having responded so beautifully to Provera and then getting a positive OPK, I felt I could get away with an extra day of exercise with a bit more intensity. Well, I didn't ovulate, which proved to me that I absolutely CANNOT revert back to old exercise habits.

May 18, 2012—I was talking to my supervisor today, she's about 35 and has a rockin', cute, curvy body. I asked her what her workout routine was like; she said that three times a week is perfect for her. Why can't I think that way??!! That is her normal and I have to just forget how I used to exercise because that simply was *not* normal, it was excessive and unhealthy.

June 8, 2012—I had an appointment with a new ob-gyn today and I absolutely love her. I really feel that she has my best interests at heart and she said she'll do all she can to help us get pregnant. The attention to my needs and concerns and the intimacy was awesome; nothing like my other doctor. Since today is CD 12 she did an ultrasound and confirmed that I have PCOS and that my HA was masking it. The ultrasound showed *tons* of follicles—none about to take off, but hopefully I'll be ovulating later in the cycle. She said she's confident that I will respond wonderfully to Clomid or if we take a break I could very well get pregnant naturally. And if Clomid doesn't work she's willing to try Femara—yay!

June 28, 2012—Yesterday when I was weighed at the doctors I saw a number I never thought I'd reach. At first I was like "Holy smokes I'll be enormous when I'm pregnant!!!" I had to quickly snap my mind out of spiraling into those negative thoughts and remind myself "It's for a baby, it's for a baby." That fat and weight gain is so *very* important for us and that it means ESTROGEN!! Twenty pounds ago I didn't respond to Provera whatsoever, had very low estrogen, and zero lining. Now at this weight, I've had three periods and had a 7mm lining at my ultrasound yesterday—very good for a HAer and only possible after my weight gain. It is so hard to gain the weight and accept the new curves that come with each week and month. But they will bring you that much closer to getting pregnant. Don't get discouraged, stay strong, *you can do this*!!

July 5, 2012—So sorry ladies I've been MIA but I just needed a break as I was very depressed and upset these last couple weeks. It's been rough since getting my low progesterone results, which indicated I didn't ovulate. I've had many "Why me's?" and crying sessions every other day but am feeling much better today. Anyway, I ended up finding yet another doctor. She did an ultrasound and I definitely have polycystic ovaries (she described them as a "string of pearls") although she doesn't have my blood work to confirm PCOS. She's pretty confident that metformin coupled with Femara and a trigger shot will work for me, so we'll most likely go that route. The metformin apparently regulates insulin levels, which then helps you ovulate.

August 7, 2012—I (finally!) have some awesome news—today I went for my CD 14 ultrasound and my lining was 8mm, trilaminar, and there was a 19mm follicle!! So I take the trigger shot tonight, the doctor recommended we have sex tonight and then we'll do an IUI. It's so very relieving to know Femara is the ticket to making my body respond and even if this doesn't end in pregnancy, I'm just so happy and excited to any minute have a chance at pregnancy, yay yay yay!! But boy, doing that trigger shot was no walk in the park. I had some serious troubles getting all the solution up into the needle and kept squirting it back into the vial to do it over again—I hope I didn't mess it up! Thankfully my husband came in and saved the day and got every last drop into the vial and injected me, which didn't hurt at all. Oh and I'll test two weeks from tomorrow will be the 22nd, the day we're leaving for my husband's best friend's wedding and to visit with his parents so it'd be pretty darn awesome if I get a positive that morning and then we can tell his parents in person. It would make for one awesome celebratory trip!

August 15, 2012—Since my late teens I've been addicted to exercise. In my 20s I was a Spinning and Group Power/Body Pump instructor; exercise was a big part of my identity. After I did a Spin class I would then run or strength train for another 30 to 60 minutes. No matter what my workouts *had* to be 1.5 to 2 hours and if not, I would leave the gym unsatisfied. Each day that the scale went down brought a new high—my identity was to be skinny and super fit. What kind of life is that?? I look back and wonder how I did it. On top of it all, I would severely undereat. I did embrace food again over time but exercise still had that pull on me and it was only when I joined this Board that I broke free. I have finally woken up this past year. It's an AMAZING feeling to be out of that jail. I wouldn't be where I am today without all these amazing women, Nico in particular, who told me first in all no nonsense honesty what I needed to do to not only get pregnant, but to be healthy and free from all those obsessions. I will forever be grateful to God for bringing her and the other women here into my life. Sure, there's still a part of me that cannot wait to do a sweat pumping workout after I have babies, but being free from the feeling that I *have* to is the most important part and I will never get back to that place. Walking and being at a happy fertile weight has brought me such peace and I am truly happier now, all 35 more pounds of me.

August 19, 2012—My pregnancy test was negative today, so I'm praying it may be too early (11 DPO) and that it turns into a positive soon. If it is negative, I'm just thankful I've responded to treatment and had my first chance at pregnancy I'm going to test again later this week but won't be able to get a beta until we get back from NY.

August 20, 2012—Positive!!!!!!!!! I was going to hold out until Wednesday but just couldn't. Today is 12 DPO and my pregnancy test is pretty faint, so I took a digital just to be sure and it says "Pregnant"!! I am still in shock, shaking, crying, excited, and nervous—I can't believe this is happening, it feels so surreal. Thank you all SO much for all your prayers, love and support. I could not have gotten through this without all you amazing women and just love you all so very much!! I'll go in for a beta tomorrow since we're heading out to NY early Wednesday morning. Praying for a strong beta and a sweet sticky bean.

Shayla nursed her son for four months, regained cycles at three months postpartum, and has been cycling naturally ever since. She is currently pregnant again, naturally conceived on her first cycle trying.

Category 6: Bones

Bone density is a concern in anyone who has HA, particularly depending on the length of time a person has been without a period. It is important to understand the ramifications of low bone density; Jessica V. spoke to many different doctors because of her diagnosis of severe osteopenia. She ultimately had two children and was able to nurse both, although at points in time she was not sure she'd be able to do either. Jess also describes some of the steps she has taken in addition to recovering from HA, in order to further rebuild bone density.

Jessica V—Exercise and Undereating (bone and recovery focus)

Please note: this is one woman's experience with HA causing bone density issues and advice she was given by her doctors. If you likewise have low bone density, please speak with a knowledgeable endocrinologist for advice tailored to your specific situation, taking into account your bone density, nutrition, supplements and past fracture history. The advice given to Jessica is not necessarily correct for anyone else.

February 26, 2011—I'm 31 years old, and was on birth control pills from about age 18 to 29. I remember missing periods during my last few years on the pill, but doctors told me it was normal. When I finally went off the pill, I discovered that my body was not ovulating and had no periods. I went to various doctors, who either told me to go back on the pill or to simply eat more. After feeling like I was the only one in this situation and there was no hope for me, I was finally referred on to a specialist who diagnosed me with HA.

For most of my adult life, I've undereaten and overexercised. For many years, I avoided fat and carbs altogether because I didn't realize that my body needed them. I got a high from eating as few calories as possible, and wore size zero clothes. I used to run an hour every day, for years and years.

The doctors referred me to a nutritionist, whom I saw several times. She really helped me to rethink my destructive patterns. I've been making a concerted effort to eat healthy fats, carbs and protein. It's been an amazing discovery to find that I can eat in a normal way and not get tremendously huge. I gained six pounds and went from BMI 20 to 22. This doesn't sound like a big difference in weight, but previously I was having a lot of sugar and alcohol (probably because my body wanted the calories), which I've basically cut out completely and replaced with healthy foods. Doctors and the nutritionist have told me that I don't need to gain more weight. I've reduced my running to 45 minutes daily. I know this might still be too much, and I'm willing to cut this out completely if necessary.

The doctors scanned my bones and found that I have osteopenia in my back (my T score was -2.2). For that reason, they put me onto Hormone Replacement Therapy (HRT), which puts the hormones that I'm not producing into my body.

The problem is that for as long as I'm on HRT it's highly unlikely that I'll become pregnant; as something about HRT stops pregnancy from happening. So, even though I really would love to have a baby, I'm basically on birth control. I'm going back to the doctor at the end of the month, and will ask to be taken off HRT for a period of time so I can see if my periods come back naturally. If they do not, then I'll give up running completely to see if that helps.

I also started going to acupuncture three months ago and have been drinking a special herbal tea from that clinic. Since the HRT is making my body have periods, I don't know whether the acupuncture has been effective in helping me to ovulate naturally. I've also been taking vitex for ages, although I don't think it's had much of an impact.

I'm an American who is temporarily living in England. This means that I get free medical care (including fertility treatment since I have a diagnosed fertility problem). I am very lucky to have this intervention for free, but on the down side, the doctor appointments are few and far between, and I do not get the kind of comprehensive information and frequent visits that other women have posted about.

The fertility doctor has offered to start me on Menopur, which would be my first intervention for having a baby. After giving it a lot of consideration, I decided that I would like to try some natural techniques to get my body ovulating again before trying treatments. It's been a difficult decision, but I think it's the right one for me at this time.

March 1, 2011—Well, here is the moment that I knew was coming. The RE today agreed that I can go off the HRT patch and try for a normal cycle, so now it's time to seriously cut down on the exercise. We agreed to a three-month trial period, and if there is no natural cycle at that point we'll revisit the idea of Menopur. Because of my osteopenia, it wouldn't be safe for me to be off HRT for too long if I'm not producing sufficient hormones naturally. She's also referring me to an obstetrician who will tell me whether it's a good idea for me to be pregnant at all right now, given that being pregnant would mean giving the baby priority on consuming any calcium that I eat, which could further impact my bones. Fingers crossed that he gives me the green light!

Since about the age of thirteen, I've been an avid daily runner. But starting tomorrow there will be no more running. I am going to look into some lighter exercise a few days per week, and walk about 30 minutes daily as part of my work commute. Everyone who knows me can't believe that I'm actually going to stop running, but reading posts on this board and knowing that others are dealing with the same issues has been so helpful in making me feel mentally ready to take this step.

The good news is that the RE also told me that results from my HSG came out normal, in addition to my pelvic ultrasound, sperm analysis, and that my uterus is a good size and has good sized follies. So if I can get these natural ovulation and osteopenia things sorted out, everything else looks good to go.

March 13, 2011—While on my walk yesterday (because I'm not running even though it's killing me), I was thinking about how a few people posted recently that they are "too scared" to find out whether they have osteopenia. I usually take the view that more information is better, as being afraid to find out something about our own bodies leaves us unable to take positive action.

I just want to mention a bit about the information that I was given after my diagnosis: as I understand it, osteopenia is reversible. Doctors do not scan your bones just to tell you that you have low bone density and then send you on your way. If you have low bone density, they can prescribe you a high dose calcium + vitamin D tablet (that dissolves in water so it's fizzy like orange soda pop) to take daily. This is supposed to at least keep your body from depleting any further calcium from your bones. I don't want to lecture anybody, but it seems that this board is all about learning from our own mistakes and making positive changes to get ourselves back on track. A lot of us damaged our bodies due to not fully understanding the impact of our actions. Now that we have more information, we can do something about it. Information is your friend.

April 18, 2011—A bit of excitement over here. No, not that kind of excitement. I'm not trying to get pregnant quite yet, although I hope to start in the next month or so. But. Last week, I had what definitely seemed to be EWCM. Due to an extended time on BCP, I haven't had a natural ovulation since high school (I'm now 31) so this is all uncharted waters. I think I'm in a two week wait and actually HOPING to get my period at the end of it. Not exactly as exciting as the kind of two week waits that many of you ladies are in, but momentous enough for me right now.

April 30, 2011—For now, I want to share my great news—a few days ago, I had a natural period!! For the past six weeks, I've stopped running altogether although I still do yoga/Pilates/exercise videos for a total of four hours weekly. I don't even have words to describe how difficult it was to stop running, but now I really do feel that it has been worthwhile.

For those who are still considering whether to cut back on exercise, I was terrified about the changes in my body, but my husband says that I actually look better with the weight that I gained. Yes, he is a very nice guy and would probably tell me that anyway but I actually agree with him!

I had HA at a BMI of 21, and it was hard for me to accept that I was just not cut out to be super skinny. However, now that I have a BMI closer to 23 or 24 I have so much more energy than I did before and have discovered that not running becomes easier a time goes on.

May 2, 2011—"Reduce exercise, increase fats... repeat, repeat, repeat." Reading that message so many times was so powerful and gave me the impetus to change. Interestingly, my doctors had been telling me basically the same thing for nearly a year, but just hearing that message once every few months from a doctor had nowhere near the same impact as hearing it daily on this Board.

May 5, 2011—I had a preconception appointment with an ob-gyn a few days ago. I had requested the appointment because of the osteopenia in my spine and wanted to know if becoming pregnant right now could lead to permanent damage. I was really anticipating that the doctor would tell me that it would be fine for me to go ahead and start trying to conceive. Unfortunately, that was not his advice. The doctor told me that while being pregnant and breastfeeding really deplete a woman's bone mineral density, the bones have a strange mechanism for recovering their density very quickly after pregnancy and doctors don't entirely understand how that happens. *However*, the risk is that all women's bone mineral density falls to some extent while they are pregnant and since I am already in the osteopenia range, I would be at greater risk of developing a fracture *during* pregnancy than a woman with average bone density. The damage that results from a fracture can be permanent. So, the doctor said that I should wait another six months until my bone mass is built up a bit more. Frustrating news after I have waited so long to try to conceive and am finally ovulating on my own. But on the other hand, what's another six months after all this waiting?

May 15, 2011—For almost the duration of my twenties, I was running for an hour each day and eating a very restricted diet. The outcome of all that was that I was only about eight pounds lighter than I am now, when I am not running and eating healthy amounts including fats. Why did I think that basic rules of nutrition like eating carbs and healthy fats did not apply to me? Now I have much more energy and my BMI only went up a few points. What a waste.

May 25, 2011—I was expecting my second natural period on Monday, but it still has not arrived. I'm not temping and had a bit of CM "down there" throughout the cycle but I'm not entirely sure when or even if I may have ovulated. I have two possible ovulation dates written on my calendar, one of which would have projected my period for today and another which predicts it would happen in a few more days. I was so thrilled after my first natural period a month ago, now I feel a bit like I've been punched in the stomach. I'm so afraid that my period won't come again and last month's was a total fluke.

May 30, 2011—Like one hour after posting about no second natural period, it arrived! I'm thrilled that it started five weeks after the last one. Not quite the most ideal cycle length, but a heck of a lot better than none at all.

June 19, 2011—I was looking at some of my wedding photos from four years ago, and I felt so sad seeing how horribly skinny I was. I remember thinking that I looked really good back then and taking real pride in wearing a size 4 wedding dress that still had to be taken in. But I looked positively skeletal and my body was starving inside. I think it must have been very hard for my family and friends to see me looking so unhealthy and running so much and eating in such a restricted way.

I'm also so appreciative of my husband. He has never ever told me off or seemed the slightest bit angry that my fertility was impacted by my own actions. For the longest time, he told me that he didn't really mind if we adopted or had children naturally. Now that I've started cycling again, I can see how excited he is, which makes me appreciate even more how he suppressed his desire to have children so as to not put pressure on me. Although I wish I could, I seriously doubt that I would be able to accommodating and understanding if our roles were reversed.

July 5, 2011—Natural period #3 started today. It always starts just when I completely lose hope. Last cycle was 35 days; this time it was 37 days. I thank my lucky stars that I have been fortunate enough to resume cycling, but I am a bit nervous my periods seem to be further and further apart (although by very small amounts) and wonder whether this is healthy and normal. In particular, I am concerned that I might still be overdoing it in the exercise department. I am doing five hours weekly of Pilates and other floor exercises, with two rest days each week. I suspect that my BMI is hovering around 22, although I don't own a scale so I'm not certain.

July 14, 2011—My estrogen was so low with HA that I did not even have withdrawal bleeds on birth control pills. I have managed to regain my cycles by increasing by fat intake and stopping running altogether. Even women who make lifestyle changes but don't regain their cycles straight away will still respond much better to any fertility treatment because of their increased BMI. I so wish that I could go back in time and address this issue when I was in my twenties. Maybe then I wouldn't have osteopenia (which in my case was brought on by the combination of undernutrition and low estrogen). I'm so scared about having the bones of a much older person, and it becomes harder to increase bone mass as you age, so if you're younger, you should really take advantage of being able to do something about your lifestyle now! I also think back to how much more emotionally stable I would have been during my twenties if I had been eating properly and giving my body the rest that it needed. You are probably discovering from reading these posts that we cannot just turn on our fertility with sudden lifestyle changes once we are ready to try for babies. Best to deal with it when you're younger so your body is ready when you are!

September 8, 2011—I managed to get bone scan results from the clinic. Not good news. Actually, very bad news. It seems that I had a false reading when I had my scan last year, and I am still extremely close to osteoporosis, with no significant change in bone density after two years of taking calcium and vitamin D supplements.

Today's results reveal that my bone density is actually worse than the ob-gyn thought it was six months ago when he told me to wait six months before trying to get pregnant. The risk is that if I became pregnant I could suffer a fracture to my spine, which can never be healed. The other risk is that I could be a hunchback at an early age because my bones aren't improving, whether I ever get pregnant or not. I'm so disappointed and sad. I cried at work for the first time today, and I'm not a big crier at all. I really don't know what to do, go for it and risk a permanent fracture or just throw in the towel and never have children and still probably have problems? There's just no good answer.

I know that the new reading was accurate because I followed the advice that I have seen on many reputable websites and abstained from taking calcium supplements for 48 hours prior to the scan. When I had the previous scan, I kept taking everything and got what I can now tell was a false reading.

September 2, 2011—I'm very selfishly going to have to take a break from the board for a while. Somehow, reading all of these posts is making me want to try and get pregnant very badly (imagine that!) and I really need to be patient and wait until I have a chance to consult with a doctor. As some of you mentioned, there are varying degrees of osteopenia. Mine is unfortunately dangerously near osteoporosis and I need to consult a specialist to find out whether I would risk a permanent fracture with pregnancy. The stakes are really too high for me to stick my head in the sand.

I've been fortunate enough to find a lot of information about things that I can to do to improve my bone health. After learning more, it's become apparent to me that I experienced an unlucky combination of HA + eating disorder + medications that depleted my bone density all at once. So most of you are probably not in the same boat as me. The good news is, mine was detected before a fracture. I definitely encourage all of you to have bone scans also, so you too can be so lucky.

Now that my HA is resolved, I'm devoting my time and energy to solving this bone thing. There is a lot that I have to learn about diet and exercise. My husband told me that I will definitely find a way to improve my health, as he pointed out that rallying and obsessing until change happens is what I do well (thank you HA personality). They shouldn't call us Type A; we should be known as Type HA = Driven women on a mission.

I've got a new mission to devote myself to, so off I go on mine and I wish you all the very best on yours! Maybe I'll be in a position to try for a baby fairly soon, maybe in a year, maybe I'll just adopt and be thankful for my health. I have to say that, whether or not I have children, regaining my periods and normality in my body has been well worth all the changes. I have more energy, I feel more alive, look better, and I know that I am much healthier.

October 9, 2011—After a dramatic exit from the board several weeks ago, I did a lot of research and decided to start trying to get pregnant. I learned that breastfeeding can cause much more depletion of bone density than pregnancy. So I probably won't be able to breastfeed; but happily I am going to try for a baby. I haven't consulted a doctor, because referrals to specialists take ages in the UK. But seriously, what am I going to do? Wait even longer? It's hard to imagine what a doctor could tell me that would make me not go ahead and try to become pregnant.

So, now I'm 11 DPO on my first ever two week wait. Wow, does the possibility of being pregnant ever make you obsess. I was missing out on all the, um, fun! I don't think this will be the cycle for me, given that my husband and I only decided to start trying while I was ovulating and the tension of that decision gave him some performance issues during the crucial window. We did manage to do it the following day, so I figure maybe there's a slim chance. But really I haven't had any symptoms, except that I went to the dentist yesterday and my gums were bleeding really a LOT. However, Doctor Google says that generally only happens during the second or third trimester. So this probably won't be the cycle for me. Looks like my LP's have varied between 12 and 15 days, so I'm not sure when my period should arrive, which doesn't make this wait any easier!

October 10, 2011—I was going to wait until tomorrow morning to take my test but you all know how tempting it is when the stick is RIGHT THERE... I raced home and did it straight away. There was a faint second line, I can hardly believe it!!

June 5, 2012—I became pregnant in October 2011, and am expecting my baby in three weeks! My ob-gyn has me on a lot of calcium and vitamin D supplementation, because the baby will deplete calcium from your bones if you don't get enough in your diet. (Although discuss this with your doctor first, since it might not be advised in the first trimester). I don't know what my current bone density is, and I'm feeling nervous about breastfeeding, which I've heard tends to diminish bone density in the short term (you gain it back, but are vulnerable to fractures in the meantime). My plan is to start breastfeeding and then see what happens.

June 24, 2013—At long last, I had my bone density scan. The last one I had was two years ago. It turns out that nothing's really changed. I'm not sure whether this is good or bad, since I did have a baby and nurse for six months in the past two years. Spine is -2.2, hip is around -.5, neck is around -.3 (I think) so my spine is the only one in the osteopenia zone. Accounting for margin of error, I think this is essentially where it's been since I started getting scans around three years ago. So I guess I'm relieved that pregnancy and nursing didn't make it worse, but also disappointed that it's not better after all the weight bearing exercise, calcium supplements, vitamin D, natto, etc. I've been doing for the past two years. Kind of makes me wonder whether I can really do much to increase it.

August 30, 2013—My endocrinologist told me that I could nurse for six to nine months (but urged me to stay closer to the six-month mark). He said that after that time I would start losing bone so I shouldn't go longer. I also had to supplement with a LOT of calcium to try to avoid my body taking the calcium from my bones to give to my baby. It was super hard, both emotionally and physically, to wean at six months, but I'm grateful that I had that time to nurse. My only caution would be that my endo gave this advice to me specifically, knowing that my bone density is in the osteopenia range, so I'm not sure if it's applicable across situations. I did not have a decrease in bone density, if anything, I had a slight increase, but there are a lot of other variables that could account for that: I've done lots of diet and exercise work to try to improve my bone density. I do think it's worth noting that the National Osteoporosis Foundation forums have quite a few accounts from younger women who didn't realize they had low bone density until they experienced a fracture while nursing. So, if you have osteopenia or osteoporosis it is definitely worth consulting a specialist before making a decision about nursing. But I've heard/read that bone density tends to rebuild very quickly after weaning, so any increased fracture risk is only while and immediately after nursing. In the long term, there shouldn't be any risk of bone density lowering as a result of nursing. Just be sure to supplement your own calcium intake very well so that your body isn't using up calcium from your bones in order to make milk for your baby.

The return of Jessica's cycles after weaning at six months postpartum was masked by Asherman's syndrome. Three months after corrective surgery, she conceived her second child naturally. She was able to nurse her son for six months also.

Category 7: HA as a Result of a Medical Condition

In the vast majority of people with HA, the condition is due to some combination of undereating, exercise, stress, and genetics. In a small subset, however, there are other reasons that lead to under eating—various medical conditions that make getting sufficient nutrients difficult. Tracy, for example, suffers from Crohn's disease, but was able through dietary changes, to keep her disease in remission for almost two years while she was trying to conceive.

Tracy—Crohn's disease (recovery focus, then pregnancy, miscarriage, ultimately pregnant with IVF)

March 29, 2012—I'm 28 years old and haven't had a period since I came off the pill a year ago. My fertility specialist has recently diagnosed me with HA after having blood work done (showing "quiet" hormones) and a pelvic ultrasound to rule out PCOS. I don't have a history of an eating disorder or over exercising, but I do have active Crohn's Disease. I have had two bad flare-ups since July 2010, and each time I dropped 20 lb *fast*. (For those that don't know, Crohn's is an inflammatory bowel disease characterized by diarrhea, weight loss, fever, and bloody stools). My normal BMI is 19.5, but each time I flared I went down to a BMI of 17.5. It only took a few weeks to gain the weight back (with the help of some nasty steroids to decrease the inflammation), but I'm putting the puzzle pieces together and have figured out that this unhealthy weight loss is likely what triggered my body to develop HA.

I'd definitely like to have a baby soon, but haven't been actively trying since I'm not menstruating. My fertility doc laid out a game plan as follows: try Clomid first (but not to get my hopes up as she said it doesn't usually work for women with HA). If/when that fails we'll move on to injectable gonadotropins. If that doesn't work out, then it's onto IVF.

The more I read on here the more I'm starting to warm up to the idea of trying to gain weight, but I think it will be very difficult because of my Crohn's. I eat a pretty restricted diet (no gluten, grains, lactose, soy, legumes, very limited sugar) so it's tough to overindulge. Plus, my digestion is all screwed up so everything I eat goes right through me and fast! But I could definitely try to increase my healthy fats and see what happens...

April 6, 2012—The other day I had an appointment with my GI doc regarding my Crohn's. He was aware that I have been amenorrheic for the past year and I told him my new plan was to gain weight in hopes of kick starting my cycle (or at least getting to the point where I'd be responsive to fertility meds), and he laughed at me! Said that he didn't think I needed to gain weight but rather needed to get my Crohn's better controlled and then my period would likely come back on its own. I mean it's probably all related but I dunno... It's confusing. It sucks for anyone to have to deal with HA, but ladies please take comfort in the fact that you're dealing with HA alone and not in combination with an inflammatory bowel disease at the same time!! It's just making things extra hard. Sorry for the pity party but my point is just to make you lovely ladies feel better about your own situation.

April 12, 2012—I've just been plugging along, trying to shove those calories down my throat. I must admit, it's been kind of fun! I have quite the sweet tooth, so not feeling guilty about indulging has been nice. According to the scale I've only gained a pound or two … but I definitely feel softer. It could just be in my head but I don't think so.

April 27, 2012—The weight gain hasn't been terribly successful for me thus far, and I'm starting to face the reality that it may just not be a possibility for me due to my digestive issues. That said, I'm definitely going to continue to try, and even though the number on the scale isn't changing maybe my body will be able to realize I'm overfeeding it and things will start happening. I have actually noticed some CM lately, and even some definite EWCM the other day, which is a total first for me! I was pretty pumped when I saw it.

June 28, 2012—Clover, so you used to have GI issues too? I'm so glad you've gotten over them! It's really quite terrible, but I always think there are much worse things out there that people have to deal with, so I try to stay positive. I do well with fats like coconut, avocado and olive oil, but the jury is still out with regards to dairy. It really seems to upset my stomach almost immediately, and I also tend to get more acne when I eat dairy, so I try to keep it to a minimum.

> **Clover**: I agree that there are far worse sufferings among us but the reality is bloating, constipation, diarrhea—oh and all at the same time—just suck… My stomach actually started digesting better on this weight gain quest. I had to cut out most fruit and vegetables, which is when I noticed my digestive issues decreasing. I am a sweet potato, olive oil, avocado, ice cream girl now.

June 29, 2012—I had my appointment with my RE today and I'm *so excited*! I went in with a copy of the Clomid Extended Protocol study to give to her, but before I even had a chance to say anything she brought it up. I had mentioned it briefly at my last appointment, at which time she said she hadn't heard about it. I guess she looked into it on her own after that, so she was all "It looks promising—I'd like to try it with you if you're willing." YES! So I got a script to do five days of 50 mg Clomid and five days of 100 mg. And I'm going to be monitored this first cycle.

As excited as I am to get started, I have to be realistic that my BMI is still too low, so I may not respond. But I'm going to give it a go and see what happens. I have to take BCP to get a bleed first, so obviously I'll keep eating like crazy and trying to gain as much as I can in the meantime. (I went out for gluten-free pizza last night and I ate the *whole* thing... and it wasn't small!)

July 3, 2012—Thank you all for your input regarding my GI issues!! I have been experimenting and not eating salads or raw veggies for the past few days and I've been feeling *great*! I hope it's not just coincidence.

July 18, 2012—I was getting a bit worried but my period finally arrived—it took a good 3.5 days after I finished the BCP. Tomorrow is CD 3, and I'll be starting Clomid EP. I phoned the nurse today and she said I'll go for blood work on CD 10. If that shows my estrogen is still low, we'll just keep doing blood work every couple days until it gets higher. She said ovulation doesn't usually happen until estrogen is around 1000 pmol/L, so once it starts rising more we'll do a scan to see what's happening. I'm excited to get going with this! Really, *really*, hoping for a good response, or at the very least any response!

July 30, 2012—Ugh, ladies it appears that the Clomid EP isn't working for me. I had blood work done today, CD 15, and my E_2 is still "less than 20." It hasn't risen at all! If it's not rising by now, then it's safe to assume there is no follicle action going on. The next step is blood work again next Tuesday, which will be CD 23. I guess if it hasn't risen this cycle will be a bust.

August 5, 2012—After I told you all that it didn't seem like the Clomid EP was working for me a few of you asked how the weight gain was going. Well... not great to be honest. I was feeling so good digestive-wise for a few weeks there, and I gained a quick seven pounds, which was awesome. Since then, I've been feeling pretty good but have had a few Crohn's symptoms reappear, which means inflammation in my GI tract so not absorbing nutrients properly. That said, I'm still feeling pretty good, so I won't complain!! But my BMI is holding steady at 19.5. To be honest, I'm not sure how much more weight I'll be able to gain. I seriously eat like a horse and do practically no exercise!!! It's just the stupid GI problems that have messed up my system. But I will keep on keepin' on!

Some good news though: I've been having hot flashes!!! That must mean something is happening, right??

August 13, 2012—I'm responding!!! So excited! Nurse just called and said my E_2 is at 187 pg/mL (US units)! This is CD 29, and E_2 up from 42 last week. Instructions to have sex every two days starting tomorrow. Then blood work again on Wednesday.

August 30, 2012—I *think* I might be pregnant!!!!! I'm excited but don't want to get *too* excited yet because the second line is very faint. It's definitely there, but not dark at all. I remember some of you ladies saying "a line is a line", so that's what I'm hoping! But when I showed my husband he was very skeptical! I tried explaining that if there's a line that means there is hCG in my system, and it's still earlyish at 12 DPO, so it is likely the real deal. But I'm not even 100% sure about that—just hoping.

September 11, 2012—My beta results today were not good. My number was only 226. If it was doubling every 48 hours, it should have been about 1800 by today. I think deep down I knew this was going to be the outcome.

I got the phone call at work, so had to put on a happy face right after and finish up my work. I did pretty well at putting it out of my thoughts, but as soon as I got into my car the tears started flowing. I thought I got it out of my system by the time I got home, but then as soon as I came in I saw a vase of flowers with an "I love you" heart-shaped note stuck on the side. And the waterworks began once again. I just love my husband so much and am so incredibly blessed to have him by my side.

Anyway I am very thankful and still shocked that I even got this far this quickly. I wasn't expecting to ovulate on my first medicated cycle, let alone get pregnant... I just pray that my Crohn's will stay in remission so that I can conceive feeling well again. I am grateful that my body responded, and that's what I need to keep reminding myself.

September 18, 2012—I had a nice weekend with my husband in Vancouver. We stayed in a beautiful hotel, did some shopping, sight-seeing, and lots of eating. I started cramping late on Saturday evening once we got back to the hotel. It was odd—they weren't sharp pains, but deep cramping that was coming in waves every couple of minutes. And then, some bleeding. Luckily I was beat from a busy day of activities, so closed my eyes and fell asleep shortly thereafter. When I woke up the cramping was gone, so I must have slept through it. I felt pretty good Sunday, and only light bleeding. Then at work today the same deep cramping came back. I had *lots* of bleeding today too—ugh. *No fun* while at work, having to put on a smiley face for everyone! I took a couple of extra strength Tylenol, and by the late afternoon was feeling better, just tired.

October 2, 2012—Just wanted to update you all on my RE appointment today. Moving forward, the plan is to do the Clomid EP once again. I have almost finished the first of two weeks of BCP, so will be starting back up with Clomid around mid-October. She was very compassionate about the early miscarriage and made a point of asking how both my husband and I were handling it all. She said I could take away one good thing from it, that it is a very strong predictor of future success.

I also mentioned that I had gained a good 10 to 15 pounds since June, as my Crohn's has been in control and I have been able to properly digest and absorb my food. She sounded happy about that and said it will only help matters.

So I'm feeling hopeful.

March 17, 2013—Just popping on for an update… 11 DPO and negative pregnancy test. I know there's still a slight chance it's too early, but I'm pretty sure I'm out this time. It's fine though, I will carry on. I am going to take a bit of a break from the Board. I'll still be around reading when I can, but feel like it's time for me to step away for a while. I plan to continue with the Clomid+injects combo, and I will make sure to let you all know if anything exciting happens. I'm rooting for each and every one of you!!

Tracy had a longer road to pregnancy after miscarriage than most; two more Clomid cycles, three cycles of Clomid + injectables, and one cycle of injectables alone that did not result in pregnancy were finally followed by successful IVF. Her Crohn's disease remained in remission throughout the first and second trimesters of her pregnancy but came back with a vengeance during the third trimester. She gave birth to a healthy baby girl but is currently still struggling with active Crohn's disease.

Parting Thoughts

We hope that the stories in this chapter, of people just like you, will provide motivation and inspiration during the difficult times as you work to recover from HA. The plan for recovery is so simple—eat more, exercise less, and reduce stress—yet so hard. During the times when you feel down about yourself, discouraged about the possibilities of ever making it to the other side, or sad about what you have lost, check back in on this chapter and remind yourself of the multitude of reasons this journey is absolutely worth taking.

Appendix

The Survey

A comprehensive three-part survey was devised that asked each participant about her journey from sickness to health. Out of approximately 550 people who were asked to take the survey, 329 answered the first series of questions. Later, 256 provided information in the second survey, which asked for information on natural and treatment cycles. The third survey was taken by 208, who provided information about their pregnancy and postpartum periods as well as conceiving again.

Most studies published on this topic in medical literature include only about 10 to 30 subjects; gathering information from the Board's much larger number and publishing it in a form accessible to all will fill a void in the existing information.

The surveys were retrospective and asked respondents to recall information like:

- how much they were exercising at different times
- what types of exercise they were doing
- how much they weighed when they experienced amenorrhea
- what their eating habits were like at various points
- whether they decided to make changes to their diets and exercise
- how long it took for these lifestyle changes to take effect
- how they felt before and after making changes
- blood test results before, during, and after recovery

Appendix cont.

- information about cycles and treatments while trying to conceive
- how long it took until natural cycles resumed postpartum
- the conception of siblings

With such a breadth of information being requested—in many cases from years' prior—the results are subject to recall bias. As a result, we recognize that individual results are not 100% reliable, though the overall pattern is completely consistent with our arguments. In a few cases, such as determining the percentage of multiple pregnancies resulting from use of oral or injectable medications, information from the survey was insufficient. Therefore, we occasionally use data collected by Nico, tracking all pregnancies conceived in people posting on the Board between 2007 and 2013.

In general, we have provided the average or median (if there are data points that are outliers and skew the average) of the results we collected, as well as percentages of survey respondents experiencing various scenarios when applicable. Statistical tests include a student's t-test to compare continuous variables, a chi-square test or Fisher's exact test for contingency tables, or a sign test to compare ranked results. If this is all Greek to you, don't worry—the details aren't super important. The next paragraph includes an example, but it's not an easy concept to understand. It's also not necessary to fully comprehend the nitty gritty to grasp our points since we have simplified the results in each chapter.

Interpreting Statistics

> *Steph*: While editing this section, Nico tried to explain the statistics to me—I found it extremely complicated. So instead, I simplified it in a way that made sense for me, and maybe it will help you too. I would summarize this section as: the smaller the *p*-value the more likely the conclusion is correct.

In various places you will notice annotations such as, "$p < 1 \times 10^{-5}$"; these are called "*p*-values." The *p*-value is the result of the statistical test performed and essentially tells you how likely the difference you are looking at is to have happened by chance if in fact there is no real difference.

Your basic assumption, called the "null hypothesis," is that there is no difference between the two (or more) groups being compared. One example, which we discuss in chapter 22, is whether there is any difference in response to oral fertility medications depending on BMI.

Appendix cont.

BMI and response to oral fertility drugs

BMI category	Number of respondents	Number of respondents ovulating	Percentage of respondents ovulating
< 20	45	29	64
20 – 21	23	18	78
≥ 21	58	52	90

Our null hypothesis is that there is no association between BMI and ovulation status; or, put another way, that there is no difference in ovulation percentages between the three BMI groups. The statistical test we chose to perform is called "Fisher's exact test," which is used to compare data from two different classifications (here, BMI and ovulation) to determine whether there is an association. In this case, the p-value is 0.00892, which you can multiply by 100 to translate into a percentage. This p-value tells us that if the null hypothesis—there is no association between BMI and response to oral medications—is true, there is a 0.892% chance that results as extreme as what you see in the table would have been obtained. Usually p-values less than 0.05 (5%) are considered significant; that is, your null hypothesis is likely to be incorrect. As the p-value gets smaller, you become increasingly confident that your null hypothesis is not accurate and that the alternate hypothesis—that there is an association—is likely to be valid. In short, the very small p-value for this test suggests that there is in fact an association between BMI and success of oral meds.

However, *it is important to understand that statistical significance does not imply causation.* In our example, it could be that low BMI prevents ovulation, or there could be another factor in common among those with low BMI, such as a low fat intake, low leptin levels, or a smoking habit that causes both the low BMI and non-response to oral fertility medications.

List of Abbreviations

ACTH	adrenocorticotropic hormone
ALC	acetyl-l-carnitine
AMH	anti-mullerian hormone
ASAP	as soon as possible
BBT	basal body temperature
BCP	birth control pills
BF	breastfeed
BMI	body mass index
bpm	beats per minute
cal	calorie (technically, a kilocalorie)
carbs	carbohydrates
CBT	cognitive behavioral therapy
CCK	cholecystokinin
CD	cycle day
CM	cervical mucus
CP	cervical position
CRH	corticotropin releasing hormone
CVD	cardiovascular disease
D&C	dilation and curretage
DBT	dialectical behavioral therapy
DHEA	dehydroepiandrosterone
dL	deciliter
DNA	deoxy ribo nucleic acid: the genetic code
DOR	diminished ovarian reserve
DPO	days past ovulation
DXA	dual x-ray absorptiometry
E_2	estradiol
EP	extended protocol
EWCM	egg-white cervical mucus
FAI	free androgen index
FDA	federal drug administration
FET	frozen embryo transfer
FG	Ferrimen-Gallwey hirsutism index
FMD	flow mediated dilation
FSH	follicle stimulating hormone
g	gram

GI	gastrointestinal
GnRH	gonadotropin releasing hormone
HA	hypothalamic amenorrhea
HAer	someone with ha
hCG	human chorionic gonadotropin: the pregnancy hormone
HDL	high-density lipoprotein
HRT	hormone replacement therapy
HSG	hysterosalpingogram
IBS	irritable bowel syndrome
IM	intramuscular
IOM	Institute of Medicine
IU	international unit
IUI	intra-uterine insemination
IVF	in vitro fertilization
kcal	kilocalorie; what we normally call a calorie
kg	kilogram
L	liter
lb	pound
LBM	lean body mass: entire body except adipose (fat) tissue.
LDL	low-density lipoprotein
LH	luteinizing hormone
LMP	last menstrual period
LOL	laughing out loud
LP	luteal phase
LPD	luteal phase defect
mg	milligram
MIA	missing in action
MIT	Massachusetts Institute of Technology
mm	millimeter
MRI	magnetic resonance imaging
NA	not applicable
ng	nanogram
NR	not reported
OB	obstetrician
ob-gyn	obstetrician/gynecologist
OHSS	ovarian hyperstimulation syndrome
OMG	oh my god/gosh/goodness
OPK	ovulation prediction kit
p	p-value, see appendix

P90X	home exercise regimen
PCOS	polycystic ovarian syndrome
pg	picogram
PMS	pre-menstrual syndrome
PYY	peptide yy
RE	reproductive endocrinologist
SI	soy isoflavones
T	testosterone
temp	temperature
TLC	tender loving care
TMI	too much information
ug	microgram
VEGF	vascular endothelial growth factor

References

Chapter 1—No Period?

1. **Liu JH, Patel B, Collins G.** "Central Causes of Amenorrhea." Endotext. Updated Mar. 1, 2016. http://www.endotext.org/chapter/central-causes-of-amenorrhea/4/
2. **Legro RS.** "Evaluation and Treatment of Polycystic Ovarian Syndroms" Endotext. Updated Sep. 19, 2009. http://www.endotext.org/chapter/evaluation-and-treatment-of-polycystic-ovary-syndrome/
3. **Wade GN, Jones JE.** "Neuroendocrinology of Nutritional Infertility." *American Journal of Physiology: Regulatory, Integrative and Comparative Physiology.* 287(6) 2004: R1277-1296. doi: 10.1152/ajpregu.00475.2004
4. **Mountjoy M, et al.** "International Olympic Committee (IOC) Consensus Statement on Relative Energy Deficiency in Sport (RED-S): 2018 Update." International Journal of Sport Nutition and Exercise Metabolism. 28(4) 2018: 316-331. doi: 10.1123/ijsnem.2018-0136
5. **Wade GN, Jones JE.** 2004. doi: 10.1152/ajpregu.00475.2004
6. **Berga SL, et al.** "Recovery of Ovarian Activity in Women with Functional Hypothalamic Amenorrhea Who Were Treated with Cognitive Behavior Therapy." *Fertility and Sterility.* 80(4) 2003: 976-81. doi: 10.1016/S0015-0282(03)01124-5
7. **Ibid.**
8. **Tschugguel W, Berga SL.** "Treatment of Functional Hypothalamic Amenorrhea with Hypnotherapy." *Fertility and Sterility.* 80(4) 2003: 982-85. doi: 10.1016/S0015-0282(03)01012-4
9. **Horvath PJ, et al.** "The Effects of Varying Dietary Fat on the Nutrient Intake in Male and Female Runners." *Journal of the American College of Nutrition.* 19(1) 2000: 42-51. doi: 10.1080/07315724.2000.10718913
10. **Hill EE, et al.** "Exercise and Circulating Cortisol Levels: The Intensity Threshold Effect." *Journal of Endocrinological Investigation.* 31(7) 2008: 587-91. doi: 10.1007/BF03345606;
    Loucks AB, et al. "Alterations in the Hypothalamic-Pituitary-Ovarian and the Hypothalamic-Pituitary-Adrenal Axes in Athletic Women." *The Journal of Clinical Endocrinology & Metabolism.* 68(2) 1989: 402-11. doi: 10.1210/jcem-68-2-402;
    Mastorakos GM, et al. "Exercise and the Stress System." *Hormones.* 4(2) 2005: 73-89. http://www.hormones.gr/57/article/article.html
11. **Loucks AB, Verdun M, Heath EM.** "Low Energy Availability, Not Stress of Exercise, Alters LH Pulsatility in Exercising Women." *Journal of Applied Physiology.* 84(1) 1998: 37-46. http://jap.physiology.org/content/84/1/37.long
12. **Ibid.;**
    Martins CL, et al. "Effects of Exercise on Gut Peptides, Energy Intake and Appetite." *Journal of Endocrinology.* 193(2) 2007: 251-58. doi: 10.1677/JOE-06-0030;
    Stubbs RJ, et al. "Rate and Extent of Compensatory Changes in Energy Intake and Expenditure in Response to Altered Exercise and Diet Composition in Humans." *AJP: Regulatory, Integrative and Comparative Physiology.* 286(2) 2004: 350R-58.

Chapter 1 References cont.

doi: 10.1152/ajpregu.00196.2003;
Williams NI, Berga SL, Cameron JL. "Synergism between Psychosocial and Metabolic Stressors: Impact on Reproductive Function in Cynomolgus Monkeys." *American Journal of Physiology: Endocrinology and Metabolism.* 293(1) 2007: E270-276. doi: 10.1152/ajpendo.00108.2007

13. Stubbs RJ, et al. 2004. doi: 10.1152/ajpregu.00196.2003
14. Horne BD, Muhlestein JB, Andersen JL. "Health effects of intermittent fasting: hormesis or harm? A systematic review." *American Journal of Clinical Nutrition* 102(2) 2015: 464-70. doi: 10.3945/ajcn.115.109553
15. Farenholtz IL, et al. "Within-day energy deficiency and reproductive function in female endurance athletes." *Scandinavian Journal of Medicine & Science in Sports* 28(3) 2018: 1139-46. doi: 10.1111/sms.13030
16. Hill EE, et al. 2008. doi: 10.1007/BF03345606
17. Bullen BA, et al. "Induction of Menstrual Disorders by Strenuous Exercise in Untrained Women." *The New England Journal of Medicine.* 312(21) 1985: 1349-353. doi: 10.1056/NEJM198505233122103
18. Biller MK, et al. "Abnormal Cortisol Secretion and Responses to Corticotropin-Releasing Hormone in Women with Hypothalamic Amenorrhea." *Journal of Clinical Endocrinology & Metabolism.* 70(2) 1990: 311-17. doi: 10.1210/jcem-70-2-311;
    Brundu B. "Increased Cortisol in the Cerebrospinal Fluid of Women with Functional Hypothalamic Amenorrhea." *Journal of Clinical Endocrinology & Metabolism.* 91(4) 2006: 1561-565. doi: 10.1210/jc.2005-2422;
    Mastorakos G, et al. 2005. http://www.hormones.gr/57/article/article.html
19. Caronia LM, et al. "A Genetic Basis for Functional Hypothalamic Amenorrhea." *The New England Journal of Medicine.* 364(3) 2011: 215-25. doi: 10.1056/NEJMoa0911064
20. Williams NI, Berga SL, Cameron JL. 2007. doi: 10.1152/ajpendo.00108.2007
21. Viswanathan MA, et al. "Outcomes of Maternal Weight Gain." *Evidence Reports/Technology Assessments.* 168 (2008): 1-223. http://www.ncbi.nlm.nih.gov/pubmedhealth/PMH0007502/
22. Archer DF, Thomas RL. "The fallacy of the postpill amenorrhea syndrome." *Clinical Obstetrics and Gynecology.* 24(3) 1981:943-50

Chapter 2—Factors in HA: What You Eat

1. "Balancing Calories to Manage Weight." In Dietary Guidlines for Americans, 2010. 7th Edition ed. Washington, D.C.: U.S. Department of Agriculture and U.S. Department of Health and Human Services, 2010. http://www.fns.usda.gov/sites/default/files/Chapter2.pdf

Chapter 3—Factors in HA: Exercise and Stress

1. Griffiths MD, Szabo A, Terry A. "The Exercise Addiction Inventory: A Quick and Easy Screening Tool for Health Practitioners." *British Journal of Sports Medicine.* 39(6) 2005. doi: 10.1136/bjsm.2004.017020. For the Exercise Addiction Inventory, a score between 13 and 23 indicates that you are at risk of exercise addiction, and a score of 24 or above suggests that you do have an addiction.

Chapter 3 References cont.

2. http://jkthompson.myweb.usf.edu/oeqweb.htm There are no validated cutoffs for the Obsessive Exercise Questionaire, but a score above 40 is cause for concern.

3. **Loucks AB.** "Energy Availability, Not Body Fatness, Regulates Reproductive Function in Women." *Exercise and Sport Sciences Reviews.* 31.3 (2003): 144-48. http://journals.lww.com/acsm-essr/Fulltext/2003/07000/Energy_Availability,_Not_Body_Fatness,_Regulates.8.aspx

4. "Balancing Calories to Manage Weight." In Dietary Guidlines for Americans, 2010. 7th Edition ed. Washington, D.C.: U.S. Department of Agriculture and U.S. Department of Health and Human Services, 2010. http://www.fns.usda.gov/sites/default/files/Chapter2.pdf

5. **Mastorakos G, et al.** "Exercise and the Stress System." *Hormones.* 4(2) 2005: 73-89. http://www.hormones.gr/57/article/article.html;
Whirledge S, Cidlowski JA. "Glucocorticoids, Stress, and Infertility." *Minerva Endocrinologica.* 35(2) 2010: 109-25. http://www.ncbi.nlm.nih.gov/pmc/articles/PMC3547681/

6. **Hill EE, et al.** "Exercise and Circulating Cortisol Levels: The Intensity Threshold Effect." *Journal of Endocrinological Investigation* 31(7) 2008: 587-91. doi: 10.1007/BF03345606

7. **Edozien LC.** "Mind over Matter: Psychological Factors and the Menstrual Cycle." *Current Opinion in Obstetrics and Gynecology.* 18(4) 2006: 452-56. doi: 10.1097/01.gco.0000233942.67049.ad

8. **Nattiv A, et al.** "American College of Sports Medicine Position Stand. The Female Athlete Triad." *Medicine & Science in Sports & Exercise.* 39(10) 2007: 1867-882. doi: 10.1249/mss.0b013e318149f111

9. **Mountjoy M, et al.** "The IOC consensus statement: beyond the Female Athlete Triad--Relative Energy Deficiency in Sport (RED-S)." British Journal of Sports Medicine. 48(7) 2014: 491-7. doi: 10.1136/bjsports-2014-093502

Chapter 4—Diagnosis

1. **Klein DA, Poth MA.** "Amenorrhea: An Approach to Diagnosis and Management." *American Family Physician.* 87(11) 2013: 781-88. http://www.aafp.org/afp/2013/0601/p781.html;
Practice Committee of the American Society of Reproductive Medicine. "Current evaluation of amenorrhea." *Fertility and Sterility.* 90(5) 2008:S219 - S225. doi: 10.1016/j.fertnstert.2008.08.038

2. **Klein DA, Poth MA.** 2013. http://www.aafp.org/afp/2013/0601/p781.html

3. **Ibid.**

4. **Bradbury, RA, Lee PC, Smith HC.** "Elevated anti-Mullerian hormone in lean women may not indicate polycystic ovarian syndrome." The Australian and New Zealand Journal of Obstetrics and Gynaecology. 57(5) 2017: 552-557. doi: 10.1111/ajo.12647

5. **Klein DA, Poth MA**. 2013. http://www.aafp.org/afp/2013/0601/p781.html

6. **Meczekalski B, et al.** "Functional Hypothalamic Amenorrhea: Current View on Neuroendocrine Aberrations." *Gynecological Endocrinology.* 24(1) 2008: 4-11. doi: 10.1080/09513590701807381;

Chapter 4 References cont.

    Vuong C, et al. "The Effects of Opioids and Opioid Analogs on Animal and Human Endocrine Systems." *Endocrine Reviews.* 31(1) 2010: 98-132. doi: 10.1210/er.2009-0009

7. The American Thyroid Association Taskforce on Thyroid Disease During Pregnancy and Postpartum. "Guidelines of the American Thyroid Association for the Diagnosis and Management of Thyroid Disease During Pregnancy and Postpartum." *Thyroid.* 21(10) 2011: 1081–1125. doi: 10.1089/thy.2011.0087

8. **Leyendecker G, Wildt L.** "Induction of Ovulation with Chronic Intermittent (pulsatile) Administration of Gn-RH in Women with Hypothalamic Amenorrhoea." *The Journal of the Sociatey for Reproduction and Fertility.* 69(1) 1983: 397-409. doi: 10.1530/jrf.0.0690397

9. **Panidis D, et al.** "Serum Anti-Müllerian Hormone (AMH) Levels Are Differentially Modulated by Both Serum Gonadotropins and Not Only by Serum Follicle Stimulating Hormone (FSH) Levels." *Medical Hypotheses.* 77(4) 2011: 649-53. doi: 10.1016/j.mehy.2011.07.005

Chapter 5—Hypothalama-WHAT??

1. **Berga SL, Naftolin F.** "Neuroendocrine Control of Ovulation." *Gynecological Endocrinology.* 28(Suppl 1) 2012: 9-13. doi: 10.3109/09513590.2012.651929;
Tracy AL, et al. "Regulation of Energy Intake in Humans." Endotext. Updated Aug. 5, 2013. http://www.endotext.org/chapter/factors-influencing-obesity/regulation-of-energy-intake-in-humans/

2. **Lechan RM, Toni R.** "Functional Anatomy of the Hypothalamus and Pituitary". Updated Feb. 22, 2013. http://www.endotext.org/chapter/functional-anatomy-of-the-hypothalamus-and-pituitary/9/

3. "1806 The Hypothalamus-Pituitary Complex" by OpenStax College - Anatomy & Physiology, Connexions. http://cnx.org/content/col11496/1.6/, Jun 19, 2013. Licensed under CC BY 3.0 via Wikimedia Commons http://creativecommons.org/licenses/by/3.0/legalcode https://commons.wikimedia.org/wiki/File:1806_The_Hypothalamus-Pituitary_Complex.jpg

4. **Berga SL, Naftolin F.** doi: 10.3109/09513590.2012.651929;
Tracy AL, et al. http://www.endotext.org/chapter/factors-influencing-obesity/regulation-of-energy-intake-in-humans/

5. "Figure 28 02 07" by OpenStax College - Anatomy & Physiology, Connexions. http://cnx.org/content/col11496/1.6/, Jun 19, 2013. Licensed under CC BY 3.0 via Wikimedia Commons http://creativecommons.org/licenses/by/3.0/legalcode http://commons.wikimedia.org/wiki/File:Figure_28_02_07.jpg

6. **Tracy AL, et al.** http://www.endotext.org/chapter/factors-influencing-obesity/regulation-of-energy-intake-in-humans/

7. **Scheid JL, De Souza MJ.** "Menstrual Irregularities and Energy Deficiency in Physically Active Women: The Role of Ghrelin, PYY and Adipocytokines." *Medicine and Sport Science.* 55; 2010: 82-102. doi: 10.1159/000321974;
Schneider L, Monaco S, Warren M. "Elevated Ghrelin Level in Women of Normal Weight with Amenorrhea Is Related to Disordered Eating." *Fertility and Sterility.* 90(1) 2008: 121-28. doi: 10.1016/j.fertnstert.2007.06.002

Chapter 5 References cont.

8. **Tracy AL, et al.** http://www.endotext.org/chapter/factors-influencing-obesity/regulation-of-energy-intake-in-humans/
9. **Ibid.**
10. **Ibid.**
11. **Moran TH, Ladenheim EE.** "Adiposity Signaling and Meal Size Control." *Physiology & Behavior.* 103(1) 2011: 21-24. doi: 10.1016/j.physbeh.2010.11.013
12. **Poretsky L, Kalin MF.** "The Gonadotropic Function of Insulin." *Endocrine Reviews.* 8(2) 1987: 132-41. doi: 10.1210/edrv-8-2-132
13. **Codner E, Merino PM, Tena-Sempere M.** "Female Reproduction and Type 1 Diabetes: From Mechanisms to Clinical Findings." *Human Reproduction Update.* 18(5) 2012: 568-85. doi: 10.1093/humupd/dms024
14. **Marx J.** "Cellular Warriors at the Battle of the Bulge." *Science.* 299(5608) 2003: 846-49. doi: 10.1126/science.299.5608.846
15. **Khan SM, et al.** "Leptin as a Modulator of Neuroendocrine Function in Humans." *Yonsei Medical Journal.* 53(4) 2012: 671. doi: 10.3349/ymj.2012.53.4.671
16. **Moran TH, Ladenheim EE.** 2011. doi: 10.1016/j.physbeh.2010.11.013
17. **Routh VH.** "Glucose Sensing Neurons in the Ventromedial Hypothalamus." *Sensors.* 10(10) 2010: 9002-025. doi: 10.3390/s101009002
18. **Zhang CM, et al.** "Gonadotropin-Releasing Hormone Neurons Express KATP Channels That Are Regulated by Estrogen and Responsive to Glucose and Metabolic Inhibition." *Journal of Neuroscience.* 27(38) 2007: 10153-0164. doi: 10.1523/JNEUROSCI.1657-07.2007
19. **Edozien LS.** "Mind over Matter: Psychological Factors and the Menstrual Cycle." *Current Opinion in Obstetrics and Gynecology.* 18(4) 2006: 452-56. doi: 10.1097/01.gco.0000233942.67049.ad
20. **Mastorakos G, et al.** "Exercise and the Stress System." *Hormones.* 4(2) 2005: 73-89. http://www.hormones.gr/57/article/article.html
21. **O'connor TM.** "The Stress Response and the Hypothalamic-pituitary-adrenal Axis: From Molecule to Melancholia." *Quarterly Journal of Medicine.* 93(6) 2000: 323-33. doi: 10.1093/qjmed/93.6.323
22. **Biller BM, et al.** "Abnormal Cortisol Secretion and Responses to Corticotropin-Releasing Hormone in Women with Hypothalamic Amenorrhea." *The Journal of Clinical Endocrinology & Metabolism.* 70(2) 1990: 311-17. doi: 10.1210/jcem-70-2-311;
Loucks AB, et al. "Alterations in the Hypothalamic-Pituitary-Ovarian and the Hypothalamic-Pituitary-Adrenal Axes in Athletic Women." *The Journal of Clinical Endocrinology & Metabolism.* 68(2) 1989: 402-11. doi: 10.1210/jcem-68-2-402
23. **Brundu B.** "Increased Cortisol in the Cerebrospinal Fluid of Women with Functional Hypothalamic Amenorrhea." *The Journal of Clinical Endocrinology & Metabolism.* 91(4) 2006: 1561-565. doi: 10.1210/jc.2005-2422
24. **Berga SL, et al.** "Recovery of Ovarian Activity in Women with Functional Hypothalamic Amenorrhea Who Were Treated with Cognitive Behavior Therapy." *Fertility and Sterility.* 80(4) 2003: 976-81. doi: 10.1016/S0015-0282(03)01124-5
25. **Loucks AB, et al.** 1989. doi: 10.1210/jcem-68-2-402

Chapter 5 References cont.

26. **Hill EE, et al.** "Exercise and Circulating Cortisol Levels: The Intensity Threshold Effect." *Journal of Endocrinological Investigation.* 31(7) 2008: 587-91. doi: 10.1007/BF03345606
27. **Whirledge S, Cidlowski JA.** "Glucocorticoids, Stress, and Infertility." *Minerva Endocrinologica.* 35(2) 2010: 109-25. http://www.ncbi.nlm.nih.gov/pmc/articles/PMC3547681/
28. **Mastorakos G, et al.** 2005. http://www.hormones.gr/57/article/article.html **O'connor TM.** 2000. doi: 10.1093/qjmed/93.6.323
29. **De Souza MJ, et al.** "Luteal Phase Deficiency in Recreational Runners: Evidence for a Hypometabolic State." *Journal of Clinical Endocrinology & Metabolism.* 88(1) 2003: 337-46. doi: 10.1210/jc.2002-020958;
    De Souza MJ, et al. "High Prevalence of Subtle and Severe Menstrual Disturbances in Exercising Women: Confirmation Using Daily Hormone Measures." *Human Reproduction.* 25(2) 2010: 491-503. doi: 10.1093/humrep/dep411
30. **Ibid.**
31. **Berga SL, Naftolin F.** 2012. doi: 10.3109/09513590.2012.651929
32. **Whirledge S, Cidlowski JA.** 2010. http://www.ncbi.nlm.nih.gov/pmc/articles/PMC3547681/
33. **Zhang CM, et al.** 2007. doi: 10.1523/JNEUROSCI.1657-07.2007
34. **Berga SL, Naftolin F.** 2012. doi: 10.3109/09513590.2012.651929
35. **Garcia-Garcia RM.** "Integrative Control of Energy Balance and Reproduction in Females." *ISRN Veterinary Science.* 2012; 2012: 1-13. doi: 10.5402/2012/121389
36. **Berga SL, Naftolin F.** 2012. doi: 10.3109/09513590.2012.651929;
    Ciccone NA, Kaiser UB. "The Biology of Gonadotroph Regulation." *Current Opinion in Endocrinology, Diabetes and Obesity.* 16(4) 2009: 321-27. doi: 10.1097/med.0b013e32832d88fb;
    Marshall JC, Eagleson CA, Mccartney CR. "Hypothalamic Dysfunction." *Molecular and Cellular Endocrinology.* 183(1-2) 2001: 29-32. doi: 10.1016/S0303-7207(01)00611-6;
    Roland AV, Moenter SM. "Regulation of Gonadotropin-releasing Hormone Neurons by Glucose." *Trends in Endocrinology & Metabolism.* 22(11) 2011: 443-49. doi: 10.1016/j.tem.2011.07.001;
    Whirledge S, Cidlowski JA. 2010. http://www.ncbi.nlm.nih.gov/pmc/articles/PMC3547681/;
    Zhang CM, et al. 2007. doi: 10.1523/JNEUROSCI.1657-07.2007
37. **Berga SL, Naftolin F.** 2012. doi: 10.3109/09513590.2012.651929
38. **Pinto S, et al.** "Rapid Rewiring of Arcuate Nucleus Feeding Circuits by Leptin." Science. 304(5667) 2004:110-5. doi: 10.1126/science.1089459
39. **Mastorakos G, et al.** 2005. http://www.hormones.gr/57/article/article.html
40. **Garcia-Garcia RM.** "Integrative Control of Energy Balance and Reproduction in Females." *ISRN Veterinary Science.* 2012; 2012: 1-13. doi: 10.5402/2012/121389. Licensed under CC BY 3.0 http://creativecommons.org/licenses/by/3.0/legalcode
41. **Berga SL, Naftolin F.** 2012. doi: 10.3109/09513590.2012.651929

Chapter 6—The HA/PCOS Conundrum

1. **Azziz R, et al.** "The Prevalence and Features of the Polycystic Ovary Syndrome in an Unselected Population." *The Journal of Clinical Endocrinology & Metabolism.* 89(6) 2004: 2745-749. doi: 10.1210/jc.2003-032046;
   March WA, et al. "The Prevalence of Polycystic Ovary Syndrome in a Community Sample Assessed under Contrasting Diagnostic Criteria." *Human Reproduction.* 25(2) 2010: 544-51. doi: 10.1093/humrep/dep399
2. **Lauritsen MP, et al.** "Revised criteria for PCOS in WHO Group II anovulatory infertility - a revival of hypothalamic amenorrhoea?" Clinical Endocrinology. 82(4) 2015: 584-91. doi: 10.1111/cen.12621
3. **Azziz R, et al.** 2004. doi: 10.1210/jc.2003-032046
4. **Johnson TRB, et al.** "Evidence-Based Methodology Workshop on Polycystic Ovary Syndrome." Bethesda, Maryland: National Institutes of Health, 2012. http://prevention.nih.gov/workshops/2012/pcos/docs/FinalReport.pdf
5. Rotterdam ESHRE/ASRM-Sponsored PCOS Consensus Workshop Group. "Revised 2003 Consensus on Diagnostic Criteria and Long-term Health Risks Related to Polycystic Ovary Syndrome (PCOS)." *Human Reproduction.* 19(1) 2004: 41-47. doi: 10.1093/humrep/deh098
6. **Ibid.**
7. **Balen AH, et al.** "Ultrasound Assessment of the Polycystic Ovary: International Consensus Definitions." *Human Reproduction Update.* 9(6) 2003: 505-14. doi: 10.1093/humupd/dmg044;
   Dewailly D, et al. "Definition and Significance of Polycystic Ovarian Morphology: A Task Force Report from the Androgen Excess and Polycystic Ovary Syndrome Society." *Human Reproduction Update.* 20(3) 2014: 334-52. doi: 10.1093/humupd/dmt061
8. **Dewailly D, et al.** 2014. doi: 10.1093/humupd/dmt061;
   Lujan ME, et al. "Updated Ultrasound Criteria for Polycystic Ovary Syndrome: Reliable Thresholds for Elevated Follicle Population and Ovarian Volume." *Human Reproduction.* 28(5) 2013: 1361-368. doi: 10.1093/humrep/det062
9. **Pigny P, et al.** "Comparative assessment of five serum antimüllerian hormone assays for the diagnosis of polycystic ovary syndrome." *Fertility and Sterility.* 105(4) 2016: 1063-69.e3. doi: 10.1016/j.fertnstert.2015.12.023
10. **Liang SJ, et al.** "Clinical and Biochemical Presentation of Polycystic Ovary Sydrome in Women between the Ages of 20 and 40." *Human Reproduction.* 26(12) 2011: 3443-449. doi: 10.1093/humrep/der302;
    Azziz R, et al. 2004. doi: 10.1210/jc.2003-032046;
    Azziz R, et al. "Criteria for Defining Polycystic Ovary Syndrome as a Predominantly Hyperandrogenic Syndrome: An Androgen Excess Society Guideline." *The Journal of Clinical Endocrinology & Metabolism.* 91(11) 2006: 4237-245. doi: 10.1210/jc.2006-0178;
    Sivayoganathan D, et al. "Full Investigation of Patients with Polycystic Ovary Syndrome (PCOS) Presenting to Four Different Clinical Specialties Reveals Significant Differences and Undiagnosed Morbidity." *Human Fertility.* 14(4) 2011: 261-65. doi: 10.3109/14647273.2011.632058

Chapter 6 References cont.

11. **Liang SJ, et al. 2011.** doi: 10.1093/humrep/der302;
    Sivayoganathan D, et al. 2011. doi: 10.3109/14647273.2011.632058;
    Fauser BC, et al. "Consensus on Women's Health Aspects of Polycystic Ovary Syndrome (PCOS): The Amsterdam ESHRE/ASRM-Sponsored 3rd PCOS Consensus Workshop Group." *Fertility & Sterility.* 97(1) 2012: 28-38. doi: 10.1016/j.fertnstert.2011.09.024
12. **Sivayoganathan D, et al.** 2011. doi: 10.3109/14647273.2011.632058
13. Ibid.
14. **Ferriman D, Gallwey JD.** "Clinical Assessment Of Body Hair Growth In Women." *The Journal of Clinical Endocrinology & Metabolism.* 21(11) 1961: 1440-447. doi: 10.1210/jcem-21-11-1440.
    Khan A, et al. "Polycystic Ovarian Syndrome: Correlation between clinical hyperandrogenism, anthropometric, metabolic and endocrine parameters." *Pakistani Journal of Medical Science.* 35(5) 2018:1227-1232. doi: 10.12669/pjms.35.5.742.
15. **Kar, S.** "Anthropometric, Clinical, and Metabolic Comparisons of the Four Rotterdam PCOS Phenotypes: A Prospective Study of PCOS Women." *Journal of Human Reproductive Sciences.* 6(3) 2013: 194. doi: 10.4103/0974-1208.121422
16. Rotterdam ESHRE/ASRM-Sponsored PCOS Consensus Workshop Group. 2004. doi: 10.1093/humrep/deh098
17. **Robin G, et al.** "Polycystic Ovary-Like Abnormalities (PCO-L) in Women with Functional Hypothalamic Amenorrhea." *The Journal of Clinical Endocrinology & Metabolism.* 97(11) 2012: 4236-243. doi: 10.1210/jc.2012-1836;
    Falsetti, L. "Long-term Follow-up of Functional Hypothalamic Amenorrhea and Prognostic Factors." *The Journal of Clinical Endocrinology & Metabolism.* 87(2) 2002: 500-05. doi: 10.1210/jcem.87.2.8195
18. **Bradbury RA, Lee P, Smith HC.** "Elevated anti-Mullerian hormone in lean women may not indicate polycystic ovarian syndrome." The Australian and New Zealand Journal of Obstetrics and Gynecology. 57(5) 2017: 552-7. doi: 10.1111/ajo.12647
19. **Moret M, et al.** "Insulin Modulation of Luteinizing Hormone Secretion in Normal Female Volunteers and Lean Polycystic Ovary Syndrome Patients." *Neuroendocrinology.* 89(2) 2009: 131-39. doi: 10.1159/000160911;
    Taylor AE, et al. "Determinants of Abnormal Gonadotropin Secretion in Clinically Defined Women with Polycystic Ovary Syndrome." *The Journal of Clinical Endocrinology & Metabolism.* 82(7) 1997: 2248-256. doi: 10.1210/jcem.82.7.4105
20. **Azziz R, et al.** 2006: 4237-245. doi: 10.1210/jc.2006-0178
21. **Bradbury RA, Lee P, Smith HC.** 2017. doi: 10.1111/ajo.12647
22. **Loucks AB, Thuma JR.** "Luteinizing Hormone Pulsatility Is Disrupted at a Threshold of Energy Availability in Regularly Menstruating Women." *The Journal of Clinical Endocrinology & Metabolism.* 88(1) 2003: 297-311. doi: 10.1210/jc.2002-020369
23. **Wang JG, Lobo RA.** "The Complex Relationship between Hypothalamic Amenorrhea and Polycystic Ovary Syndrome." *The Journal of Clinical Endocrinology & Metabolism.* 93(4) 2008: 1394-397. doi: 10.1210/jc.2007-1716;
    Robin G, et al. 2012. doi: 10.1210/jc.2012-1836

Chapter 6 References cont.

24. **Carmina E, Fruzzetti F, Lobo RA.** "Features of polycystic ovary syndrome (PCOS) in women with functional hypothalamic amenorrhea (FHA) may be reversible with recovery of menstrual function." *Gynecological Endocrinology.* 34(4) 2018: 301-4. doi: 10.1080/09513590.2017.1395842

25. **Haqq L, et al.** "Effect of lifestyle intervention on the reproductive endocrine profile in women with polycystic ovarian syndrome: a systematic review and meta-analysis." *Endocrine Connections.* 3(1) 2014: 36-46. doi: 10.1530/EC-14-0010

26. **Wang JG, Lobo RA.** 2008. doi: 10.1210/jc.2007-1716;
Robin G, et al. 2012. doi: 10.1210/jc.2012-1836;
Sum M, Warren MP. "Hypothalamic Amenorrhea in Young Women with Underlying Polycystic Ovary Syndrome." *Fertility and Sterility.* 92(6) 2009. doi: 10.1016/j.fertnstert.2009.05.063

27. **Wang JG, Lobo RA.** 2008. doi: 10.1210/jc.2007-1716;
Sum M, Warren MP. 2009. doi: 10.1016/j.fertnstert.2009.05.063

28. **Thompson IA, Kaiser, UB.** "GnRH Pulse Frequency-dependent Differential Regulation of LH and FSH Gene Expression." Molecular and Cellular Endocrinology. 385(1-2) 2014: 28-35. doi: 10.1016/j.mce.2013.09.012

29. **Haqq L, et al.** 2014 doi: 10.1530/EC-14-0010

30. **Jakubowicz D, et al.** "Effects of Caloric Intake Timing on Insulin Resistance and Hyperandrogenism in Lean Women with Polycystic Ovary Syndrome." *Clinical Science.* 125(9) 2013: 423-32. doi: 10.1042/CS20130071

31. **Minozzi M, Nordio M, Pajalich R.** "The Combined Therapy Myo-inositol plus D-Chiro-inositol, in a Physiological Ratio, Reduces the Cardiovascular Risk by Improving the Lipid Profile in PCOS Patients." *European Review for Medical and Pharmacological Sciences.* 17(4) 2013: 537-40. http://www.europeanreview.org/wp/wp-content/uploads/537-540.pdf;
Isabella R, Raffone E. "Does Ovary Need D-chiro-inositol?" *Journal of Ovarian Research.* 5(1) 2012: 14-20. doi: 10.1186/1757-2215-5-14;
Iuorno MJ, et al. 2002. doi: 10.4158/EP.8.6.417

32. **Nordio M, Basciani S, Camajani E.** "The 40:1 myo-inositol/D-chiro-inositol plasma ratio is able to restore ovulation in PCOS patients: comparison with other ratios." *Eur Rev Med Pharmacol Sci.* 23(12) 2019: 5512-5521. doi: 10.26355/eurrev_201906_18223;
Roseff S, Montenegro M. "Inositol Treatment for PCOS Should Be Science-Based and Not Arbitrary." *Int J Endocrinol.* 2020 Mar 27: 6461254. doi: 10.1155/2020/6461254;
Monastra G et al. "Combining treatment with myo-inositol and D-chiro-inositol (40:1) is effective in restoring ovary function and metabolic balance in PCOS patients." *Gynecol Endocrinol.* 33(1) 2019:1-9. doi: 10.1080/09513590.2016.1247797

33. Nordio M, Basciani S, Camajani E. 2019. doi: 10.26355/eurrev_201906_18223

34. Roseff S, Montenegro M. 2020. doi: 10.1155/2020/6461254

35. **Jakubowicz D, et al.** 2013. doi: 10.1042/CS20130071

36. **Baillargeon J, et al.** "Effects of Metformin and Rosiglitazone, Alone and in Combination, in Nonobese Women with Polycystic Ovary Syndrome and Normal Indices of Insulin Sensitivity." *Fertility and Sterility.* 82(4) 2004: 893-902. doi: 10.1016/j.fertnstert.2004.02.127

Chapter 6 References cont.

37. **Iuorno MJ, et al.** "Effects Of D-Chiro-Inositol In Lean Women With The Polycystic Ovary Syndrome." *Endocrine Practice*. 8(6) 2002: 417-23. doi: 10.4158/EP.8.6.417
38. **Shroff R, et al.** "Risk of Metabolic Complications in the New PCOS Phenotypes Based on the Rotterdam Criteria." *Fertility and Sterility*. 88(5) 2007: 1389-395. doi: 10.1016/j.fertnstert.2007.01.032
39. **Bates GW, Legro RS.** "Longterm Management of Polycystic Ovarian Syndrome (PCOS)." *Molecular and Cellular Endocrinology*. 373(1-2) 2013: 91-97. doi: 10.1016/j.mce.2012.10.029;
    Rotterdam ESHRE/ASRM-Sponsored PCOS Consensus Workshop Group. 2004. doi: 10.1093/humrep/deh098;
    Fauser BC, et al. 2012: 28-38. doi: 10.1016/j.fertnstert.2011.09.024
40. **Fauser BC, et al.** 2012: 28-38. doi: 10.1016/j.fertnstert.2011.09.024
41. Kamenov Z, Gateva A. "Inositols in PCOS." *Molecules*. 2020; 25(23):5566. doi: 10.3390/molecules25235566;
    Kim, CH, Chon, SJ & Lee, SH. "Effects of lifestyle modification in polycystic ovary syndrome compared to metformin only or metformin addition: A systematic review and meta-analysis." *Sci Rep* 2020 10: 7802 doi: 10.1038/s41598-020-64776-w
42. **Haoula Z, Salman M, Atiomo W.** "Evaluating the Association between Endometrial Cancer and Polycystic Ovary Syndrome." *Human Reproduction* 27(5) 2012: 1327-331. doi: 10.1093/humrep/des042
43. **Hardiman P, Pillay OS, Atiomo W.** "Polycystic Ovary Syndrome and Endometrial Carcinoma." *The Lancet* 361(9371) 2003: 1810-812. doi: 10.1016/S0140-6736(03)13409-5
44. **Ibid.**
45. Dr. Phoebe Holmes-Juck email to Dr. Nicola Sykes (Rinaldi) on January 20, 2014

Chapter 7—Brittle Bones and Other Health Consequences of HA

1. **Khosla S, Melton LJ, Riggs BL.** "The Unitary Model for Estrogen Deficiency and the Pathogenesis of Osteoporosis: Is a Revision Needed?" *Journal of Bone and Mineral Research*. 26(3) 2011: 441-51. doi: 10.1002/jbmr.262
2. **Seifert-Klauss V, Prior JC.** "Progesterone and Bone: Actions Promoting Bone Health in Women", Journal of Osteoporosis, vol. 2010, Article ID 845180, 18 pages, 2010. doi: 10.4061/2010/845180.
3. **Charatcharoenwitthaya N, et al.** "Effect of Blockade of TNF-α and Interleukin-1 Action on Bone Resorption in Early Postmenopausal Women." *Journal of Bone and Mineral Research*. 22(5) 2007: 724-29. doi: 10.1359/jbmr.070207
4. **Clarke BL, Khosla S.** "Female Reproductive System and Bone." *Archives of Biochemistry and Biophysics*. 503(1) 2010: 118-28. doi: 10.1016/j.abb.2010.07.006;
    Kovacs CS, Kronenberg HM. "Maternal-Fetal Calcium and Bone Metabolism During Pregnancy, Puerperium, and Lactation." *Endocrine Reviews*. 18(6) 1997: 832-72. doi: 10.1210/edrv.18.6.0319
5. **Kovacs CS, Kronenberg HM.** 1997. doi: 10.1210/edrv.18.6.0319
6. **Ibid.**

7. **Bruni V, et al.** "Body Composition Variables and Leptin Levels in Functional Hypothalamic Amenorrhea and Amenorrhea Related to Eating Disorders." *Journal of Pediatric and Adolescent Gynecology.* 24(6) 2011: 347-52. doi: 10.1016/j.jpag.2011.06.004;
Gibson JH, et al. "Determinants of Bone Density and Prevalence of Osteopenia among Female Runners in Their Second to Seventh Decades of Age." *Bone.* 26(6) 2000: 591-98. doi: 10.1016/S8756-3282(00)00274-X;
Gibson JH, et al. "Nutritional and Exercise-related Determinants of Bone Density in Elite Female Runners." *Osteoporosis International.* 15(8) 2004: 611-18;
Grinspoon SK, et al. "Effects of a Triphasic Combination Oral Contraceptive Containing Norgestimate/Ethinyl Estradiol on Biochemical Markers of Bone Metabolism in Young Women with Osteopenia Secondary to Hypothalamic Amenorrhea." *The Journal of Clinical Endocrinology & Metabolism.* 88(8) 2003: 3651-656. doi: 10.1210/jc.2003-030033;
Keen AD, Drinkwater BL. "Irreversible Bone Loss in Former Amenorrheic Athletes." *Osteoporosis International.* 7(4) 1997: 311-15;
Miller KK, et al. "Determinants of Skeletal Loss and Recovery in Anorexia Nervosa." *The Journal of Clinical Endocrinology & Metabolism.* 91(8) 2006: 2931-937. doi: 10.1210/jc.2005-2818;
Mencken ML, Chesnut CH, Drinkwater BL. "Bone Density at Multiple Skeletal Sites in Amenorrheic Athletes." *JAMA: The Journal of the American Medical Association.* 276(3) 1996: 238-40. doi: 10.1001/jama.1996.03540030072035

8. **Miller KK, et al.** 2006. doi: 10.1210/jc.2005-2818

9. **Petre, BM.** http://emedicine.medscape.com/article/1948532-overview#showall, updated July 18, 2013

10. **Clarke BL, Khosla S.** 2010. doi: 10.1016/j.abb.2010.07.006;
Kalkwarf HJ, et al. "The Bone Mineral Density in Childhood Study: Bone Mineral Content and Density According to Age, Sex, and Race" *The Journal of Clinical Endocrinology & Metabolism.* 92(6) 2007: 2087-99. doi: 10.1210/jc.2006-2553

11. **Kemper HCG, et al.** "A Fifteen-year Longitudinal Study in Young Adults on the Relation of Physical Activity and Fitness with the Development of the Bone Mass: The Amsterdam Growth and Health Longitudinal Study." *Bone.* 27(6) 2000: 847-53. doi: 10.1016/S8756-3282(00)00397-5

12. **Khosla S, Melton LJ, Riggs BL.** 2011. doi: 10.1002/jbmr.262

13. **Doren, M., J. A. Nilsson, and O. Johnell.** "Effects of Specific Post-menopausal Hormone Therapies on Bone Mineral Density in Post-menopausal Women: A Meta-analysis." *Human Reproduction.* 18(8) 2003: 1737-746. doi: 10.1093/humrep/deg315

14. **Khosla S, Melton LJ, Riggs BL.** 2011. doi: 10.1002/jbmr.262

15. **Ihle R, Loucks AB.** "Dose-Response Relationships Between Energy Availability and Bone Turnover in Young Exercising Women." *Journal of Bone and Mineral Research.* 19(8) 2004: 1231-240. doi: 10.1359/JBMR.040410

16. **Duckham RL, et al.** "Risk Factors for Stress Fracture in Female Endurance Athletes: A Cross-sectional Study." BMJ Open 2(6) 2012: E001920. doi: 10.1136/bmjopen-2012-001920;
Frusztajer NT, et al. "Nutrition and the Incidence of Stress Fractures in Ballet Dancers." *American Journal of Clinical Nutrition.* 51(5) 1990: 779-83. http://ajcn.

Chapter 7 References cont.

nutrition.org/content/51/5/779.long;
Marx RG, et al. "Stress Fracture Sites Related to Underlying Bone Health in Athletic Females." *Clinical Journal of Sport Medicine.* 11(2) 2001: 73-76

17. **Loucks AB, Thuma JR.** "Luteinizing Hormone Pulsatility Is Disrupted at a Threshold of Energy Availability in Regularly Menstruating Women." *The Journal of Clinical Endocrinology & Metabolism.* 88(1) 2003: 297-311. doi: 10.1210/jc.2002-020369;
Ihle R, Loucks AB. 2004. doi: 10.1359/JBMR.040410
18. Ibid.
19. Ibid.
20. Ibid.
21. Ibid.
22. **Foo JP, Hamnvik OR, Mantzoros CS.** "Optimizing Bone Health in Anorexia Nervosa and Hypothalamic Amenorrhea: New Trials and Tribulations." *Metabolism.* 61(7) 2012: 899-905. doi: 10.1016/j.metabol.2012.01.003;
Vescovi JD, Jamal SA, De Souza MJ. "Strategies to Reverse Bone Loss in Women with Functional Hypothalamic Amenorrhea: A Systematic Review of the Literature." *Osteoporosis International.* 19(4) 2008: 465-78. doi: 10.1007/s00198-007-0518-6
23. **Fredericson M, Kent K.** "Normalization of Bone Density in a Previously Amenorrheic Runner with Osteoporosis." *Medicine & Science in Sports & Exercise.* 37(9) 2005: 1481-486. doi: 10.1249/01.mss.0000177561.95201.8f
24. **Grinspoon SK, et al.** 2003. doi: 10.1210/jc.2003-030033
25. **Ackerman KE et al.** "Oestrogen replacement improves bone mineral density in oligo-amenorrhoeic athletes: a randomised clinical trial." *British Journnal of Sports Medicine.* 53(4) 2019:1–9. doi:10.1136/bjsports-2018-099723
26. **Gibson JH, et al.** 2000. doi: 10.1016/S8756-3282(00)00274-X
27. **Miller KK, et al.** 2006. doi: 10.1210/jc.2005-2818
28. Ibid.
29. **Khosla S, Melton LJ, Riggs BL.** 2011. doi: 10.1002/jbmr.262
30. **Misra M, et al.** "Weight Gain and Restoration of Menses as Predictors of Bone Mineral Density Change in Adolescent Girls with Anorexia Nervosa-1." *The Journal of Clinical Endocrinology & Metabolism.* 93(4) 2008: 1231-237. doi: 10.1210/jc.2007-1434
31. **Schulze UM, et al.** "Bone Mineral Density in Partially Recovered Early Onset Anorexic Patients - a Follow-up Investigation." *Child & Adolescesnt Psychiatry & Mental Health.* 4(1) 2010: 20. doi: 10.1186/1753-2000-4-20
32. **Zanker CL, et al.** "Annual Changes of Bone Density over 12 Years in an Amenorrheic Athlete." *Medicine & Science in Sports & Exercise.* 36(1) 2004: 137-42. http://journals.lww.com/acsm-msse/Fulltext/2004/01000/Annual_Changes_of_Bone_Density_over_12_Years_in_an.23.aspx
33. **Fredericson M, Kent K.** 2005. doi: 10.1249/01.mss.0000177561.95201.8f

34. **Hind K.** "Recovery of Bone Mineral Density and Fertility in a Former Amenorrheic Athlete." *Journal of Sports Science and Medicine.* 7(3) 2008): 415-18. http://www.ncbi.nlm.nih.gov/pmc/articles/PMC3761891/

35. **Egan E.** "Bone Mineral Density among Female Sports Participants." *Bone.* 38(2) 2006: 227-33. doi: 10.1016/j.bone.2005.08.024;
    Nichols JF, et al. "Bone Mineral Density in Female High School Athletes: Interactions of Menstrual Function and Type of Mechanical Loading." *Bone.* 41(3) 2007: 371-77. doi: 10.1016/j.bone.2007.05.003;
    Saraví FD, Sayegh F. "Bone Mineral Density and Body Composition of Adult Premenopausal Women with Three Levels of Physical Activity." *Journal of Osteoporosis.* 2013(2013): 1-7. doi: 10.1155/2013/953271;
    Taaffe DR, et al. "High-Impact Exercise Promotes Bone Gain in Well-Trained Female Athletes." *Journal of Bone and Mineral Research.* 12(2) 1997: 255-60. doi: 10.1359/jbmr.1997.12.2.255

36. **Heinonen A, et al.** "Effects of High-Impact Training and Detraining on Femoral Neck Structure in Premenopausal Women: A Hip Structural Analysis of an 18-Month Randomized Controlled Exercise Intervention with 3.5-Year Follow-Up." *Physiotherapy Canada.* 64(1) 2012: 98-105. doi: 10.3138/ptc.2010-37

37. **Kontulainen S, et al.** "Former Exercisers of an 18-month Intervention Display Residual ABMD Benefits Compared with Control Women 3.5 Years Post-intervention: A Follow-up of a Randomized Controlled High-impact Trial." *Osteoporosis International.* 15(3) 2004): 248-51. doi: 10.1007/s00198-003-1559-0

38. **Gibson JH, et al.** 2000. doi: 10.1016/S8756-3282(00)00274-X;
    Keen AD, Drinkwater BL. 1997

39. **Miller KK, et al.** 2006. doi: 10.1210/jc.2005-2818

40. **Lambrinoudaki I, Papadimitriou D.** "Pathophysiology of Bone Loss in the Female Athlete." *Annals of the New York Academy of Sciences.* 1205(1) 2010: 45-50. doi: 10.1111/j.1749-6632.2010.05681.x

41. **Michaelsson KH, et al.** "Long Term Calcium Intake and Rates of All Cause and Cardiovascular Mortality: Community Based Prospective Longitudinal Cohort Study." *British Medical Journal.* 346; 2013: F228. doi: 10.1136/bmj.f228

42. **Wallace, TC.** "Dried Plums, Prunes and Bone Health: A Comprehensive Review." Nutrients. 9(4) 2017: pii:E401. doi: 10.3390/nu9040401

43. **Rondanelli M, et al.** "Pivotal role of boron supplementation on bone health: A narrative review." *J Trace Elem Med Biol.* 62 2020:126577. doi: **10.1016/j.jtemb.2020.126577**.

44. **Hoch AZ, et al.** "Athletic Amenorrhea and Endothelial Dysfunction." *Wisconsin Medical Journal.* 106(6) 2007: 301-06. https://www.wisconsinmedicalsociety.org/_WMS/publications/wmj/pdf/106/6/301.pdf

45. **Rivera CM, et al.** "Increased Mortality for Neurological and Mental Diseases following Early Bilateral Oophorectomy." *Neuroepidemiology.* 33(1) 2009: 32-40. doi: 10.1159/000211951

46. **Hamelin BA, et al.** "Influence of the Menstrual Cycle on the Timing of Acute Coronary Events in Premenopausal Women." *The American Journal of Medicine.* 114(7) 2003: 599-602. doi: 10.1016/S0002-9343(03)00051-2;
    Lloyd GW, et al. "Does Angina Vary with the Menstrual Cycle in Women

Chapter 7 References cont.

with Premenopausal Coronary Artery Disease?" *Heart*. 84(2) 2000: 189-92. doi: 10.1136/heart.84.2.189

47. **Hanke H, et al.** "Estradiol Concentrations in Premenopausal Women with Coronary Heart Disease.*" Coronary Artery Diseases*. 8(8-9) 1997: 511-15;
Bairey Merz CN, et al. "Hypoestrogenemia of Hypothalamic Origin and Coronary Artery Disease in Premenopausal Women: A Report from the NHLBI-sponsored WISE Study.*" Journal of the American College of Cardiologists*. 41(3) 2003): 413-19. doi: 10.1016/S0735-1097(02)02763-8

48. **Casiero D, Frishman, EH.** "Cardiovascular Complications of Eating Disorders." *Cardiology in Review*. 14(5) 2006: 227-31. doi: 10.1097/01.crd.0000216745.96062.7c

49. **Hoch AZ, et al.** 2007. https://www.wisconsinmedicalsociety.org/_WMS/publications/wmj/pdf/106/6/301.pdf;
Rickenlund A, et al. "Oral Contraceptives Improve Endothelial Function in Amenorrheic Athletes *The Journal of Clinical Endocrinology & Metabolism*. 90(6) 2005: 3162-167.doi: 10.1210/jc.2004-1964;
Yoshida N, et al. "Impaired Endothelium-dependent and -independent Vasodilation in Young Female Athletes with Exercise-associated Amenorrhea." *Arteriosclerosis, Thrombosis, and Vascular Biology*. 26(1) 2006: 231-32. doi: 10.1161/01.ATV.0000199102.60747.18

50. **Ibid.**

51. **Yoshida, N, et al.** 2006. doi: 10.1161/01.ATV.0000199102.60747.18

52. **Hamelin BA, et al.** 2003. doi: 10.1016/S0002-9343(03)00051-2;
O'donnell EJ, Goodman M, Harvey PJ. "Cardiovascular Consequences of Ovarian Disruption: A Focus on Functional Hypothalamic Amenorrhea in Physically Active Women." *The Journal of Clinical Endocrinology & Metabolism*. 96(12) 2011: 3638-648. doi: 10.1210/jc.2011-1223.

53. **Hoch AZ, et al.** 2007. https://www.wisconsinmedicalsociety.org/_WMS/publications/wmj/pdf/106/6/301.pdf;
Rickenlund A, et al. 2005. doi: 10.1210/jc.2004-1964;
Yoshida, N, et al. 2006. doi: 10.1161/01.ATV.0000199102.60747.18

54. **O'donnell EJ, Goodman M, Harvey PJ.** 2011. doi: 10.1210/jc.2011-1223;
Rickenlund A, et al. 2005. doi: 10.1210/jc.2004-1964;
Soleimany G, et al. "Bone Mineral Changes and Cardiovascular Effects among Female Athletes with Chronic Menstrual Dysfunction." *Asian Journal of Sports Medicine*. 3(1) 2012: 53-58. http://www.ncbi.nlm.nih.gov/pmc/articles/PMC3307967/
Rickenlund A, et al., "Amenorrhea in Female Athletes Is Associated with Endothelial Dysfunction and Unfavorable Lipid Profile," *The Journal of Clinical Endocrinology & Metabolism*, 90(3), 2005:1354–1359, doi: 10.1210/jc.2004-1286.

55. **Hoch AZ, et al.** 2007. https://www.wisconsinmedicalsociety.org/_WMS/publications/wmj/pdf/106/6/301.pdf;
Rickenlund A, et al. 2005. doi: 10.1210/jc.2004-1964;
Yoshida, N., et al. 2006. doi: 10.1161/01.ATV.0000199102.60747.18

56. **Zhang Y, et al.** "Bone Mineral Density and Verbal Memory Impairment: Third National Health and Nutrition Examination Survey." *American Journal of Epidemiology*. 154(9) 2001: 795-802. doi: 10.1093/aje/154.9.795

57. **Ibid.**

58. **Vegeto E, Benedusi V, Maggi A.** "Estrogen Anti-inflammatory Activity in Brain: A Therapeutic Opportunity for Menopause and Neurodegenerative Diseases." *Frontiers in Neuroendocrinology.* 29(4) 2008: 507-19. doi: 10.1016/j.yfrne.2008.04.001;
Giatti S, et al. "Neuroactive Steroids, Their Metabolites, and Neuroinflammation." *Journal of Molecular Endocrinology.* 49(3) 2012: R125-134. doi: 10.1530/JME-12-0127

59. **Rocca WA, et al.** "Increased Risk of Cognitive Impairment or Dementia in Women Who Underwent Oophorectomy before Menopause." *Neurology.* 69f(11) 2007: 1074-083. doi: 10.1212/01.wnl.0000276984.19542.e6;
Rocca WA, et al. "Increased Risk of Parkinsonism in Women Who Underwent Oophorectomy before Menopause." *Neurology.* 70(3) 2008: 200-09. doi: 10.1212/01.wnl.0000280573.30975.6a

60. **Rivera CM., et al.** "Increased Mortality for Neurological and Mental Diseases following Early Bilateral Oophorectomy." *Neuroepidemiology.* 33(1) 2009: 32-40. doi: 10.1159/000211951

61. **Scott E, et al.** "Estrogen Neuroprotection and the Critical Period Hypothesis." *Frontiers in Neuroendocrinology.* 33(1) 2012: 85-104. doi: 10.1016/j.yfrne.2011.10.001

62. **Hesson, J.** "Cumulative Estrogen Exposure and Prospective Memory in Older Women." *Brain and Cognition.* 80(1) 2012: 89-95. doi: 10.1016/j.bandc.2012.05.001;
Smith CA, et al. "Lifelong Estrogen Exposure and Cognitive Performance in Elderly Women." *Brain and Cognition.* 39(3) 1999: 203-18. doi: 10.1006/brcg.1999.1078

63. **Hesson, J.** 2012. doi: 10.1016/j.bandc.2012.05.001

64. **Yaffe K, et al.** "Association between Bone Mineral Density and Cognitive Decline in Older Women." *Journal of the American Geriatric Society.* 47(10) 1999: 1176-182;
Zhang, Y., et al. 2001. doi: 10.1093/aje/154.9.795

Chapter 8—You Want Me to Eat WHAT?? The HA Recovery Plan

1. **Medicine, Institute Of.** "Energy." In Dietary Reference Intakes for Energy, Carbohydrate, Fiber, Fat, Fatty Acids, Cholesterol, Protein, and Amino Acids, 107-264. Washington, D.C.: National Academies Press, 2005. http://books.nap.edu/openbook.php?record_id=10490

2. **Loucks AB, Kiens B, Wright HA.** "Energy Availability in Athletes." *Journal of Sports Sciences.* 29(Sup 1) 2011: S7-S15. doi: 10.1080/02640414.2011.588958

3. **Medicine, Institute Of.** 2005. http://books.nap.edu/openbook.php?record_id=10490

4. **Ibid.**

5. **Ibid.**;
Redman LM, et al. "Energy Requirements in Nonobese Men and Women: Results from CALERIE." *American Journal of Clinical Nutrition.* 99(1) 2013: 71-78. doi: 10.3945/ajcn.113.065631

6. "Balancing Calories to Manage Weight." In Dietary Guidelines for Americans, 2010. 7th Edition ed. Washington, D.C.: U.S. Department of Agriculture and U.S. Department of Health and Human Services, 2010. http://www.fns.usda.gov/sites/default/files/Chapter2.pdf

Chapter 8 References cont.

7. **Medicine, Institute Of.** 2005. http://books.nap.edu/openbook.php?record_id=10490
8. **Ibid.;**
   Redman LM, et al. 2013. doi: 10.3945/ajcn.113.065631
9. **Medicine, Institute Of.** "Energy." 2005. http://books.nap.edu/openbook.php?record_id=10490;
   Westerterp KR. "Physical Activity and Physical Activity Induced Energy Expenditure in Humans: Measurement, Determinants, and Effects." *Frontiers in Physiology.* 4(90) 2013. doi: 10.3389/fphys.2013.00090
10. **Loucks AB, Kiens B, Wright HA.** "Energy Availability in Athletes." *Journal of Sports Sciences.* 29(Sup 1) 2011: S7-S15. doi: 10.1080/02640414.2011.588958;
    Nattiv A, et al. "American College of Sports Medicine Position Stand. The Female Athlete Triad." *Medicine & Science in Sports & Exercise.* 39(10) 2007: 1867-882. doi: 10.1249/mss.0b013e318149f111
11. **Ten Haaf T, Weijs PJM.** "Resting Energy Expenditure Prediction in Recreational Athletes of 18–35 Years: Confirmation of Cunningham Equation and an Improved Weight-Based Alternative." *PLoS One.* 9(10) 2014: E108460. doi: 10.1371/journal.pone.0108460
12. **Falsetti L.** "Long-term Follow-up of Functional Hypothalamic Amenorrhea and Prognostic Factors." *The Journal of Clinical Endocrinology & Metabolism.* 87(2) 2002: 500-05. doi: 10.1210/jcem.87.2.8195
13. **Ibid.**
14. **Arends JC, et al.** "Restoration of Menses with Nonpharmacologic Therapy in College Athletes with Menstrual Disturbances: A 5-year Retrospective Study." *International Journal of Sport Nutrition and Exercise Metabolism.* 22(2) 2012:98-108. http://www.ncbi.nlm.nih.gov/pubmed/22465870
15. **Misra M, et al.** "Weight Gain and Restoration of Menses as Predictors of Bone Mineral Density Change in Adolescent Girls with Anorexia Nervosa-1." *The Journal of Clinical Endocrinology & Metabolism.* 93(4) 2008: 1231-237. doi: 10.1210/jc.2007-1434
16. **Berga SL, et al.** "Recovery of Ovarian Activity in Women with Functional Hypothalamic Amenorrhea Who Were Treated with Cognitive Behavior Therapy." *Fertility and Sterility.* 80(4) 2003: 976-81. doi: 10.1016/S0015-0282(03)01124-5

Chapter 9—Putting Recovery Into Practice

1. **Chavarro JE, et al.** "A Prospective Study of Dairy Foods Intake and Anovulatory Infertility." *Human Reproduction.* 22(5) 2007: 1340-347. doi: 10.1093/humrep/dem019
2. **Zhang CM, et al.** "Gonadotropin-Releasing Hormone Neurons Express KATP Channels That Are Regulated by Estrogen and Responsive to Glucose and Metabolic Inhibition." *Journal of Neuroscience.* 27(38) 2007: 10153-0164. doi: 10.1523/JNEUROSCI.1657-07.2007
3. **Poretsky L, Kalin MF.** "The Gonadotropic Function of Insulin." *Endocrine Reviews.* 8(2) 1987: 132-41
4. **Chavarro JE, et al.** 2007. doi: 10.1093/humrep/dem019

Chapter 9 References cont.

5. **Hartmann S, Lacorn M, Steinhart H.** "Natural Occurrence of Steroid Hormones in Food." *Food Chemistry.* 62(1) 1998: 7-20. doi: 10.1016/S0308-8146(97)00150-7

6. **Ibid.**

7. **Fahrenholtz IL, et al.** "Within-day energy deficiency and reproductive function in female endurance athletes." *Scandinavian Journal of Medicine & Science in Sports.* 28(3) 2018: 1139-46. doi: 10.1111/sms.13030

8. **Loucks AB, Thuma JR.** "Luteinizing Hormone Pulsatility Is Disrupted at a Threshold of Energy Availability in Regularly Menstruating Women." *The Journal of Clinical Endocrinology & Metabolism.* 88(1) 2003: 297-311. doi: 10.1210/jc.2002-020369

Chapter 10—What to Expect…

1. **Miller KK, et al.** "Determinants of Skeletal Loss and Recovery in Anorexia Nervosa." *The Journal of Clinical Endocrinology & Metabolism.* 91(8) 2006: 2931-937. doi: 10.1210/jc.2005-2818;
   Misra M, et al. "Weight Gain and Restoration of Menses as Predictors of Bone Mineral Density Change in Adolescent Girls with Anorexia Nervosa-1." *The Journal of Clinical Endocrinology & Metabolism.* 93(4) 2008: 1231-237. doi: 10.1210/jc.2007-1434;
   Schulze, UM, et al. "Bone Mineral Density in Partially Recovered Early Onset Anorexic Patients - a Follow-up Investigation." *Child & Adolescent Psychiatry & Mental Health.* 4(1) 2010): 20. doi: 10.1186/1753-2000-4-20

2. **Mallinson RJ, et al.** "A Case Report of Recovery of Menstrual Function following a Nutritional Intervention in Two Exercising Women with Amenorrhea of Varying Duration." *Journal of the International Society of Sports Nutrition.* 10(1) 2013: 34. doi: 10.1186/1550-2783-10-34

3. **Rigaud D, et al.** "Body Fluid Retention and Body Weight Change in Anorexia Nervosa Patients during Refeeding." *Clinical Nutrition.* 29(6) 2010: 749-55. doi: 10.1016/j.clnu.2010.05.007

4. **Mayer, LE, et al.** "Adipose Tissue Distribution after Weight Restoration and Weight Maintenance in Women with Anorexia Nervosa." *American Journal of Clinical Nutrition.* 90(5) 2009: 1132-137. doi: 10.3945/ajcn.2009.27820

5. **Speakman, JR, et al.** "Set points, settling points and some alternative models: theoretical options to understand how genes and environments combine to regulate body adiposity." Disease Models and Mechanisms. 4(6) 2011: 733-745. doi: 10.1242/dmm.008698

6. **Ibid.**

7. **Keesey RE, Hirvonen MD.** "Body Weight Set-points: Determination and Adjustment." *The Journal of Nutrition.* 127(9) 1997: 1875S-883S. http://jn.nutrition.org/content/127/9/1875S.long

Chapter 12—The HA Recovery Plan: Exercise Changes

1. **Bullen BA, et al.** "Induction of Menstrual Disorders by Strenuous Exercise in Untrained Women." *New England Journal of Medicine.* 312(21) 1985: 1349-353. doi: 10.1056/NEJM198505233122103

Chapter 12 References cont.

2. **Ibid.**
3. **De Souza MJ, et al.** "High Frequency of Luteal Phase Deficiency and Anovulation in Recreational Women Runners: Blunted Elevation in Follicle-stimulating Hormone Observed during Luteal-follicular Transition." *The Journal of Clinical Endocrinology & Metabolism.* 83(12) 1998: 4220-232. doi: 10.1210/jcem.83.12.5334
4. **De Souza MJ, et al.** "High Prevalence of Subtle and Severe Menstrual Disturbances in Exercising Women: Confirmation Using Daily Hormone Measures." *Human Reproduction.* 25(2) 2010: 491-503. doi: 10.1093/humrep/dep411
5. **Mallinson RJ, et al.** "A Case Report of Recovery of Menstrual Function following a Nutritional Intervention in Two Exercising Women with Amenorrhea of Varying Duration." *Journal of the International Society of Sports Nutrition.* 10(1) 2013: 34. doi: 10.1186/1550-2783-10-34
6. **Wise LA, et al.** "A Prospective Cohort Study of Physical Activity and Time-to-pregnancy." *Fertility and Sterility.* 97(5) 2012: 1136-142. doi: 10.1016/j.fertnstert.2012.02.025
7. **Hill EE, et al.** "Exercise and Circulating Cortisol Levels: The Intensity Threshold Effect." *Journal of Endocrinological Investigation.* 31(7) 2008: 587-91. doi: 10.1007/BF03345606
8. **Gibson JH, et al.** "Nutritional and Exercise-related Determinants of Bone Density in Elite Female Runners." *Osteoporosis International.* 15(8) 2004: 611-18; **De Souza MJ, et al.** 1998. doi: 10.1210/jcem.83.12.5334; **De Souza MJ, et al.** 2010. doi: 10.1093/humrep/dep411

Chapter 13—There Is More to Life Than Exercise

1. **Linehan, Marsha.** Skills Training Manual for Treating Borderline Personality Disorder. New York: Guilford Press, 1993
2. Chapter 15—Partners in Recovery
1. **Mountjoy M, et al.** "International Olympic Committee (IOC) Consensus Statement on Relative Energy Deficiency in Sport (RED-S): 2018 Update." International Journal of Sport Nutition and Exercise Metabolism. 28(4) 2018: 316-331. doi: 10.1123/ijsnem.2018-0136

Chapter 16—Recovering Natural Cycles

1. **Baerwald AR, Adams GP, Pierson RA.** "Ovarian Antral Folliculogenesis during the Human Menstrual Cycle: A Review." *Human Reproduction Update.* 18(1) 2011: 73-91. doi: 10.1093/humupd/dmr039
2. **Baerwald AR.** "Characterization of Ovarian Follicular Wave Dynamics in Women." *Biology of Reproduction.* 69(3) 2003: 1023-031. doi: 10.1095/biolreprod.103.017772
3. Dana Byrd, facebook message to Dr. Nicola Sykes (Rinaldi) April 15, 2014
4. **Wise LA, et al.** "A Prospective Cohort Study of Physical Activity and Time-to-pregnancy." *Fertility and Sterility.* 97(5) 2012: 1136-142. doi: 10.1016/j.fertnstert.2012.02.025

5. **De Laet C et al.** "Body mass index as a predictor of fracture risk: A meta-analysis." *Osteoporosis International.* 16(11) 2005: 1330–1338. doi:10.1007/s00198-005-1863-y

Chapter 17—Tracking Ovulation and Family Planning

1. **Elliott-Sale KJ et al.** "Examining the role of oral contraceptive users as an experimental and/or control group in athletic performance studies." Contraception. 88(3) 2013:408-12. doi: 10.1016/j.contraception.2012.11.023
2. **Prior, JC.** "Progesterone for the prevention and treatment of osteoporosis in women." Climacteric, 21(4) 2018: 366-374. doi: 10.1080/13697137.2018.1467400
3. **Dunson DB, et al.** "Day-specific Probabilities of Clinical Pregnancy Based on Two Studies with Imperfect Measures of Ovulation." *Human Reproduction.* 14(7) 1999: 1835-839. doi: 10.1093/humrep/14.7.1835;
Dunson DB, Columbo B, Baird DD. "Changes with Age in the Level and Duration of Fertility in the Menstrual Cycle." *Human Reproduction.* 17(5) 2002: 1399-403. doi: 10.1093/humrep/17.5.1399;
Stanford JB, Dunson DB. "Effects of Sexual Intercourse Patterns in Time to Pregnancy Studies." *American Journal of Epidemiology.* 165(9) 2007: 1088-095. doi: 10.1093/aje/kwk111;
Wilcox AJ, Weinberg CR, Baird DD. "Timing of Sexual Intercourse in Relation to Ovulation — Effects on the Probability of Conception, Survival of the Pregnancy, and Sex of the Baby." *New England Journal of Medicine.* 333(23) 1995: 1517-521. doi: 10.1056/NEJM199512073332301
4. **Dunson DB et al.** 1999. doi: 10.1093/humrep/14.7.1835;
Dunson DB, Columbo B, Baird DD. 2002. doi: 10.1093/humrep/17.5.1399;
Wilcox AJ, Weinberg CR, Baird DD.) 1995. doi: 10.1056/NEJM199512073332301
5. **Gould JE.** "Assessment of Human Sperm Function after Recovery from the Female Reproductive Tract." *Biology of Reproduction.* 31(5) 1984: 888-94. doi: 10.1095/biolreprod31.5.888
6. **Levitas E, et al.** "Relationship between the Duration of Sexual Abstinence and Semen Quality: Analysis of 9,489 Semen Samples." *Fertility and Sterility.* 83(6) 2005: 1680-686. doi: 10.1016/j.fertnstert.2004.12.045
7. **Gould JE** 1984. doi: 10.1095/biolreprod31.5.888
8. **Mcgovern PG, et al.** "Absence of Secretory Endometrium after False-positive Home Urine Luteinizing Hormone Testing." *Fertility and Sterility.* 82(5) 2004: 1273-277. doi: 10.1016/j.fertnstert.2004.03.070.
9. **Dunson DB, et al.** 1999. doi: 10.1093/humrep/14.7.1835;
Dunson DB, Columbo B, Baird DD. 2002. doi: 10.1093/humrep/17.5.1399;
Wilcox AJ, Weinberg CR, Baird DD. 1995. doi: 10.1056/NEJM199512073332301
10. **Häggström M.** "Reference Ranges for Estradiol, Progesterone, Luteinizing Hormone and Follicle-stimulating Hormone during the Menstrual Cycle." *Wikiversity Journal of Medicine.* 1(25) 2014. doi: 10.15347/wjm/2014.001
11. **Hull, MGR, et al.** "The Value of a Single Serum Progesterone Measurement in the Midluteal Phase as a Criterion of a Potentially Fertile Cycle ("ovulation")

Chapter 17 References cont.

Derived from Treated and Untreated Conception Cycles." *Fertility and Sterility*. 37(3) 1982: 355-60

12. **Forman RG, Chapman MC, Steptoe PC.** "The Effect of Endogenous Progesterone on Basal Body Temperature in Stimulated Ovarian Cycles." *Human Reproduction*. 2(8) 1987: 631-34.

Chapter 18—Still No Period?!

1. **Berga SL, et al.** "Recovery of Ovarian Activity in Women with Functional Hypothalamic Amenorrhea Who Were Treated with Cognitive Behavior Therapy." *Fertility and Sterility*. 80(4) 2003: 976-81. doi: 10.1016/S0015-0282(03)01124-5
2. **Tschugguel W, Berga SL.** "Treatment of Functional Hypothalamic Amenorrhea with Hypnotherapy." *Fertility and Sterility*. 80(4) 2003: 982-85. doi: 10.1016/S0015-0282(03)01012-4
3. **Acosta-Martínez M.** "PI3K: An Attractive Candidate for the Central Integration of Metabolism and Reproduction." *Frontiers in Endocrinology*. 2(110) 2012. doi: 10.3389/fendo.2011.00110
4. **Senashova O, et al.** "The Effect of Citalopram on Midbrain CRF Receptors 1 and 2 in a Primate Model of Stress-Induced Amenorrhea." *Reproductive Sciences*. 19(6) 2012: 623-32. doi: 10.1177/1933719111430992
5. **Herod SM, Pohl CM, Cameron JL.** "Treatment with a CRH-R1 Antagonist Prevents Stress-induced Suppression of the Central Neural Drive to the Reproductive Axis in Female Macaques." *AJP: Endocrinology and Metabolism*. 300(1) 2010. doi: 10.1152/ajpendo.00224.2010
6. **Daniels TL, Berga SL.** "Resistance of Gonadotropin Releasing Hormone Drive to Sex Steroid-Induced Suppression in Hyperandrogenic Anovulation." *The Journal of Clinical Endocrinology & Metabolism*, 82(12) 1997: 4179–4183. doi: 10.1210/jcem.82.12.4402
7. **WebMD, LLC.** "ACETYL-L-CARNITINE: Uses, Side Effects, Interactions and Warnings - WebMD." WebMD. Accessed September 23, 2015. http://www.webmd.com/vitamins-supplements/ingredientmono-834-ACETYL-L-CARNITINE.aspx?activeIngredientId=834&activeIngredientName=ACETYL-L-CARNITINE
8. **Genazzani AD et al.** "Acetyl-l-carnitine as Possible Drug in the Treatment of Hypothalamic Amenorrhea." *Acta Obstetricia et Gynecologica Scandinavica*. 70(6) 1991: 487-92. doi: 10.3109/00016349109007165.
Genazzani AD et al. "Acetyl-L-carnitine (ALC) Administration Positively Affects Reproductive Axis in Hypogonadotropic Women with Functional Hypothalamic Amenorrhea." *Journal of Endocrinological Investigation*. 34(4) 2011: 287-91. doi: 10.1007/BF03347087.
Genazzani AD et al. "Modulatory effects of l-carnitine plus l-acetyl-carnitine on neuroendocrine control of hypothalamic functions in functional hypothalamic amenorrhea (FHA)." *Gynecol Endocrinol*. 33(12) 2017:963-967. doi: 10.1080/09513590.2017.1332587
9. **Genazzani AD, et al.** 1991: 487-92. doi: 10.3109/00016349109007165;
Genazzani AD, et al. 2011: 287-91. doi: 10.3275/6997
10. **Phipps WR et al.** "Effect of flax seed ingestion on the menstrual cycle." *J Clin Endocrinol Metab*. 77(5) 1993:1215-9. doi: 10.1210/jcem.77.5.8077314

11. Ibid.
12. **Naveen S et al.** "Anti-depressive effect of polyphenols and omega-3 fatty acid from pomegranate peel and flax seed in mice exposed to chronic mild stress." *Psychiatry Clin Neurosci.* 67(7) 2013:501-8. doi: 10.1111/pcn.12100.
    Phipps WR et al. 1993. doi: 10.1210/jcem.77.5.8077314
13. **Adolphe J et al.** "Health effects with consumption of the flax lignan secoisolariciresinol diglucoside." *British Journal of Nutrition*, 103(7) 2010:929-938. doi:10.1017/S0007114509992753
14. **Phipps WR et al.** 1993. doi: 10.1210/jcem.77.5.8077314
15. **George GJM** et al. "Interaction of Estrogenic Chemicals and Phytoestrogens with Estrogen Receptor β." *Endocrinology*, 139(10) 1998:4252–63, doi: 10.1210/endo.139.10.6216
16. **George GJM** et al. 1998. doi: 10.1210/endo.139.10.6216;
    Sasson S. "Equilibrium binding analysis of estrogen agonists and antagonists: relation to the activation of the estrogen receptor." *Pathol Biol (Paris).* 39(1) 1991:59-69. PMID: 2011412.
    Katzenellenbogen BS, Miller MA, Eckert RL, Sudo K. "Antiestrogen pharmacology and mechanism of action." *J Steroid Biochem.* 19(1A) 1983:59-68. PMID: 6887873.
    Clark JH, Markaverich BM. "The agonistic-antagonistic properties of clomiphene: a review." *Pharmacol Ther.* 15(3) 1981:467-519. doi: 10.1016/0163-7258(81)90055-3
17. **Borges LE, et al.** "New Protocol of Clomiphene Citrate Treatment in Women with Hypothalamic Amenorrhea." *Gynecological Endocrinology.* 23(6) 2007: 343-46. doi: 10.1080/09513590701327620
18. **Beate K, et al.** "Genetics of Isolated Hypogonadotropic Hypogonadism: Role of GnRH Receptor and Other Genes." *International Journal of Endocrinology.* 2012: 1-9. doi: 10.1155/2012/147893;
    Caronia LM, et al. "A Genetic Basis for Functional Hypothalamic Amenorrhea." *The New England Journal of Medicine.* 364(3) 2011: 215-25. doi: 10.1056/NEJMoa0911064
19. **Wildt L, Leyendecker G.** "Induction Of Ovulation By The Chronic Administration Of Naltrexone In Hypothalamic Amenorrhea." *The Journal of Clinical Endocrinology & Metabolism.* 64(6) 1987: 1334-335. doi: 10.1210/jcem-64-6-1334
20. Ibid.
21. **Remorgida V, et al.** "Naltrexone in Functional Hypothalamic Amenorrhea and in the Normal Luteal Phase." *Obstetrics and Gynecology.* 76(6) 1990: 1115-120
22. **Genazzani AD, et al.** "Naltrexone Administration Modulates the Neuroendocrine Control of Luteinizing Hormone Secretion in Hypothalamic Amenorrhoea." *Human Reproduction.* 10(11) 1995: 2868-871. http://humrep.oxfordjournals.org/content/10/11/2868.long
23. **Remorgida V, et al.** 1990
24. Ibid.
25. **Genazzani AD, et al.** 1995. http://humrep.oxfordjournals.org/content/10/11/2868.long

Chapter 18 References cont.

26. **Welt CK, et al.** "Recombinant Human Leptin in Women with Hypothalamic Amenorrhea." *New England Journal of Medicine.* 351(10) 2004: 987-97. doi: 10.1056/NEJMoa040388
27. **Chou SH, et al.** "Leptin Is an Effective Treatment for Hypothalamic Amenorrhea." *Proceedings of the National Academy of Sciences.* 108(16) 2011: 6585-590. doi: 10.1073/pnas.1015674108
28. **Jayasena CN, et al.** "Increasing LH Pulsatility in Women with Hypothalamic Amenorrhoea Using Intravenous Infusion of Kisspeptin-54." *The Journal of Clinical Endocrinology & Metabolism.* 99(6) 2014: E953-961. doi: 10.1210/jc.2013-1569
29. **Borges LE et al.** 2007. doi: 10.1080/09513590701327620
30. **Ismail AM et al.** "Adding L-carnitine to clomiphene resistant PCOS women improves the quality of ovulation and the pregnancy rate. A randomized clinical trial." *Eur J Obstet Gynecol Reprod Biol.* 180 2014:148-52. doi: 10.1016/j.ejogrb.2014.06.008.

Chapter 19—Luteal Phase

1. **American Society of Reproductive Medicine.** "Progesterone Supplementation during the Luteal Phase and in Early Pregnancy in the Treatment of Infertility: An Educational Bulletin." *Fertility and Sterility.* 90(5S) 2008: S150-153. doi: 10.1016/j.fertnstert.2008.08.064
2. **Wuttke W, et al.** "LH Pulses and the Corpus Luteum: The Luteal Phase Deficiency LPD." *Vitamins and Hormones.* 63 (2001): 131-58
3. **Henmi H, et al.** "Effects of Ascorbic Acid Supplementation on Serum Progesterone Levels in Patients with a Luteal Phase Defect." *Fertility and Sterility.* 80(2) 2003: 459-61. doi: 10.1016/S0015-0282(03)00657-5
4. **Andersen CY, Andersen KV.** "Improving the Luteal Phase after Ovarian Stimulation: Reviewing New Options." *Reproductive BioMedicine Online.* 28(5) 2014:552-9. doi: 10.1016/j.rbmo.2014.01.012
5. **Wuttke W, et al.** 2001
6. **Strott CA, et al.** "The Short Luteal Phase." *The Journal of Clinical Endocrinology & Metabolism.* 30(2) 1970: 246-51. doi: 10.1210/jcem-30-2-246
7. **Downs KA, Gibson M.** "Clomiphene Citrate Therapy for Luteal Phase Defect." *Fertility and Sterility.* 39(1) 1983: 34-38
8. **Cook CL, et al.** "Induction of Luteal Phase Defect with Clomiphene Citrate." *American Journal of Obstetrics and Gynecology.* 149(6) 1984: 613-16
9. **Hill MJ, et al.** "Progesterone Luteal Support after Ovulation Induction and Intrauterine Insemination: A Systematic Review and Meta-analysis." *Fertility and Sterility.* 100(5) 2013: 1373-380.e6. doi: 10.1016/j.fertnstert.2013.06.034;
Miralpeix EM, et al. "Efficacy of Luteal Phase Support with Vaginal Progesterone in Intrauterine Insemination: A Systematic Review and Meta-analysis." *Journal of Assisted Reproduction and Genetics.* 31(1) 2014: 89-100. doi: 10.1007/s10815-013-0127-6
10. **Williams NI, et al.** "Effects of Short-term Strenuous Endurance Exercise upon Corpus Luteum Function." *Medicine & Science in Sports & Exercise.* 31(7) 1999: 949-58
11. **Wuttke W, et al.** 2001

Chapter 19 References cont.

12. Ibid.
13. Ibid.
14. Ibid.
15. **American Society of Reproductive Medicine.** 2008. doi: 10.1016/j.fertnstert.2008.08.064
16. Ibid.;
    Miles RA, et al. "Pharmacokinetics and Endometrial Tissue Levels of Progesterone after Administration by Intramuscular and Vaginal Routes: A Comparative Study." *Fertility and Sterility.* 62(3) 1994: 485-90
17. **Archer DF, et al.** "Initial and Steady-state Pharmacokinetics of a Vaginally Administered Formulation of Progesterone." *American Journal of Obstetrics and Gynecology.* 173(2) 1995: 471-78. doi: 10.1016/0002-9378(95)90268-6
18. **Henmi H, et al.** 2003.doi: 10.1016/S0015-0282(03)00657-5
19. **Phipps WR et al.** "Effect of flax seed ingestion on the menstrual cycle." Journal of Clinical Endocrinology and Metabolism. 77(5) 1993: 1215-19. doi: 10.1210/jcem.77.5.8077314
20. **Westphal LM, et al.** "A Nutritional Supplement for Improving Fertility in Women: A Pilot Study." *Journal of Reprodcutive Medicine.* 49(4) 2004: 289-93
21. **Carey BJ, et al.** "A Study to Evaluate Serum and Urinary Hormone Levels following Short and Long Term Administration of Two Regimens of Progesterone Cream in Postmenopausal Women." *BJOG: An International Journal of Obstetrics and Gynaecology.* 107(6) 2000: 722-26. doi: 10.1111/j.1471-0528.2000.tb13331.x
22. **Stanczyk FZ, Paulson RJ, Roy S.** "Percutaneous Administration of Progesterone: Blood Levels and Endometrial Protection." *Menopause.* 12(2) 2005: 232-37. doi: 10.1097/00042192-200512020-00019
23. **Andersen CY and Andersen KV.** 2014. doi: 10.1016/j.rbmo.2014.01.012
24. **Hull, MGR, et al.** "The Value of a Single Serum Progesterone Measurement in the Midluteal Phase as a Criterion of a Potentially Fertile Cycle ("ovulation") Derived from Treated and Untreated Conception Cycles." *Fertility and Sterility.* 37(3) 1982: 355-60
25. **Henmi H, et al.** 2003.doi: 10.1016/S0015-0282(03)00657-5
26. **American Society of Reproductive Medicine.** 2008. doi: 10.1016/j.fertnstert.2008.08.064
27. **Siemienowicz KJ, et al.** "Early pregnancy maternal progesterone administration alters pituitary and testis function and steroid profile in male fetuses." *Sci Rep.* 10(1) 2020:21920. doi: 10.1038/s41598-020-78976-x
    Davidovitch M, et al. "Infertility treatments during pregnancy and the risk of autism spectrum disorder in the offspring." *Prog Neuropsychopharmacol Biol Psychiatry.* 86 2018:175-179. doi: 10.1016/j.pnpbp.2018.05.022.
28. **Duncan WC.** "The inadequate corpus luteum." *Reprod Fertil.* 2:(1) 2021:C1-C7. doi: 10.1530/RAF-20-0044
29. **Kyrou D, et al.** "Does cessation of progesterone supplementation during early pregnancy in patients treated with recFSH/GnRH antagonist affect ongoing pregnancy rates? A randomized controlled trial." *Hum Reprod.* 26(5) 2011:1020-4. doi:

Chapter 19 References cont.

10.1093/humrep/der012

Mizrachi Y, Raziel A, Weissman A. "When Can We Safely Stop Luteal Phase Support in Fresh IVF Cycles? A Literature Review." *Front Reprod Health.* 2 2020:610532. doi: 10.3389/frph.2020.610532

30. **Lisova KM, et al.** "Changes in the level of fetoplacental complex hormones in pregnant women with miscarriage." *J Med Life.* 14(4) 2021:487-491. doi: 10.25122/jml-2021-0089

    Devall AJ, et al. "Progestogens for preventing miscarriage: a network meta-analysis." *Cochrane Database Syst Rev.* 4(4) 2021:CD013792. doi: 10.1002/14651858.CD013792.pub2

Chapter 20—When You Need a Jump-Start

1. **González RR, et al.** "Leptin and Leptin Receptor Are Expressed in the Human Endometrium and Endometrial Leptin Secretion Is Regulated by the Human Blastocyst." *The Journal of Clinical Endocrinology & Metabolism.* 85(12) 2000: 4883-888. doi: 10.1210/jcem.85.12.7060

2. **Cervero A, et al.** "The Leptin System during Human Endometrial Receptivity and Preimplantation Development." *The Journal of Clinical Endocrinology & Metabolism.* 89(5) 2004: 2442-451. doi: 10.1210/jc.2003-032127

3. **González, R. R., et al.** 2000. doi: 10.1210/jcem.85.12.7060

4. **Zhou X, Liu F, Zhai S.** "Effect of L-carnitine And/or L-acetyl-carnitine in Nutrition Treatment for Male Infertility: A Systematic Review." *Asia Pacific Journal of Clinical Nutrition.* 16(S1) 2007: 383-90. http://apjcn.nhri.org.tw/server/APJCN/16%20Suppl%201//383.pdf

5. **Ross C, et al.** "A Systematic Review of the Effect of Oral Antioxidants on Male Infertility." *Reproductive Biomedicine Online.* 20(6) 2010: 711-23

6. **Ahmad G, et al.** "Mild Induced Testicular and Epididymal Hyperthermia Alters Sperm Chromatin Integrity in Men." *Fertility and Sterility.* 97(3) 2012: 546-53. doi: 10.1016/j.fertnstert.2011.12.025;

    Jurewicz J, et al. "Lifestyle Factors and Sperm Aneuploidy." *Reproductive Biology.* 14(3) 2014: 190-99. doi: 10.1016/j.repbio.2014.02.002;

    Povey AC, et al. "Modifiable and Non-modifiable Risk Factors for Poor Semen Quality: A Case-referent Study." *Human Reproduction.* 27(9) 2012: 2799-806. doi: 10.1093/humrep/des183

7. **Venturella R, et al.** "OvAge: A New Methodology to Quantify Ovarian Reserve Combining Clinical, Biochemical and 3D-ultrasonographic Parameters." *Journal of Ovarian Research.* 8(21) 2015. doi: 10.1186/s13048-015-0149-z

8. **Ibid**.

9. **Lehmann P, et al.** "Anti-Müllerian Hormone (AMH): A Reliable Biomarker of Oocyte Quality in IVF." *Journal of Assisted Reproduction and Genetics.* 31(4) 2014: 493-98. doi: 10.1007/s10815-014-0193-4

10. **Venturella, R., et al.** 2015. doi: 10.1186/s13048-015-0149-z

11. **Panidis D, et al.** "Serum Anti-Müllerian Hormone (AMH) Levels Are Differentially Modulated by Both Serum Gonadotropins and Not Only by Serum Follicle Stimulating Hormone (FSH) Levels." *Medical Hypotheses.* 77(4) 2011: 649-53. doi: 10.1016/j.mehy.2011.07.005

12. **Gleicher N and Barad DH.** "Dehydroepiandrosterone (DHEA) Supplementation in Diminished Ovarian Reserve (DOR)." *Reproductive Biology and Endocrinology.* 9(1) 2011: 67. doi: 10.1186/1477-7827-9-67
13. **Ibid.**

Chapter 21—Popping Pills to Ovulate: Oral Medications

1. **Messinis IE.** "Ovarian Feedback, Mechanism of Action and Possible Clinical Implications." *Human Reproduction Update.* 12(5) 2006: 557-71. doi: 10.1093/humupd/dml020;
   Welt CK, et al. "Control of Follicle-Stimulating Hormone by Estradiol and the Inhibins: Critical Role of Estradiol at the Hypothalamus during the Luteal-Follicular Transition." *The Journal of Clinical Endocrinology & Metabolism.* 88(4) 2003: 1766-771. doi: 10.1210/jc.2002-021516

2. **Welt CK, et al.** 2003. doi: 10.1210/jc.2002-021516

3. **Shaw ND, et al.** "Estrogen Negative Feedback on Gonadotropin Secretion: Evidence for a Direct Pituitary Effect in Women." *The Journal of Clinical Endocrinology & Metabolism.* 95(4) 2010: 1955-961. doi: 10.1210/jc.2009-2108

4. **Kerin JF, et al.** "Evidence for a Hypothalamic Site of Action of Clomiphene Citrate in Women." *The Journal of Clinical Endocrinology & Metabolism.* 61(2) 1985: 265-68. doi: 10.1210/jc.2009-2108;
   Welt CK, et al. 2003. doi: 10.1210/jc.2002-021516

5. **Kerin JF, et al.** 1985. doi: 10.1210/jc.2009-2108

6. **Gielen SC, et al.** "Signaling by Estrogens and Tamoxifen in the Human Endometrium." *The Journal of Steroid Biochemistry and Molecular Biology.* 109(3-5) 2008: 219-23. doi: 10.1016/j.jsbmb.2008.03.021;
   Katzenellenbogen BS, Katzenellenbogen JA. "Biomedicine: Defining the "S" in SERMs." *Science.* 295(5564) 2002: 2380-1. doi: 10.1126/science.1070442

7. **Armeanu MC, Moss RJ, Schoemaker J.** "Ovulation Induction with a Single-blind Treatment Regimen Comparing Naltrexone, Placebo and Clomiphene Citrate in Women with Secondary Amenorrhea." *European Journal of Endocrinology.* 126.5 (1992): 410-15. doi: 10.1530/acta.0.1260410;
   Borges LE, et al. "New Protocol of Clomiphene Citrate Treatment in Women with Hypothalamic Amenorrhea." *Gynecological Endocrinology.* 23(6) 2007: 343-46. doi: 10.1080/09513590701327620;
   Djurovic M, et al. "Gonadotropin Response to Clomiphene and Plasma Leptin Levels in Weight Recovered but Amenorrhoeic Patients with Anorexia Nervosa." *Journal of Endocrinological Investigation.* 27(6) 2004: 523-27. doi: 10.1007/BF03347473

8. **Gnoth C, et al.** "Time to Pregnancy: Results of the German Prospective Study and Impact on the Management of Infertility." *Human Reproduction.* 18(9) 2003: 1959-966. doi: 10.1093/humrep/deg366

9. **Fouda UM, Sayed AM.** "Extended Letrozole Regimen versus Clomiphene Citrate for Superovulation in Patients with Unexplained Infertility Undergoing Intrauterine Insemination: A Randomized Controlled Trial." *Reproductive Biology and Endocrinology.* 9(1) 2011: 84. doi: 10.1186/1477-7827-9-84;
   Franik S, et al. "Aromatase Inhibitors for Subfertile Women with Polycystic Ovary Syndrome." *The Cochrane Database of Systematic Reviews.* 2014. doi:

Chapter 21 References cont.

    10.1002/14651858.CD010287.pub2;
Liu A, et al. "Letrozole versus Clomiphene Citrate for Unexplained Infertility: A Systematic Review and Meta-analysis." The *Journal of Obstetrics and Gynaecology Research*. 40(5) 2014: 1205-216. doi: 10.1111/jog.12393;
Roy K, et al. "A Prospective Randomized Trial Comparing the Efficacy of Letrozole and Clomiphene Citrate in Induction of Ovulation in Polycystic Ovarian Syndrome." *Journal of Human Reproductive Sciences*. 5(1) 2012: 20. doi: 10.4103/0974-1208.97789

10. **Gerhard I, Runnebaum B.** "Comparison between Tamoxifen and Clomiphene Therapy in Women with Anovulation." *Archives of Gynecology*. 227(4) 1979: 279-88;
Steiner AZ, Terplan M, Paulson RJ. "Comparison of Tamoxifen and Clomiphene Citrate for Ovulation Induction: A Meta-analysis." *Human Reproduction*. 20(6) 2005: 1511-515. doi: 10.1093/humrep/deh840

11. **Franik, S., et al.** 2014. doi: 10.1002/14651858.CD010287.pub2;
Liu, A., et al. 2014. doi: 10.1111/jog.12393

12. **Fouda UM, Sayed AM.** 2011. doi: 10.1186/1477-7827-9-84;
Franik, S., et al. 2014. doi: 10.1002/14651858.CD010287.pub2;
Liu, A., et al. 2014. doi: 10.1111/jog.12393;
Roy K, et al. 2012. doi: 10.4103/0974-1208.97789

13. **Takasaki A, et al.** "A Pilot Study to Prevent a Thin Endometrium in Patients Undergoing Clomiphene Citrate Treatment." *Journal of Ovarian Research*. 6(1) 2013: 94. doi: 10.1186/1757-2215-6-94

14. **Biljan MM, Hemmings R, Brassard N.** "The Outcome of 150 Babies Following the Treatment With Letrozole or Letrozole and Gonadotropins." *Fertility and Sterility*. 84(S1) 2005: S95. doi: 10.1016/j.fertnstert.2005.07.230

15. **Gill SK, Moretti M, Koren G.** "Is the Use of Letrozole to Induce Ovulation Teratogenic?" *Canadian Family Physician*. 54(3) 2008: 353-54. http://www.ncbi.nlm.nih.gov/pmc/articles/PMC2278348;
Sharma S, et al. "Congenital Malformations among Babies Born Following Letrozole or Clomiphene for Infertility Treatment." *PLoS ONE*. 9(10) 2014. doi: 10.1371/journal.pone.0108219;
Tulandi T, et al. "Congenital Malformations among 911 Newborns Conceived after Infertility Treatment with Letrozole or Clomiphene Citrate." *Fertility and Sterility*. 85(6) 2006: 1761-765. 10.1016/j.fertnstert.2006.03.014

16. **Klement AH, Casper RF.** "The Use of Aromatase Inhibitors for Ovulation Induction." *Current Opinion in Obstetrics and Gynecology*. 27(3) 2015: 206-09. doi: 10.1097/GCO.0000000000000163

17. **Gerhard I, Runnebaum B.** 1979;
Steiner AZ, Terplan M, Paulson RJ. 2005. doi: 10.1093/humrep/deh840

18. **Dhaliwal LK, et al.** "Tamoxifen: An Alternative to Clomiphene in Women with Polycystic Ovary Syndrome." *Journal of Human Reproductive Sciences*. 4(2) 2011: 76-79. doi: 10.4103/0974-1208.86085

19. **Ibid.**

20. **Borges LE, et al.** 2007. doi: 10.1080/09513590701327620;
Djurovic M, et al. 2004. doi: 10.1007/BF03347473

21. **Badawy A, et al.** "Extended Letrozole Therapy for Ovulation Induction in Clomiphene-resistant Women with Polycystic Ovary Syndrome: A Novel Protocol." *Fertility and Sterility.* 92(1) 2009: 236-39. doi: 10.1016/j.fertnstert.2008.04.065;
    Fouda UM, Sayed AM. 2011. doi: 10.1186/1477-7827-9-84;
    Kjeld JM, et al. "Hormonal Responses To A First Course Of Clomiphene Citrate In Women With Amenorrhoea." *British Journal of Obstetrics and Gynaecology.* 82(5) 1975: 397-404. abstract only;
    Lobo RA, et al. "An Extended Regimen of Clomiphene Citrate in Women Unresponsive to Standard Therapy." *Fertility and Sterility.* 37(6) 1982: 762-66. Abstract only

22. **Hurst BS, et al.** "Novel Clomiphene "stair-step" Protocol Reduces Time to Ovulation in Women with Polycystic Ovarian Syndrome." *American Journal of Obstetrics and Gynecology.* 200(5) 2009: 510.e1-10.e4. doi: 10.1016/j.ajog.2008.10.031

23. **Göl K, et al**. "The Effects of 3-day Clomiphene Citrate Treatment on Endocrine and Ovulatory Responses." *Gynecological Endocrinology.* 10(3) 1996: 171-76

24. **Hajishafiha M, et al.** "Combined Letrozole and Clomiphene versus Letrozole and Clomiphene Alone in Infertile Patients with Polycystic Ovary Syndrome." *Drug Design, Development and Therapy.* 7 2013: 1427-431. doi: 10.2147/DDDT.S50972

25. **Badawy A, Metwally M, Fawzy M**. "Randomized Controlled Trial of Three Doses of Letrozole for Ovulation Induction in Patients with Unexplained Infertility." *Reproductive Biomedicine Online.* 14(5) 2007: 559-62;
    Pritts EA, et al. "The Use of High Dose Letrozole in Ovulation Induction and Controlled Ovarian Hyperstimulation." *ISRN Obstetrics and Gynecology.* 2011. doi: 10.5402/2011/242864

26. **Pritts EA, et al.** 2011. doi: 10.5402/2011/242864

27. **Badawy A, et al.** 2009. doi: 10.1016/j.fertnstert.2008.04.065

28. **Kjeld JM, et al**. 1975. abstract only

29. **Borges LE, et al.** 2007. doi: 10.1080/09513590701327620

30. **Ibid**.

31. **Ibid**.

32. **Badawy A, et al.** 2009. doi: 10.1016/j.fertnstert.2008.04.065

33. **Hurst BS, et al.** 2009. doi: 10.1016/j.ajog.2008.10.031

34. **Baerwald AR.** "Characterization of Ovarian Follicular Wave Dynamics in Women." *Biology of Reproduction.* 69(3) 2003: 1023-031. doi: 10.1095/biolreprod.103.017772

35. **Diamond MP, et al.** "Endometrial Shedding Effect on Conception and Live Birth in Women With Polycystic Ovary Syndrome." *Obstetrical & Gynecological Survey.* 67(9) 2012: 548-49. doi: 10.1097/01.ogx.0000421452.19985.8f;
    Casper RF. "Detrimental Effect of Induced or Spontaneous Menses Before Ovulation Induction on Pregnancy Outcome in Patients With Polycystic Ovary Syndrome." *Obstetrics & Gynecology.* 119(5) 2012: 886-87. doi: 10.1097/aog.0b013e318251a076

36. **Diamond MP, et al.** 2012. doi: 10.1097/01.ogx.0000421452.19985.8f

37. **Casper RF.** 2012. doi: 10.1097/aog.0b013e318251a076

Chapter 21 References cont.

38. **Badawy A, et al.** "Luteal Phase Clomiphene Citrate for Ovulation Induction in Women with Polycystic Ovary Syndrome: A Novel Protocol." *Fertility and Sterility.* 91(3) 2009: 838-41. doi: 10.1016/j.fertnstert.2008.01.016;
    Biljan MM, et al. "Prospective Randomized Double-blind Trial of the Correlation between Time of Administration and Antiestrogenic Effects of Clomiphene Citrate on Reproductive End Organs." *Fertility and Sterility.* 71(4) 1999: 633-38. doi: 10.1016/S0015-0282(98)00534-2;
    Göl K, et al. 1996;
    Takasaki A, et al. 2013. doi: 10.1186/1757-2215-6-94

39. **Biljan MM, et al.** 1999. doi: 10.1016/S0015-0282(98)00534-2

40. **Badawy A, et al.** 2009. doi: 10.1016/j.fertnstert.2008.01.016

41. **Takasaki A, et al.** 2013. doi: 10.1186/1757-2215-6-94

42. **Göl K, et al.** 1996

43. **Gerli S, et al.** "Use of Ethinyl Estradiol to Reverse the Antiestrogenic Effects of Clomiphene Citrate in Patients Undergoing Intrauterine Insemination: A Comparative, Randomized Study." *Fertility and Sterility.* 73(1) 2000: 85-89. doi: 10.1016/s0015-0282(99)00447-1;
    Satirapod C, et al. "Effect of Estradiol Valerate on Endometrium Thickness during Clomiphene Citrate-stimulated Ovulation." *The Journal of Obstetrics and Gynaecology Research.* 40(1) 2014: 96-101. doi: 10.1111/jog.12130;
    Shahin AY, et al. "Adding Phytoestrogens to Clomiphene Induction in Unexplained Infertility Patients – a Randomized Trial." *Reproductive BioMedicine Online.* 16(4) 2008: 580-88. doi: 10.1016/s1472-6483(10)60465-8

44. http://dailymed.nlm.nih.gov/dailymed/drugInfo.cfm?setid=a683e58a-63ea-44b8-a326-1a99a537bcf2&audience=consumer;
    Silverberg KM, et al. "Follicular Size at the Time of Human Chorionic Gonadotropin Administration Predicts Ovulation Outcome in Human Menopausal Gonadotropin-stimulated Cycles." *Fertility and Sterility.* 56(2) 1991: 296-300

45. **Palatnik A, et al.** "What Is the Optimal Follicular Size before Triggering Ovulation in Intrauterine Insemination Cycles with Clomiphene Citrate or Letrozole? An Analysis of 988 Cycles." *Fertility and Sterility.* 97(5) 2012: 1089-94. doi: 10.1016/j.fertnstert.2012.02.018

46. **Imani B, et al.** "Predictors of Chances to Conceive in Ovulatory Patients during Clomiphene Citrate Induction of Ovulation in Normogonadotropic Oligoamenorrheic Infertility." *The Journal of Clinical Endocrinology & Metabolism.* 84(5) 1999: 1617-22. doi: 10.1210/jcem.84.5.5705

47. **Fouda UM, Sayed AM.** 2011. doi: 10.1186/1477-7827-9-84;
    Franik S, et al. . 2014. doi: 10.1002/14651858.CD010287.pub2;
    Liu A, et al. 2014. doi: 10.1111/jog.12393;
    Roy K, et al. 2012. doi: 10.4103/0974-1208.97789

Chapter 22—Shooting up: Injectables

1. **Shalom-Paz E, et al.** "Does Optimal Follicular Size in IUI Cycles Vary between Clomiphene Citrate and Gonadotrophins Treatments?" *Gynecological Endocrinology.* 30(2) 2014: 107-10. doi: 10.3109/09513590.2013.860126;
    Silverberg KM, et al. "Follicular Size at the Time of Human Chorionic

Gonadotropin Administration Predicts Ovulation Outcome in Human Menopausal Gonadotropin-stimulated Cycles." *Fertility and Sterility.* 56(2) 1991: 296-300

2. **Bedaiwy MA, et al.** "Cost-effectiveness of Aromatase Inhibitor Co-treatment for Controlled Ovarian Stimulation." *Human Reproduction.* 21(11) 2006: 2838-844. doi: 10.1093/humrep/del273;
Noriega-Portella L, et al. "Effect of Letrozole at 2.5 Mg or 5.0 Mg/day on Ovarian Stimulation with Gonadotropins in Women Undergoing Intrauterine Insemination." *Fertility and Sterility.* 90(5) 2008: 1818-825. doi: 10.1016/j.fertnstert.2007.08.060;
Ozdemir U, et al. "Letrozole Usage Adjuvant to Gonadotropins for Ovulation Induction for Patients with Clomiphene Citrate Failure." *Archives of Gynecology and Obstetrics.* 288(2) 2013: 445-48. doi: 10.1007/s00404-013-2780-5

3. **Silverberg KM, et al.** 1991

4. **Bedaiwy MA, et al.** 2006. doi: 10.1093/humrep/del273;
Noriega-Portella L, et al. 2008. doi: 10.1016/j.fertnstert.2007.08.060

5. **Ozdemir U, et al.** 2013. doi: 10.1007/s00404-013-2780-5

6. **Balasch J, et al.** "Follicular Development and Hormone Concentrations following Recombinant FSH Administration for Anovulation Associated with Polycystic Ovarian Syndrome: Prospective, Randomized Comparison between Low-dose Step-up and Modified Step-down Regimens." *Human Reproduction.* 16(4) 2001: 652-56. doi: 10.1093/humrep/16.4.652

7. **Van Santbrink EJP, Fauser BC.** "Urinary Follicle-Stimulating Hormone for Normogonadotropic Clomiphene-Resistant Anovulatory Infertility: Prospective, Randomized Comparison between Low Dose Step-Up and Step-Down Dose Regimens." *The Journal of Clinical Endocrinology & Metabolism.* 82(11) 1997: 3597-602. doi: 10.1210/jcem.82.11.4369

8. **Silverberg KM, et al.** 1991

9. **Hill MJ, et al.** "Progesterone Luteal Support after Ovulation Induction and Intrauterine Insemination: A Systematic Review and Meta-analysis." *Fertility and Sterility.* 100(5) 2013: 1373-380. doi: 10.1016/j.fertnstert.2013.06.034

10. **Biljan MM, et al.** "Effects of Functional Ovarian Cysts Detected on the 7th Day of Gonadotropin-releasing Hormone Analog Administration on the Outcome of IVF Treatment." *Fertility and Sterility.* 74(5) 2000: 941-45. doi: 10.1016/s0015-0282(00)01555-7

Chapter 23—Medicated Ovulation and Beyond

1. **Mcgovern PG, et al.** "Absence of Secretory Endometrium after False-positive Home Urine Luteinizing Hormone Testing." *Fertility and Sterility.* 82(5) 2004: 1273-277. doi: 10.1016/j.fertnstert.2004.03.070

2. **Dunson DB, et al.** "Day-specific Probabilities of Clinical Pregnancy Based on Two Studies with Imperfect Measures of Ovulation." *Human Reproduction.* 14(7) 1999: 1835-839. doi: 10.1093/humrep/14.7.1835;
Stanford JB, Dunson DB. "Effects of Sexual Intercourse Patterns in Time to Pregnancy Studies." *American Journal of Epidemiology.* 165(9) 2007: 1088-095. doi: 10.1093/aje/kwk111

Chapter 23 References cont.

3. **Hull, MGR, et al.** "The Value of a Single Serum Progesterone Measurement in the Midluteal Phase as a Criterion of a Potentially Fertile Cycle ("ovulation") Derived from Treated and Untreated Conception Cycles." *Fertility and Sterility.* 37(3) 1982: 355-60
4. **Snick HK, Collins JA, Evers JLH.** "What Is the Most Valid Comparison Treatment in Trials of Intrauterine Insemination, Timed or Uninfluenced Intercourse? A Systematic Review and Meta-analysis of Indirect Evidence." *Human Reproduction.* 23(10) 2008: 2239-245. doi: 10.1093/humrep/den214;
Veltman-Verhulst SM, et al. "Intra-uterine Insemination for Unexplained Subfertility." *The Cochrane Database of Systematic Reviews.* 12(9) 2012. doi: 10.1002/14651858.CD001838.pub4
5. **Bensdorp A, et al.** "Intra-uterine Insemination for Male Subfertility." *The Cochrane Database of Systematic Reviews.* 2007. doi: 10.1002/14651858.CD000360.pub4;
Hashim HA, Ombar O, Elaal IA. "Intrauterine Insemination versus Timed Intercourse with Clomiphene Citrate in Polycystic Ovary Syndrome: A Randomized Controlled Trial." *Acta Obstetricia Et Gynecologica Scandinavica.* 90(4) 2011: 344-50. doi: 10.1111/j.1600-0412.2010.01063.x
6. **Polyzos NP, et al.** "Double versus Single Intrauterine Insemination for Unexplained Infertility: A Meta-analysis of Randomized Trials." *Fertility and Sterility.* 94(4) 2010: 1261-266. doi: 10.1016/j.fertnstert.2009.06.052;
Zavos A, et al. "Double versus Single Homologous Intrauterine Insemination for Male Factor Infertility: A Systematic Review and Meta-analysis." *Asian Journal of Andrology.* 15(4) 2013: 533-38. doi: 10.1038/aja.2013.4
7. **Hill MJ, et al.** "Progesterone Luteal Support after Ovulation Induction and Intrauterine Insemination: A Systematic Review and Meta-analysis." *Fertility and Sterility.* 100(5) 2013: 1373-380.e6. doi: 10.1016/j.fertnstert.2013.06.034;
Miralpeix EM, et al. "Efficacy of Luteal Phase Support with Vaginal Progesterone in Intrauterine Insemination: A Systematic Review and Meta-analysis." *Journal of Assisted Reproduction and Genetics.* 31(1) 2014: 89-100. doi: 10.1007/s10815-013-0127-6
8. **Mehri S, et al.** "Correlation between follicular diameters and flushing versus no flushing on oocyte maturity, fertilization rate and embryo quality." *Journal of Assisted Reproduction and Genetics.* 2014 Jan;31(1):73-7. doi: 10.1007/s10815-013-0124-9
9. **Zhong Y, et al.** "The efficacy of conversion from IUI to IVF-ET in infertility patients with hyper-response to ovulation induction: a retrospective study." *Biomedical Papers.* 2012 Jun;156(2):159-63. doi: 10.5507/bp.2012.044

Chapter 24—In Vitro Fertilization

1. **Veleva Z, et al.** "High and Low BMI Increase the Risk of Miscarriage after IVF/ICSI and FET." *Human Reproduction.* 23(4) 2008: 878-84. doi: 10.1093/humrep/den017
2. **González RR, et al.** "Leptin and Leptin Receptor Are Expressed in the Human Endometrium and Endometrial Leptin Secretion Is Regulated by the Human Blastocyst." *The Journal of Clinical Endocrinology & Metabolism.* 85(12) 2000: 4883-888. doi: /10.1210/jcem.85.12.7060

Chapter 24 References cont.

3. **Cervero A, et al.** "The Leptin System during Human Endometrial Receptivity and Preimplantation Development." *The Journal of Clinical Endocrinology & Metabolism.* 89(5) 2004: 2442-451. doi: 10.1210/jc.2003-032127
4. **Sazonova A, et al.** "Factors Affecting Obstetric Outcome of Singletons Born after IVF." *Human Reproduction.* 26(10) 2011: 2878-886. doi: 10.1093/humrep/der241
5. **Wise LA, et al.** "A Prospective Cohort Study of Physical Activity and Time-to-pregnancy." *Fertility and Sterility* 97(5) 2012: 1136-142. doi: 10.1016/j.fertnstert.2012.02.025
6. http://www.cdc.gov/art/artreports.htm
7. **Griesinger G, et al.** "Oral Contraceptive Pill Pretreatment in Ovarian Stimulation with GnRH Antagonists for IVF: A Systematic Review and Meta-analysis." *Fertility and Sterility.* 90(4) 2008: 1055-063. doi: 10.1016/j.fertnstert.2007.07.1354; **Smulders B, et al.** "Oral Contraceptive Pill, Progestogen or Estrogen Pre-treatment for Ovarian Stimulation Protocols for Women Undergoing Assisted Reproductive Techniques." *The Cochrane Database of Systematic Reviews.* 2010. doi: 10.1002/14651858.CD006109.pub2
8. **Barad DH, et al.** "Does Hormonal Contraception Prior to in Vitro Fertilization (IVF) Negatively Affect Oocyte Yields? - A Pilot Study." *Reproductive Biology and Endocrinology.* 11(1) 2013: 28. doi: 10.1186/1477-7827-11-28
9. **Yuan G, et al.** "Natural Products and Anti-inflammatory Activity." *Asia Pacific Journal of Clinical Nutrition* 15(2) 2006: 143-52. http://apjcn.nhri.org.tw/server/APJCN/15/2/143.pdf
10. **Grajecki D, Zyriax BC, Buhling KJ.** "The Effect of Micronutrient Supplements on Female Fertility: A Systematic Review." *Archives of Gynecology and Obstetrics.* 285(5) 2012: 1463-471. doi: 10.1007/s00404-012-2237-2
11. **Gleicher N, Barad DH.** "Dehydroepiandrosterone (DHEA) Supplementation in Diminished Ovarian Reserve (DOR)." *Reproductive Biology and Endocrinology.* 9(1) 2011: 67. doi: 10.1186/1477-7827-9-67
12. **Cheong YC, et al.** "Acupuncture and Assisted Reproductive Technology." *The Cochrane Database of Systematic Reviews.* 2013. doi: 10.1002/14651858.CD006920.pub3; **Qu F, Zhou J, Ren RX.** "Effects of Acupuncture on the Outcomes of in Vitro Fertilization: A Systematic Review and Meta-analysis." *Journal of Alternative and Complementary Medicine.* 18(5) 2012: 429-39. doi: 10.1089/acm.2011.0158
13. **Manheimer E, et al.** "The Effects of Acupuncture on Rates of Clinical Pregnancy among Women Undergoing in Vitro Fertilization: A Systematic Review and Meta-analysis." *Human Reproduction Update.* 19(6) 2013: 696-713. doi: 10.1093/humupd/dmt026; **Shen C, et al.** "The Role of Acupuncture in in Vitro Fertilization: A Systematic Review and Meta-Analysis." *Gynecologic and Obstetric Investigation.* 79(1) 2014:1-12. doi: 10.1159/000362231
14. **Villahermosa DI, et al.** "Influence of Acupuncture on the Outcomes of in Vitro Fertilisation When Embryo Implantation Has Failed: A Prospective Randomised Controlled Clinical Trial." *Acupuncture in Medicine.* 31(2) 2013: 157-61. doi: 10.1136/acupmed-2012-010269
15. **Ibid.**

Chapter 24 References cont.

16. **Abou-Setta AM, et al.** "Post-embryo transfer interventions for assisted reproduction technology cycles." *The Cochrane Database of Systematic Reviews.* 2014. doi: 10.1002/14651858.CD006567.pub3
17. **Al-Inany HG, et al.** "Gonadotrophin-releasing Hormone Antagonists for Assisted Reproductive Technology." *The Cochrane Database of Systematic Reviews.* 2011. doi: 10.1002/14651858.CD001750.pub3;
    Fiedler K, Ezcurra D. "Predicting and Preventing Ovarian Hyperstimulation Syndrome (OHSS): The Need for Individualized Not Standardized Treatment." *Reproductive Biology and Endocrinology.* 10(1) 2012: 32. doi: 10.1186/1477-7827-10-32;
    Humaidan P, Kol S, Papanikolaou E. "GnRH Agonist for Triggering of Final Oocyte Maturation: Time for a Change of Practice?" *Human Reproduction Update.* 17(4) 2011: 510-24. doi: 10.1093/humupd/dmr008
18. **Humaidan P, Kol S, Papanikolaou E.** 2011. doi: 10.1093/humupd/dmr008
19. **Haas J, et al.** "HCG (1500IU) Administration on Day 3 after Oocytes Retrieval, following GnRH-agonist Trigger for Final Follicular Maturation, Results in High Sufficient mid Luteal Progesterone Levels - a Proof of Concept." *Journal of Ovarian Research.* 7(1) 2014: 35. doi: 10.1186/1757-2215-7-35
20. **Fiedler K, Ezcurra D.** "Predicting and Preventing Ovarian Hyperstimulation Syndrome (OHSS): The Need for Individualized Not Standardized Treatment." *Reproductive Biology and Endocrinology.* 10(1) 2012: 32. doi: 10.1186/1477-7827-10-32
21. **Evans J, et al.** "Fresh versus frozen embryo transfer: backing clinical decisions with scientific and clinical evidence." *Human Reproduction Update.* 20(6) 2014:808-21. doi: 10.1093/humupd/dmu027
22. **Baumgarten M, et al.** "Do Dopamine Agonists Prevent or Reduce the Severity of Ovarian Hyperstimulation Syndrome in Women Undergoing Assisted Reproduction? A Systematic Review and Meta-analysis." *Human Fertility.* 16(3) 2013: 168-74. doi: 10.3109/14647273.2013.833348;
    Fiedler K, Ezcurra D. 2012. doi: 10.1186/1477-7827-10-32;
    Leitao VM, et al. "Cabergoline for the Prevention of Ovarian Hyperstimulation Syndrome: Systematic Review and Meta-analysis of Randomized Controlled Trials." *Fertility and Sterility.* 101(3) 2014: 664-75. doi: 10.1016/j.fertnstert.2013.11.005
23. **Gomez R, et al.** "Low-Dose Dopamine Agonist Administration Blocks Vascular Endothelial Growth Factor (VEGF)-Mediated Vascular Hyperpermeability without Altering VEGF Receptor 2-Dependent Luteal Angiogenesis in a Rat Ovarian Hyperstimulation Model." *Endocrinology.* 147(11) 2006: 5400-11. doi: 10.1210/en.2006-0657
24. **Corbett S, et al.** "The Prevention of Ovarian Hyperstimulation Syndrome." *Journal of Obstetrics and Gynaecology Canada : JOGC .* 36(11) 2014: 1024-36
25. **D'Angelo A, Brown J, Amso NN.** "Coasting (withholding Gonadotrophins) for Preventing Ovarian Hyperstimulation Syndrome." *The Cochrane Database of Systematic Reviews.* 2011. doi: 10.1002/14651858.CD002811.pub3
26. **Mayo Clinic Staff.** "Ovarian Hyperstimulation Syndrome." (OHSS) Symptoms. 14 Feb. 2014. http://www.mayoclinic.org/diseases-conditions/ovarian-hyperstimulation-syndrome-ohss/basics/symptoms/con-20033777

Chapter 25—I'm Pregnant—Now What??

1. **Siemienowicz KJ, et al.** "Early pregnancy maternal progesterone administration alters pituitary and testis function and steroid profile in male fetuses." *Sci Rep.* 10(1) 2020:21920. doi: 10.1038/s41598-020-78976-x.
   Davidovitch M, et al. "Infertility treatments during pregnancy and the risk of autism spectrum disorder in the offspring." *Prog Neuropsychopharmacol Biol Psychiatry.* 86 2018:175-179. doi: 10.1016/j.pnpbp.2018.05.022.
2. **Duncan WC.** "The inadequate corpus luteum." *Reprod Fertil.* 2:(1) 2021:C1-C7. doi: 10.1530/RAF-20-0044.
3. **Kyrou D, et al.** "Does cessation of progesterone supplementation during early pregnancy in patients treated with recFSH/GnRH antagonist affect ongoing pregnancy rates? A randomized controlled trial." *Hum Reprod.* 26(5) 2011:1020-4. doi: 10.1093/humrep/der012.
   Mizrachi Y, Raziel A, Weissman A. "When Can We Safely Stop Luteal Phase Support in Fresh IVF Cycles? A Literature Review." *Front Reprod Health.* 2 2020:610532. doi: 10.3389/frph.2020.610532.
4. **Lisova KM, et al.** "Changes in the level of fetoplacental complex hormones in pregnant women with miscarriage." *J Med Life.* 14(4) 2021:487-491. doi: 10.25122/jml-2021-0089.
   Deng W, et al. "Prediction of miscarriage in first trimester by serum estradiol, progesterone and β-human chorionic gonadotropin within 9 weeks of gestation." *BMC Pregnancy Childbirth.* 22(1) 2022:112. doi: 10.1186/s12884-021-04158-w.
5. http://www.betabase.info
6. **Institute of Medicine (US) and National Research Council (US) Committee to Reexamine IOM Pregnancy Weight Guidelines.** Weight Gain during Pregnancy: Reexamining the Guidelines. Ed. Kathleen M. Rasmussen and Ann L. Yaktine. Washington, DC: National Academies, 2009. http://iom.nationalacademies.org/Reports/2009/Weight-Gain-During-Pregnancy-Reexamining-the-Guidelines.aspx.
7. **Oster, E.** Expecting Better: Why the Conventional Pregnancy Wisdom Is Wrong—and What You Really Need to Know. New York, New York: The Penguin Press, 2013
8. **Institute of Medicine (US) and National Research Council (US) Committee to Reexamine IOM Pregnancy Weight Guidelines.** 2009. http://iom.nationalacademies.org/Reports/2009/Weight-Gain-During-Pregnancy-Reexamining-the-Guidelines.aspx
9. Ibid.
10. **Murkoff HE, Mazel S.** What to Expect When You're Expecting. New York: Workman Pub., 2008
11. **Institute of Medicine (US) and National Research Council (US) Committee to Reexamine IOM Pregnancy Weight Guidelines.** 2009. http://iom.nationalacademies.org/Reports/2009/Weight-Gain-During-Pregnancy-Reexamining-the-Guidelines.aspx;
    Viswanathan M, et al. "Outcomes of Maternal Weight Gain." *Evidence Reports/Technology Assessments.* 168 (2008): 1-223. http://www.ncbi.nlm.nih.gov/pubmedhealth/PMH0007502/

Chapter 25 References cont.

12. **Fisher, RE, Steele M, Karrow NA.** "Fetal Programming of the Neuroendocrine-Immune System and Metabolic Disease." *Journal of Pregnancy.* 2012 (2012): 1-10. doi: 10.1155/2012/792934;
    Hales C, Barker D. "Type 2 (non-insulin-dependent) Diabetes Mellitus: The Thrifty Phenotype Hypothesis." *International Journal of Epidemiology.* 42(5) 2013: 1215-222. doi: 10.1093/ije/dyt133;
    Yajnik CS. "Commentary: Thrifty Phenotype: 20 Years Later." *International Journal of Epidemiology.* 42(5) 2013: 1227-229. doi: 10.1093/ije/dyt132

13. **Hales C, Barker D.** 2013. doi: 10.1093/ije/dyt133;
    Yajnik CS. 2013. doi: 10.1093/ije/dyt132

14. **Bodnar LM, et al.** "Gestational Weight Gain in Twin Pregnancies and Maternal and Child Health: A Systematic Review." *Journal of Perinatology.* 34(4) 2014: 252-63. doi: 10.1038/jp.2013.177;
    Fox NS, et al. "The Association between Maternal Weight Gain and Spontaneous Preterm Birth in Twin Pregnancies." *Journal of Maternal-Fetal and Neonatal Medicine.* 27(16) 2014:1652-5. doi: 10.3109/14767058.2014.898058;
    Institute of Medicine (US) and National Research Council (US) Committee to Reexamine IOM Pregnancy Weight Guidelines. 2009. http://iom.nationalacademies.org/Reports/2009/Weight-Gain-During-Pregnancy-Reexamining-the-Guidelines.aspx;
    Pettit KE, et al. "The Association of Inadequate Mid-pregnancy Weight Gain and Preterm Birth in Twin Pregnancies." *Journal of Perinatology.* 35(2) 2015: 85-89. doi: 10.1038/jp.2014.160

15. **Pettit KE, et al.** 2015. doi: 10.1038/jp.2014.160

16. **Clapp JF, Cram C.** Exercising through Your Pregnancy. Omaha, Nebraska: Addicus Books, 2012

17. **Ibid.**

18. **Murkoff HE, Mazel S.** What to Expect When You're Expecting. New York: Workman Pub., 2008

19. **Hakakha M, Brown A.** Expecting 411: The Insider's Guide to Pregnancy and Childbirth: Clear Answers & Smart Advice for Your Pregnancy. Boulder, CO: Windsor Peak Press, 2014

20. **Curtis GB, Schuler J.** Your Pregnancy Week by Week. Philadelphia, PA: Da Capo Lifelong, 2011

21. **McCutcheon S, Rosegg P.** Natural Childbirth the Bradley Way. New York, NY, U.S.A.: Plume, 1996

22. http://dailymed.nlm.nih.gov

Chapter 26—Pregnancy Loss

1. **Avalos LA, Galindo C, Li D.** "A Systematic Review to Calculate Background Miscarriage Rates Using Life Table Analysis." *Birth Defects Research Part A: Clinical and Molecular Teratology.* 94(6) 2012: 417-23. doi: 10.1002/bdra.23014

2. **Goldhaber MK, Fireman BH.** "The Fetal Life Table Revisited: Spontaneous Abortion Rates in Three Kaiser Permanente Cohorts." *Epidemiology.* 2(1) 1991: 33-39

Chapter 26 References cont.

3. **Mukherjee S, et al.** "Risk of Miscarriage Among Black Women and White Women in a US Prospective Cohort Study." *American Journal of Epidemiology.* 177(11) 2013: 1271-278. doi: 10.1093/aje/kws393
4. **Wilcox AJ, et al.** "Incidence of Early Loss of Pregnancy." *New England Journal of Medicine.* 319.4 (1988): 189-94. doi: 10.1056/NEJM198807283190401
5. **Shearer BM, et al.** "Reflex Fluorescent in Situ Hybridization Testing for Unsuccessful Product of Conception Cultures: A Retrospective Analysis of 5555 Samples Attempted by Conventional Cytogenetics and Fluorescent in Situ Hybridization." *Genetics in Medicine.* 13(6) 2011: 545-52. doi: 10.1097/GIM.0b013e31820c685b
6. **Jenderny, J.** "Chromosome Aberrations in a Large Series of Spontaneous Miscarriages in the German Population and Review of the Literature." *Molecular Cytogenetics.* 7 2014:38. doi: 10.1186/1755-8166-7-38
7. **Feodor Nilsson S, et al.** "Risk Factors for Miscarriage from a Prevention Perspective: A Nationwide Follow-up Study." *BJOG.* 121(11) 2014: 1375-84. doi: 10.1111/1471-0528.12694;
Veleva Z, et al. "High and Low BMI Increase the Risk of Miscarriage after IVF/ICSI and FET." *Human Reproduction.* 23(4) 2008: 878-84. doi: 10.1093/humrep/den017
8. **Baird DD.** "The Gestational Timing of Pregnancy Loss: Adaptive Strategy?" *American Journal of Human Biology.* 21(6) 2009: 725-27. doi: 10.1002/ajhb.20935
9. **Ibid.**
10. **Armstrong BG, Mcdonald AD, Sloan M.** "Cigarette, Alcohol, and Coffee Consumption and Spontaneous Abortion." *American Journal of Public Health.* 82(1) 1992: 85-87. http://www.ncbi.nlm.nih.gov/pmc/articles/PMC1694397;
Pineles BL, Park E, Samet JM. "Systematic Review and Meta-Analysis of Miscarriage and Maternal Exposure to Tobacco Smoke During Pregnancy." *American Journal of Epidemiology.* 179(7) 2014: 807-23. doi: 10.1093/aje/kwt334
11. **Pineles BL, Park E, Samet JM.** 2014. doi: 10.1093/aje/kwt334
12. **Armstrong BG, Mcdonald AD, Sloan M.** 1992. http://www.ncbi.nlm.nih.gov/pmc/articles/PMC1694397
13. **Avalos LA, et al.** "Volume and Type of Alcohol during Early Pregnancy and the Risk of Miscarriage." *Substance Use & Misuse.* 49(11) 2014: 1437-445. doi: 10.3109/10826084.2014.912228
14. **Greenwood DC, et al.** "Caffeine Intake during Pregnancy and Adverse Birth Outcomes: A Systematic Review and Dose-response Meta-analysis." *European Journal of Epidemiology.* 29(10) 2014: 725-34. doi: 10.1007/s10654-014-9944-x
15. **Savitz, DA, et al.** "Caffeine and Miscarriage Risk." *Epidemiology.* 19(1) 2008: 55-62. doi: 10.1097/EDE.0b013e31815c09b9
16. **American College of Obstetricians and Gynecologists.** "ACOG Committee Opinion No. 462: Moderate Caffeine Consumption during Pregnancy." *Obstetrics and Gynecology.* 116(2 Pt 1) 2010: 467-68. doi: 10.1097/AOG.0b013e3181eeb2a1
17. **Rafi J, Khalil H.** "Expectant Management of Miscarriage in View of NICE Guideline 154." *Journal of Pregnancy.* 2014: 824527. doi: 10.1155/2014/824527

Chapter 26 References cont.

18. **Al-Ma'ani W, Solomayer EF, Hammadeh M.** "Expectant versus Surgical Management of First-trimester Miscarriage: A Randomised Controlled Study." *Archives of Gynecology and Obstetrics.* 289(5) 2014: 1011-5. doi: 10.1007/s00404-013-3088-1

19. **Love ER, et al.** "Effect of Interpregnancy Interval on Outcomes of Pregnancy after Miscarriage: Retrospective Analysis of Hospital Episode Statistics in Scotland." *BMJ.* 341 2010: C3967. doi: 10.1136/bmj.c3967

20. **Davanzo J, Hale L, Rahman M.** "How Long after a Miscarriage Should Women Wait before Becoming Pregnant Again? Multivariate Analysis of Cohort Data from Matlab, Bangladesh." *BMJ Open.* 2(4) 2012. doi: 10.1136/bmjopen-2012-001591

21. **Goldstein RR, Croughan MA, Robertson PA.** "Neonatal Outcomes in Immediate versus Delayed Conceptions after Spontaneous Abortion: A Retrospective Case Series." *American Journal of Obstetrics and Gynecology.* 186(6) 2002: 1230-236. doi: 10.1067/mob.2002.123741

22. **Rud B, Klünder K.** "The Course of Pregnancy following Spontaneous Abortion." *Acta Obstetricia Et Gynecologica Scandinavica.* 64(3) 1985: 277-78. doi: 10.3109/00016348509155129

23. **Wyss P, Biedermann K, Huch A.** "Relevance of the Miscarriage-new Pregnancy Interval." *Journal of Perinatal Medicine.* 22(3) 1994: 235-41

24. **Cohen J.** Coming to Term: Uncovering the Truth about Miscarriage. New Brunswick, NJ: Rutgers University Press, 2007

Chapter 27—Postpartum, Cycling, and Conceiving Again

1. **Institute of Medicine (US) and National Research Council (US) Committee to Reexamine IOM Pregnancy Weight Guidelines.** Weight Gain during Pregnancy: Reexamining the Guidelines. Ed. K.M. Rasmussen and A.L. Yaktine. Washington, DC: National Academies, 2009. http://iom.nationalacademies.org/Reports/2009/Weight-Gain-During-Pregnancy-Reexamining-the-Guidelines.aspx; **Viswanathan M, et al.** "Outcomes of Maternal Weight Gain." *Evidence Reports/Technology Assessments.* 168 (2008): 1-223. http://www.ncbi.nlm.nih.gov/pubmedhealth/PMH0007502/

2. **Hales C, Barker D.** "Type 2 (non-insulin-dependent) Diabetes Mellitus: The Thrifty Phenotype Hypothesis." *International Journal of Epidemiology.* 42(5) 2013: 1215-222. doi: 10.1093/ije/dyt133;
Yajnik CS. "Commentary: Thrifty Phenotype: 20 Years Later." *International Journal of Epidemiology.* 42(5) 2013: 1227-229. doi: 10.1093/ije/dyt132

3. **Fisher, RE, Steele M, Karrow NA.** "Fetal Programming of the Neuroendocrine-Immune System and Metabolic Disease." *Journal of Pregnancy.* 2012 (2012): 1-10. doi: 10.1155/2012/792934

4. **Valeggia C, Ellison PT.** "Interactions between Metabolic and Reproductive Functions in the Resumption of Postpartum Fecundity." *American Journal of Human Biology.* 21(4) 2009: 559-66. doi: 10.1002/ajhb.20907

5. **Ibid.**

6. **Ibid.**

7. **Berga SL, et al.** "Recovery of Ovarian Activity in Women with Functional Hypothalamic Amenorrhea Who Were Treated with Cognitive Behavior Therapy." *Fertility and Sterility.* 80(4) 2003: 976-81. doi: 10.1016/S0015-0282(03)01124-5

8. **Tschugguel W, Berga SL.** "Treatment of Functional Hypothalamic Amenorrhea with Hypnotherapy." *Fertility and Sterility.* 80(4) 2003: 982-85. doi: 10.1016/S0015-0282(03)01012-4

9. **Genazzani AD, et al.** "Acetyl-l-carnitine as Possible Drug in the Treatment of Hypothalamic Amenorrhea." *Acta Obstetricia et Gynecologica Scandinavica.* 70(6) 1991: 487-92. doi: 10.3109/00016349109007165;
   Genazzani AD, et al. "Acetyl-L-carnitine (ALC) Administration Positively Affects Reproductive Axis in Hypogonadotropic Women with Functional Hypothalamic Amenorrhea." *Journal of Endocrinological Investigation.* 34(4) 2011: 287-91. doi: 10.3275/6997

10. **Genazzani AD, et al.** 2011. doi: 10.3275/6997

11. **Borges LE, et al.** "New Protocol of Clomiphene Citrate Treatment in Women with Hypothalamic Amenorrhea." *Gynecological Endocrinology.* 23(6) 2007: 343-46. doi: 10.1080/09513590701327620

12. **Armeanu MC, Moss RJ, Schoemaker J.** "Ovulation Induction with a Single-blind Treatment Regimen Comparing Naltrexone, Placebo and Clomiphene Citrate in Women with Secondary Amenorrhea." *European Journal of Endocrinology.* 126.5 (1992): 410-15. doi: 10.1530/acta.0.1260410;
    Genazzani AD, et al. "Naltrexone Administration Modulates the Neuroendocrine Control of Luteinizing Hormone Secretion in Hypothalamic Amenorrhoea." *Human Reproduction.* 10(11) 1995: 2868-871. http://humrep.oxfordjournals.org/content/10/11/2868.long;
    Remorgida V, et al. "Naltrexone in Functional Hypothalamic Amenorrhea and in the Normal Luteal Phase." *Obstetrics and Gynecology.* 76(6) 1990: 1115-120;
    Wildt L, Leyendecker G. "Induction Of Ovulation By The Chronic Administration Of Naltrexone In Hypothalamic Amenorrhea." *The Journal of Clinical Endocrinology & Metabolism.* 64(6) 1987: 1334-335. doi: 10.1210/jcem-64-6-1334

13. http://myaleptrems.com/rems.aspx

14. **Chou SH, et al.** "Leptin Is an Effective Treatment for Hypothalamic Amenorrhea." *Proceedings of the National Academy of Sciences.* 108(16) 2011: 6585-590. doi: 10.1073/pnas.1015674108;
    Welt CK, et al. "Recombinant Human Leptin in Women with Hypothalamic Amenorrhea." *New England Journal of Medicine.* 351(10) 2004: 987-97. doi: 10.1056/NEJMoa040388

Chapter 28—Long-term Health

1. https://web.archive.org/web/20130317005511/http://www.youreatopia.com/blog/2013/2/26/insidious-activity.html

Chapter 29—Stories of Recovery

1. **De Souza MJ, et al.** "Luteal Phase Deficiency in Recreational Runners: Evidence for a Hypometabolic State." *Journal of Clinical Endocrinology & Metabolism.* 88(1) 2003: 337-46. doi: 10.1210/jc.2002-020958;

Chapter 29 References cont.

De Souza MJ, et al. "High Prevalence of Subtle and Severe Menstrual Disturbances in Exercising Women: Confirmation Using Daily Hormone Measures." *Human Reproduction.* 25(2) 2010: 491-503. doi: 10.1093/humrep/dep411

2. **Carlsen E, et al.** "History of Febrile Illness and Variation in Semen Quality." *Human Reproduction.* 18(10) 2003: 2089-92. doi: 10.1093/humrep/deg412
3. **Robin G, et al.** "Polycystic Ovary-Like Abnormalities (PCO-L) in Women with Functional Hypothalamic Amenorrhea." *Journal of Clinical Endocrinology & Metabolism.* 97(11) 2012: 4236-43

Index

A

acetyl-l-carnitine (ALC), 241–4, 249, 276, 393
acne, 56, 59–61, 117, 430, 472
acupuncture, 222–23, 336, 444
affirmations, 144, 152–53
all in, 106, 115, 126, 129, 157–58, 302
androgens, 58, 61, 67, 117
anovulatory, 160–61, 163
anti-Müllerian hormone (AMH), 40, 271–74, 335
antral follicles, 271–72, 335, 337
Appetite control hormones, 48–50

B

BBT, see temperature,
bloodwork,
   and HA, 33–34, 59–60, 236, 248, 278, 447, 451, 454, 463, 470, 486
   and PCOS, 58, 62, 69, 463, 470, 472
   and trying to conceive, 254, 274
BMI, see also weight,
   fertile 102, 104, 110, 393, 417, 446, 474, 476
   high 8, 134–35
   low 60, 80, 270, 323–24, 371, 463, 493
   pre-pregnancy 359, 379–81, 390
bone
   and birth control pills (BCP), 78–80
   breakdown 75, 77–79
   cortical 76–77
   density 28, 37, 76–84, 87–88, 407, 425, 470–79
   spinal 79–80, 84
   formation 75–79
   loss 74–77, 79, 81, 83
   trabecular 76–77, 80
breastfeeding, 87, 354, 377–86, 393–94, 449

and bone density, 75, 80, 379–83, 480, 484

C

cancellation, 306, 314, 323
carbohydrates, 48, 113–16, 122, 140, 192
CD (cycle day),
   and medications, 274, 289, 285–88, 297, 305, 303–4, 313, 456
   and menstrual cycle, 46–47, 350
   and ovulation, 211–14, 285–88, 297, 309, 350, 391, 414–15, 424
cervical mucus,
   and recovery, 208–9, 420
   and tracking ovulation, 238–39, 242–43, 288, 297
cervical position (CP), 224–5, 227, 229, 258, 297
cholesterol, 69, 85
Clomid
   extended protocol, 249, 283–84, 292, 394, 487
   vs. Femara and tamoxifen, 247, 277–79, 281–85, 299
   and getting pregnant, 223, 281, 277–79, 281–91, 299, 394
   and HA recovery, 36, 246, 281, 291, 394
   and luteal phase, 261
   response 264–65, 277–78, 286, 426–27, 438–39
cognitive behavioral therapy (CBT), 9, 105, 141–42, 175, 241, 393
corpus luteum, 46–48, 258–59, 266, 282, 372
cortisol, 10, 26, 50, 52, 117, 158, 282
cramping, 211, 313, 353
   and miscarriage, 369–70, 378, 489

C cont.

cycle day. See CD,
cycles
  abnormal 11, 161, 260
  canceled 310, 315, 325
  initial 301–2
  monitoring 231, 236, 283, 304, 301–3, 320, 323, 353
  postpartum 109, 382–89, 401
  regain / resume / return, 29, 80, 105, 109, 115, 158, 218, 237, 241–50, 283, 419
  regular xvi, 51, 182, 400
  subsequent 286, 307, 307–9
  treatment 239, 272, 305, 323, 378
cysts, 36, 55, 313, 317, 324

D

dairy, full-fat, 116–17, 122
DHEA, 279, 336
dialectical behavioral therapy (DBT), 175–77, 406
diminished ovarian reserve (DOR), 34, 40, 271–74
DXA, 77, 81–84

E

eating disorder, 10, 16–19, 28, 64, 141, 181, 303, 402, 413, 444, 452, 483
egg white cervical mucus (EWCM), 212, 222–4, 227, 229, 234, 248, 420, 453
energy deficit, 4–5, 10, 43, 66, 163, 193, 217, 261, 387, 384–85, 396
estradiol, 34–35, 47, 58, 211, 220, 236, 244–6, 282, 291, 319, 324, 338, 471
estrogen, 36–37, 46–47, 69, 80, 117, 220, 223, 259, 318–19
  low 12, 74, 77, 84–87, 431, 474, 482
  and Clomid/Femara, 282, 288, 310
  high 69, 75
exercise
  and IVF, 329, 332, 336
  high-intensity 51, 157–58, 161, 163–64, 191, 195–96, 210, 216, 360, 399
  moderate 26–27, 163, 165
extended protocol. See Clomid extended protocol,

F

fats, healthy, 114–16, 174, 428, 470, 474, 477, 481, 486
Femara, 247, 273, 275–85, 287–90, 299, 310, 317, 394, 416
fertile signs, 209–10, 218, 221–2, 236, 291
fertility medications oral, 247, 249, 394, 493, See, also, Clomid, Femara, tamoxifen
follicles
  dominant 41, 212, 307, 323
  multiple 315, 323, 333
follicle size, 306, 302–4, 320, 324
follicle stimulating hormone (FSH), 33–36, 46–47, 52, 58–60, 63, 115, 209–10, 219, 243, 272–73, 282, 291, 342
  injections 299–300, 308, 310
follicular phase, 46–47, 262
follicular recruitment waves, 226
food groups, 6, 18, 21, 113–15, 191
foods, fertility, 113, 115, 122, 217
fractures, 12, 89, 479, 475–78
FSH and LH, 243, 257–58, 296, 299–300, 304–5
full fat, 114, 117

G

gaining weight, 64, 70, 88, 106, 113, 116, 125, 131–32, 139–40, 142–43, 146, 151, 184, 197, 202, 264–65, 303, 360, 362, 444, 449, 471,
glucose, 50, 52, 56, 67–69, 115, 117, 122

G cont.

GnRH, 47, 115, 211, 219, 236, 243, 247, 248, 258–59, 282, 390
gonadotropins, see FSH and LH,

H

heart, 4, 74, 84–88, 102–3, 156, 171, 184, 408
heart disease, 68–69, 73–74, 84–85
heart rate, 27, 84, 158, 160, 166, 355–56
hirsutism, 33, 56, 59–61
hormone replacement therapy (HRT), 74, 77–80, 86–87, 243, 393, 471–72
hormones
  hunger 48–49
  male 56, 117, 335
HSG, 268–69, 305, 373
hyperandrogenism, 57–58
hypnosis, 241, 393
hypothalamus
  control of hormones, 3–4, 47, 52, 212, 219–20, 258–59, 282, 390, 393
  and hunger, 6, 43, 48–50, 52–53, 114, 190–91, 282, 400
  and luteal phase defect, 258–59
  and oral medications, 246, 276–77, 291, 295, 310, 393, 457
  and stress, 8, 50, 52, 146, 158, 172, 241, 263, 386–87, 456

I

in vitro fertilization (IVF), 62, 137, 269, 279, 285, 298, 319, 324, 323–37, 372, 372–73, 393, 395
injectable cycles, 262, 274, 297–304, 312, 314, 317, 320, 324
injectables, 62, 277–79, 299, 295–301, 310, 309–11, 319, 317–18, 326, 330, 372, 392, 394, 401
injections, 306–7, 313–14
Institute of Medicine (IOM), 102, 104, 356

insulin, 48–50, 52, 56, 65–69, 115, 117, 358, 390, 392
intercourse, 219–2, 224, 226, 229, 285, 296, 314–16
inter-pregnancy interval (IPI), 380
intrauterine insemination (IUI), 285, 314–16, 319–20

L

last menstrual period (LMP), 350
lean body mass (LBM), 102–4
leptin, 49–50, 52, 69, 248, 271, 331, 392, 394
Lisa
  and HA, 13, 16, 22, 28, 29, 37, 41, 44, 51, 70, 96, 111, 115, 122, 130, 140, 142, 152, 164, 166, 174, 177
  recovery 218, 253, 398, 409
  trying to conceive, 266, 275, 299, 317, 343, 363
luteal phase (LP), 46–47, 51, 160–3, 213–15, 220, 222, 230–2, 244, 255–62, 322, 324, 391, 428
  short 256–58, 266, 391
luteal phase defect (LPD), 160–61, 259, 257–59
  hypothalamic 258–59, 265
luteinizing hormone (LH), 33–36, 38, 46–47, 58–64, 69, 95, 115, 117, 209–10, 220, 226–7, 236, 243–4, 249, 306, 304–5, 390
  and LPD, 257–59
  surges natural, 222, 227, 296, 319, 335, 331–32

M

marathons, 16, 180, 399
maternal weight gain low, 352–54, 386
mature eggs, 34, 36, 46–7, 68, 308, 320, 324, 333
mature follicles, 291, 304–6, 314
medicated cycles, 254, 262, 272, 275–76, 286, 313–14, 331

M cont.

Menopur, 300–305
menstrual cycles see cycles,
metformin, 66–67
miscarriage, 347, 354, 361, 359–76, 395
  chance of, 366, 373
  natural 369–71
  post 372–73
  risk of, 330, 371, 373
miscarriage rates, 214, 260, 279, 309, 354, 366, 365–67
monitoring, 283, 295, 301, 304, 301–2, 310, 320, 353, 423
multiples, 284, 288, 284–85, 310, 323, 357, 435, 467

N

naltrexone, 247–9, 394
natural cycles xvi, 35, 45, 66, 88, 95, 108–9, 131, 133–34, 158, 163, 209, 210–14, 222, 226, 236, 237, 262, 265, 269, 284–86, 347, 492
nerve cells, 48, 50, 52–54, 115
Nico
  and HA xiv, 3, 19, 23, 73, 93, 118, 160, 162, 175, 210, 213, 228, 387, 409, 471
  miscarriage 365, 361–62, 370, 377
  trying to concieve, 3, 32, 162, 213, 227, 246–47, 274, 305, 322, 324, 326, 334, 347, 343–44, 362, 387, 391
normal cycles, 35, 47, 160–61, 164, 212, 282, 393, 460
  resumed 388, 393
nursing, 381–85, 422, 449, 460, 463, 478–79
nutritionist, 16, 93, 118, 430, 470, 477
nuts, 106, 114, 118–19, 122, 387, 409, 416, 422, 431

O

oral medications, 62, 213, 247, 249, 256, 269, 267–68, 275–81, 289, 296, 292–93, 316, 319, 326, 394

osteopenia/osteoporosis, 21, 28, 73, 77, 81–84, 86, 88–89, 132, 156, 190, 426, 470–74, 476–79
ovarian hyper-stimulation syndrome (OHSS), 40, 62, 323, 335, 331–34
ovarian reserve diminished, 34, 40, 270, 271–274
overstimulation, 301–2, 304–5, 314, 317, 319, 317–18, 326
ovulation
  confirmation 220, 222, 227–31, 257, 297, 314–15
  induction with medication, 246–7, 249, 282, 278–87, 289–93, 301, 304, 306, 309, 316, 313–14, 394
  and intercourse timing, 219–22, 224, 226, 229
  late 211–13, 218, 278–80, 290–91, 309, 350, 354, 371, 378, 391, 421
  and luteal phase (LP), 35, 40, 46–48, 259, 258–60, 321
  and normal cycle, 34, 46–48
  and PCOS, 56, 65–67
  postpartum 390, 394
  predicting 212, 221–6, 276, 297, 320, 432
  and pregnancy, 211, 215, 222, 226, 243, 278–81, 294
  and supplements, 242–5, 248–9, 239, 296, 393
  trigger 295, 306, 303–7, 313–18, 445, 459, 468, 475
ovulation predictor kits (OPKs), 47, 212, 221–3, 226–30, 234, 257, 296, 351, 414–15, 425–30, 449, 474

P

patience, 203, 237, 280, 396, 455
PCOS, 4, 31, 33–39, 55–71, 77, 227, 289, 308, 399, 415
  diagnosis of, 55, 57–61, 70–71
  lean 39, 56, 59, 62, 65–69
  symptoms 63, 66, 70, 447, 455, 464, 466, 468, 472

P cont.

physical exam, 33, 35, 55
piggybacking, 289, 291, 293
pituitary, 34, 45, 47, 50, 52–53, 211, 258–259, 282, 296, 307, 337
polycystic ovaries, 57–59, 62, 463
pregnancy
  natural 285, 350, 365
  subsequent 394
  underweight 355, 357
  and weight, 136, 359, 383, 381–82, 400, 449
  weight gain low, 359
pregnancy complications, 354
pregnancy loss, 366, 372, 380, 382, 395
  chemical 342, 366, 376
pregnancy rates, 68, 212–13, 221, 261–62, 276, 279, 278–81, 291, 287–88, 299, 303–4, 315, 315–16, 329–30
progesterone, 36, 40, 46–48, 70, 82, 86, 88, 220, 231, 236, 241, 243–5, 255, 255–62, 282, 322, 338, 372, 393
  prescription 264, 266
  pulses 258–59
  supplements 255, 255–58
  support 313, 317, 319, 315–16, 326, 372
prolactin, 33–34, 390
proteins, 48, 67, 83, 100, 113–16, 118, 122, 192, 356, 427, 461, 477
protocols
  extended 246–7, 249, 283–84, 292, 299, 342, 419, 442
  low and slow, 300–301, 304–5, 317
  standard 284–85, 299
  step-down 307, 311, 317
Provera, 35–36, 41, 236, 243, 248–9, 274, 284–88, 293, 325, 378, 393, 424–26, 442, 467–68

R

Recovery Plan xvi, 70, 74, 95, 98–99, 120, 125, 128, 135, 155–56, 166, 210, 216–17, 235, 237–8, 240
and fertility treatments, 108, 243, 269, 317, 332
regained cycles xvi, 61, 79, 95, 135, 164, 388, 392, 396
relaxation, 146, 171, 181, 203–5
rest days, 24–25, 29, 172, 360
running, 10, 20, 61, 81, 157–61, 163–64, 166, 172, 179–86, 239, 424–27, 434–38, 445–46, 454, 450–52, 454–55, 463, 471–76

S

snacks, 117, 120, 122, 136, 387, 399, 405
soy isoflavones (SI), 213, 242, 245, 249, 275–78, 287, 290, 289–290, 299
sperm, 211, 221, 223, 257, 272, 276, 285, 288, 296, 321, 327–28
spine, 76, 79–81, 83, 88, 480, 482, 484
Steph
  HA and recovery, 6, 10, 16, 37, 51, 57, 93, 113, 117, 140, 148, 159, 199, 209, 239, 241, 273, 389, 398, 409, 413,
  therapy 141, 149, 159, 176, 221–22, 304
  trying to conceive, 39, 57, 149, 227, 273, 294, 304, 349, 356, 384, 389
stress
  hormones 8–9, 52
  psychological 4, 9, 50, 52, 240–1, 243–4
sugar, 6, 96–97, 115–16, 122
supplements, 65, 67, 82–83, 242–5, 248–9, 261–62, 270–71, 295, 336, 384, 477, 476–79
survey respondents,
  and DOR, 278
  and HA xv–xvi, 7–8, 17–20, 25–27, 34–35, 37, 76, 95, 104
  and LPD, 258–59
  and miscarriage, 366, 371, 372–74
  and PCOS xv, 61

survey respondents cont.

and pregnancy, 283, 287, 292, 309, 309–10, 352, 359, 387, 393
and recovery xvi, 95, 97–98, 101, 104–5, 108–10, 127, 133, 135, 158, 163, 204, 213, 236–7, 240
and subsequent pregnancy, 389, 393, 396
and trying to conceive, 237–38, 272, 277–78, 287, 292, 296, 306, 309, 309–10
and weaning, 389

T

tamoxifen, 230, 239, 273, 275–78, 287, 289, 291, 394
temperature, BBT, 212, 216, 243, 243–44, 246–50, 260, 291, 297, 321, 421
therapist, 121, 141, 174, 185, 198–99, 255, 270, 304, 391, 393, 396–97, 405, 407
thyroid stimulating hormone (TSH), 33–35, 436
T-score, 77, 79, 80–82
twins, 288, 308–9, 323, 346–47, 355–56

U

ultrasound
  and HA, 4, 33, 36, 41, 434, 454, 463, 465
  and miscarriage, 365, 374, 376, 381, 460
  and polycystic ovaries, 4, 33, 36, 57, 59, 454, 462, 474
  and pregnancy, 346–47, 358
  and trying to conceive, 274, 289, 301–2, 310, 320, 456, 474
undereating, 4, 12, 17, 22, 134, 189–90, 396, 409–10
underfueling, 18, 51, 62, 95–96, 104, 110, 409–10
underweight, 7, 39, 60, 192, 231, 271, 324–25, 359, 371, 394

uterine lining, 32, 35–40, 45–46, 69–70, 259, 265, 282, 281–82, 293

V

vegetables, 122, 350–51, 447, 487
vitamins, 82–83, 261–62, 270–71, 296, 479, 482, 484
vitex, 228

W

weaning, 75, 213, 223–24, 383, 383–84, 391, 401, 422, 440, 464, 485
weighing, 148, 398–99, 407
weight
  current 5, 12, 54, 134, 217
  healthy 156, 393, 399, 421, 447, 450, 472
  normal 7, 9, 445
  postpartum 194, 359, 385
  pre-pregnancy 380–81, 391, 403, 426
  stable 51, 102, 134
  water 128, 424
weight lifting, 23–24, 158, 162
weight loss,
  after recovery/pregnancy, 109, 217, 400
  and HA, 2, 7–9, 12, 17, 33–34, 53, 61, 66–67, 93, 450, 447–48, 464

Y

yoga, 142, 146, 156–57, 159, 164, 166, 169, 171, 173, 185, 214, 233, 303, 360, 418, 424, 445, 453, 462, 465

Consult with Dr. Nicola Sykes, PhD: http://noperiod.info/appointments

Visit us at www.NoPeriodNowWhat.com
for more information and blog posts on a variety of topics.
Find our Support Group at http://noperiod.info/Support,
support for getting pregnant at http://noperiod.info/TTC,
and follow on Instagram @NoPeriodNowWhat

Made in the USA
Middletown, DE
19 May 2025